Medicine and humanism in late medieval Italy

This book is the first study to consider the extraordinary manuscript now known as the *Carrara Herbal* (British Library, Egerton 2020) within the complex network of medical, artistic and intellectual traditions from which it emerged. The manuscript contains an illustrated, vernacular copy of the thirteenth-century pharmacopeia by Ibn Sarābī, an Arabic-speaking Christian physician working in al-Andalus known in the West as Serapion the Younger. By 1290, Serapion's treatise was available in Latin translation and circulated widely in medical schools across the Italian peninsula.

Commissioned in the late fourteenth century by the prince of Padua, Francesco II 'il Novello' da Carrara (r. 1390–1405), the *Carrara Herbal* attests to the growing presence of Arabic medicine both inside and outside of the University. Its contents speak to the Carrara family's historic role as patrons and protectors of the *Studium*, yet its form – a luxury book in Paduan dialect adorned with family heraldry and stylistically diverse representations of plants – locates it in court culture. In particular, the manuscript's form connects Serapion's treatise to patterns of book collection and rhetorics of self-making encouraged by humanists and practiced by Francesco's ancestors.

Beginning with Petrarch (1304–74) and continuing with Pier Paolo Vergerio (ca. 1369–1444), humanists held privileged positions in the Carrara court, and humanist culture vied with the University's successes for leading roles in Carrara self-promotion. With the other illustrated books in the prince's collection, the *Herbal* negotiated these traditional arenas of family patronage and brought them into confluence, promoting Francesco as an ideal 'physician prince' capable of ensuring the moral and physical health of Padua. Considered in this way, the *Carrara Herbal* is the product of an intersection between the Pan-Mediterranean transmission of medical knowledge and the rise of humanism in the Italian courts, an intersection typically attributed to the later Renaissance.

Sarah R. Kyle is an associate professor of humanities at the University of Central Oklahoma, USA.

Medicine in the Medieval Mediterranean
Series Editor
Alain Touwaide
Institute for the Preservation of Medical Traditions, Washington, DC, USA

Editorial Board
Vivian Nutton
Wellcome Trust Centre for the History of Medicine at University College, London, UK

Paul Canart
Biblioteca Apostolica Vaticana, Vatican City

Marie-Hélène Congourdeau
Centre d'Histoire et Civilisation de Byzance, Paris, France

Dimitri Gutas
Yale University, USA

Medicine in the Medieval Mediterranean is a series devoted to all aspects of medicine in the Mediterranean area during the Middle Ages, from the 3rd/4th centuries to the 16th. Though with a focus on Greek medicine, diffused through the whole Mediterranean world and especially developed in Byzantium, it also includes the contributions of the cultures that were present or emerged in the area during the Middle Ages and after, and which interacted with Byzantium: the Latin West and early vernacular languages, the Syrian and Arabic worlds, Armenian, Georgian and Coptic groups, Jewish and Slavic cultures and Turkish peoples, particularly the Ottomans.

Medicine is understood in a broad sense: not only medical theory, but also the health conditions of people, nosology and epidemiology, diet and therapy, practice and teaching, doctors and hospitals, the economy of health, and the non-conventional forms of medicine from faith to magic, that is, all the spectrum of activities dealing with human health.

The series includes texts and studies. It will bring to light previously unknown, overlooked or poorly known documents interpreted with the most appropriate methods, and publish the results of cutting-edge research, so providing a wide range of scholarly and scientific fields with new data for further explorations.

Medicine and humanism in late medieval Italy

The *Carrara Herbal* in Padua

Sarah R. Kyle
University of Central Oklahoma

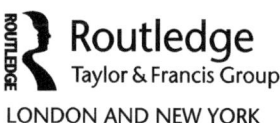

LONDON AND NEW YORK

First published 2017 by Routledge

2 Park Square, Milton Park, Abingdon, Oxfordshire OX14 4RN
52 Vanderbilt Avenue, New York, NY 10017

Routledge is an imprint of the Taylor & Francis Group, an informa business

First issued in paperback 2019

British Library Cataloguing in Publication Data
A catalogue record for this book is available from the British Library

Library of Congress Cataloging-in-Publication Data
A catalog record has been requested for this book

ISBN: 978-1-4724-4652-7 (hbk)
ISBN: 978-0-367-87984-6 (pbk)

Typeset in Times New Roman
by Apex CoVantage, LLC

For my mother and father

Contents

Illustrations

Black and white figures in text

Acknowledgements

In the years spent preparing this manuscript, many individuals have supported and guided me, generously sharing their knowledge and expertise. I take pleasure in acknowledging them here.

C. Jean Campbell encouraged me to pursue my research on the *Carrara Herbal* and provided direction and insightful criticism during the research and writing of the dissertation from which this book grew. I owe a special debt to her and to the other members of my dissertation committee, Walter Melion and Jack Zupko. I also thank Cathleen Hoeniger for first introducing me to the traditions of illustrated botanical manuscripts and Karen Reeds for engaging me in lively discussions and correspondence about the study of botany during the early Renaissance. Alain Touwaide, my editor and a respected mentor, worked diligently with me on the final stages of this project. His confidence in my work and his thoughtful recommendations have been invaluable and have helped transform a dissertation into a book. Additionally, I would like to thank the Board of the *Medicine in the Medieval Mediterranean* series for their support and for the opportunity to share my ideas with the series' diverse readership.

Colleagues and friends at the University of Central Oklahoma and at institutions further afield encouraged my research and the writing of this book. My deepest thanks to Margaret Musgrove for her perceptive comments on portions of the book and its argument and for her assiduous help in making sense of often-obscure medieval Latin texts (certain thorny passages from Paduan chronicles in particular). Darian DeBolt cheerfully assisted me with any Greek terminology I brought to his desk. Scott Samuelson thoughtfully commented on early drafts of a number of chapters and helped me to better understand, among other things, the Aristotle in Avicenna. I am deeply grateful to Gabriella Zuccolin, who shared her manuscript-in-preparation of the critical edition of Michele Savonarola's *Speculum phisionomie*, enriching my understanding of Savonarola's work enormously. Vivian Nutton graciously met with me to discuss the *Carrara Herbal* and its intersections with trends in humanism and traditions in medicine. His astute observations steered me in new directions and so saved me from several errors of omission. I also would like to thank Geraldine Brooks for her kind permission to include a line from her beautiful novel, *The People of the Book*, as the epigraph to my introduction.

In my research on manuscripts and book culture, libraries and librarians naturally have played central roles. I especially thank Susy Marcon and Elizabeth

Lugato of the Biblioteca Nazionale Marciana, Gabriele Bejor and Vincenza Donvito of the Biblioteca Civica di Padova, and Valeria Vettorato and Marco Callegari of the Museo Bottacin di Padova for their kindness, interest in my project, and guidance in navigating their institutions' respective collections. My thanks to Kathleen Doyle, Curator of Illuminated Manuscripts at the British Library, and to the staff of the British Library's Manuscript Reading Room, who made my research a joy and allowed me to spend a great deal of uninterrupted time with the *Carrara Herbal*. In addition, I am indebted to the Interlibrary Loan department at the University of Central Oklahoma for their tireless efforts in procuring (often-unwieldy) books from near and far during the final phases of this project.

Over the last several years, I have presented parts of this book to audiences at the College Art Association and the Renaissance Society of America annual conferences and at the International Congress on Medieval Studies, and I especially thank Shelley MacLaren, Allie Terry-Fritsch, Jennifer Webb, Mildred Budny, Gur Zak, Todd Richardson and John R. Decker for their thought-provoking questions and conversation in these settings. Portions of this book also have appeared in different form in *The Anthropomorphic Lens: Anthropomorphism, Microcosmism and Analogy in Early Modern Thought and Visual Arts* (Leiden: Brill, 2014) and *Mediaevalia* 35 (2015). I would like to thank Brill Publishers and SUNY Press for introducing some of my ideas to a wider audience and for permission to reproduce them here.

From its inception as a dissertation, my project has received generous financial support from several institutions. The Laney Graduate School and the Art History Department of Emory University financed research travel, and an Andrew W. Mellon Dissertation Seminar Fellowship and a graduate fellowship at the Manuscript, Archives, and Rare Book Library (MARBL) of Emory University provided support during the writing stages of the dissertation. A University of Central Oklahoma Liberal Arts College Research Grant funded a final research trip to London, and a Faculty On-Campus Regular Grant provided a much-needed course release to enable the completion of this manuscript. A Department of Humanities and Philosophy grant helped to offset the cost of images and permissions fees. I also would like to thank the Biblioteca Civica di Padova, the Museo Bottacin di Padova, the Università degli Studi di Padova, the Accademia Galileiana di Scienze, Lettere ed Arti in Padova and the Süleymaniye Kütüphanesi in Istanbul for generously waiving their fees for administration and image reproduction rights.

Last, but by no means least, I am profoundly grateful to my friends and family for their good cheer, humour and confidence in me, especially to Sarah Milan, Meme Moore, Randell Baze, Phillip Dunford, Sienna Brown, Jessica Gershultz and Graham Kepfer. I also thank Erik Tamplin. I greatly appreciate the kindness of Renée Schlueter, Ceren Ciraci, Thomas Kirk and Teodora Kirk, who, at the eleventh hour, helped me to chase down image permissions in Istanbul and Florence. Patricia Kyritsi Howell introduced me to the history and practice of herbal medicine in the Appalachian Mountains, an experience that enriched my understanding of traditions of healing and for which I am thankful. Finally, I owe a great debt to my family, especially to my mother and father, Krystyna and Gerald Kyle, for their innumerable kindnesses, love and unwavering faith in me. I dedicate this book to them, with gratitude and love.

Introduction
Medicine and metaphor
at the Carrara court

'A book is more than the sum of its materials. It is an artifact of the human mind and hand'.[1]

~ Geraldine Brooks, *People of the Book: A Novel*

On 9 May 1404, Francesco Zago made a list of books belonging to Francesco II 'il Novello' da Carrara, the last seigniorial lord of Padua (1359–1406, r. 1390–1405).[2] Zago, the official deputy of the *massaria* (the office that managed Padua's revenues), recorded titles and authors and gave brief descriptions of the contents of 57 books, and he further described the books' bindings, formats and any identifying marks (Venice, Biblioteca Marciana, lat. XIV, 93 [coll. 4530], f. 147r).[3] Remarkably, over two-thirds of the titles on Zago's list address the theory and practice of medicine, especially from the Arabic tradition, while, perhaps more expectedly, local histories, chronicles and family genealogies account for the remaining third. The collection is a curious one for the prince of a late medieval city-state, especially for a prince with no training in the discipline of medicine.[4]

While the whereabouts of most of the books on Zago's list remain unknown, a handful have been identified based on Zago's descriptions and the presence of Carrara family heraldry.[5] The sole identified medical book on the list, recorded by Zago as 'Serapiom in volgare', is known in contemporary scholarly literature as the *Carrara Herbal* (London, British Library, Egerton 2020). In addition to the pronounced Carrara heraldry on the book's frontispiece, the scribe (and perhaps translator), Frater Jacobus Philippus, identified the place of production in his excipit.[6] However, knowing the identity of this book only adds to the mystery of Francesco Novello's book collection.

The *Carrara Herbal* is an exceptional illustrated book of *materia medica* (therapeutic substances drawn from plants, animals and minerals).[7] It is exceptional in both its illustrations and its content, making it of interest to historians of art and medicine alike. The *Herbal* contains a translation into Paduan dialect of a Latin version of the mid-thirteenth-century Arabic pharmacopeia, *Kitāb al-Adwiya al-mufrada* (*The Book of Simple Medicines*), written by Ibn Sarābī,[8] a Christian physician working in al-Andalus and known in the Latin West as Serapion the Younger.[9] The treatise is Serapion's sole extant work, which Simon of Genoa (fl. late thirteenth century) and Abrāhām ben Shēm-Tōb of Tortosa (fl. late thirteenth century) translated into Latin as *Liber Serapionis aggregatus in medicinis simplicibus* (*Serapion's Book of Aggregated Simple Medicines*) around 1290, perhaps in Rome.[10] In his treatise, Serapion accumulated information about 'simples' (medical substances) drawn from earlier Greek and Arabic sources and brought them together into one volume. He noted this fact in his preface, along with his intention to amalgamate and reconcile the views of the two principal Greek medical authorities, Dioscorides (first century CE) and Galen (129–ca. 216/17 CE).[11] Further, Serapion told his readers that he intended to improve these Greek authorities with the knowledge of other Arabic physicians.[12]

In the *Carrara Herbal*, an ambitious, though unfinished, illustrative cycle accompanies Serapion's treatise.[13] Executed by an unknown artist in gouache on vellum, 56 images of individual plants range in type from the extraordinarily verisimilar (from a botanical viewpoint) to the staunchly schematic and to distinctive hybrids of the two.[14] The illustrations complicate and blend traditional and new forms of plant representation and, doing so, they echo the complex history of transmission and compilatory form of Serapion's treatise and break from the trajectory of contemporary and earlier herbal illustrations.

This study considers how the *Carrara Herbal* redefined Carrara family patronage away from *imitatio antiquorum*, with its roots in the Petrarchan humanism so central to the patronage of Francesco Novello's ancestors, and toward a celebration of contemporary medical learning and practice as taught at the University of Padua. The *Carrara Herbal* reflects this transition from an old to a new rhetoric of patronage in its novel content and, most clearly, in its multifaceted illustrations. The artist incorporated and blended visual elements from older forms of botanical illustration while he also invented new ones. Doing so, he created illustrations that not only parallel the aggregate nature of Serapion's text, they effectively parallel the transition in self-making practices mobilised by Francesco Novello's patronage choices as well. Francesco's efforts to align advances in medical knowledge with his vision of self and of Carrara-ruled Padua represent the first expression in northern Italy of an assimilation of science into a visualisation of political ideology, a practice historically associated with the later Renaissance.

In previous scholarship on the *Carrara Herbal*, the complexity of the artist's illustrative apparatus and his motives for creating it remain obscured, as do the patron's motives for commissioning the book itself. Following art historian Otto Pächt's once influential precedent, scholars have focussed on the artist's use of verisimilitude and divorced the imagery from Serapion's text.[15] Likewise, in Gustav Ineichen's masterly philological exploration of the *Carrara Herbal*, the significance of the book's imagery is left out.[16] Yet the diversity of the *Herbal*'s illustrations and their integral role in the reading experience are as relevant to any discussion of the *Herbal* as its verisimilar details or use of the Paduan vernacular. Furthermore, Carrara book-collecting practices, in general, and the *Carrara Herbal*, in particular, are predominantly absent from scholarship on the patronage of the Carrara family, which instead has focussed on the family's more public commissions (primarily their tombs and the frescoes adorning the Carrara palace and other Paduan monuments).[17] This study seeks to understand the complexity of the *Carrara Herbal* within the nexus of cultural, intellectual and artistic traditions out of which it grew, and, in doing so, to shed new light on some of these older questions and lacunae in our understanding of the Carrara and their patronage.

*

The *Carrara Herbal* contains the second book of Serapion's treatise. In this book, Serapion grouped 462 different medical substances into three large categories according to their place in the *tria regna naturae* (the three kingdoms of nature): plants (365), animals (48) and minerals (49).[18] Within these three dominant categories, Serapion grouped the *materia medica* into smaller categories according to the substances' elemental qualities and their combinations (temperate, hot/dry, hot/humid, cold/dry, and cold/humid). He then subdivided the substances within each quality according to their degree of intensity (from first to fourth), following the example of Galenic medicine, and accordingly organised them into chapters.[19]

The chapters in the *Herbal* range in length and are each dedicated to a medical simple. For every chapter, the scribe reserved upwards of two-thirds of a page for an image of the chapter's corresponding medical substance. In these images, the artist merged different illustrative techniques and representational types. By carefully recording observed details of the plant and by consciously perpetuating visual elements encountered in historic models, the artist broke from the contemporary genres of herbal illustration and created an entirely new visual experience. The use of the traditional types together with the verisimilar ones served to revive the historic models within the new context of Francesco's *Herbal*.

The artist's combination of innovation, amalgamation and experimentation is a clue to understanding the illustrations' hermeneutical role in the codex: this varied use of imagery visually parallels the form of Serapion's treatise itself, mirroring the treatise in its 'aggregation' and 'amelioration' of past imagery of *materia medica*. In other words, the artist designed his imagery in relation to the content of the *Herbal*. Moreover, the artist's composition of the illustrations interacts with the text and the available page surface to command the reader's attention in various ways. Although the majority of his images occupy the lower two-thirds of the page, the artist interspersed many illustrations between passages of their associated texts or between entries, creating breaks or continuities in the rhythm of reading.[20] The text and imagery together construct meaning.

Looking at the entire set of images and their relationship to the text, we see that the artist integrated the illustrations with the textual content of the manuscript, making the illustrations central to the process of reading and not separate from it. The artist charged the reading experience – made it memorable and unique – by moving between lifelike, fanciful and schematic types of representation: he put the experience of viewing the illustrations into conversation with the book's very words and then with the history of those words. The artist defied reader expectations of compositional consistency, and, doing so, he cultivated an engaged reading experience defined by its diverse pleasures and utilities.[21] Furthermore, the readers' active engagement with the reading experience draws their attention back to the book as an object, an object that belonged to Francesco Novello. In drawing attention back to the prince and his book collection, the role of the *Carrara Herbal* as a locus of Francesco's patronage and generative source for his self-image becomes clearer.

The *Carrara Herbal* is exceptional, in part, because of its singularity. There are no other extant vernacular, illustrated versions of Serapion's work from the end of the fourteenth century. Its singularity suggests its allure as a novel – and perhaps defining – addition to Francesco Novello's library. Yet, in addition to its novelty, the book appealed to Francesco because it enabled him to bring together aspects of his familial patronage traditions and to present them in a way unique to his own rule. Considered within Francesco Novello's library, full of medical books and family histories, the *Carrara Herbal* becomes a site of exchange: through its distinctive form and content, the book puts into conversation medical and moral wisdom celebrated at the Carrara court in Padua and visible in the historic patronage of Francesco's family.

For Francesco, possessing an illustrated version of Serapion's treatise conceptually connected the lord (and other privileged readers) to the medicine and pharmacology taught at the University of Padua, a site of civic pride and of Carrara patronage.[22] Simultaneously, the very materiality of the *Carrara Herbal* as an illustrated book connected Francesco to other patronage strategies practiced by his ancestors, especially to their book-collecting practices associated with early humanists' moralising study of civil history. The *Carrara Herbal* was both a source of innovative medical content and a touchstone for the medical metaphors central to the humanistic understanding of history's value.

In the following introductory pages, I present a broad picture of Paduan culture at the end of the fourteenth century, a culture influenced by the rise to prominence of the university, especially its medical schools, and by Petrarch (1304–1374) and his humanist successors. Within this framework, I situate ideas and themes that inform the analysis of the *Carrara Herbal* presented in the ensuing chapters, focussing on the complementary relationship between natural philosophy and ethics in the study of medicine and nature and in humanist pedagogy. Further, I introduce how this relationship manifested in the imitative patronage practices cultivated by generations of Carrara princes.

A set of 'humanist habits'

In commissioning the *Carrara Herbal*, Francesco Novello was attuned to trends in medicine and traditions in humanism and to the roles these disciplines played at court. The study and practice of medicine and its relationship to humanistic inquiry were in transition at the end of the fourteenth century.[23] By the time Francesco commissioned the *Carrara Herbal*, the traditional boundaries of humanism, as shaped by Petrarch and the earlier Paduan humanists Lovato Lovati (ca. 1237–1309) and Albertino Mussato (1261–1329), were broadening as well. While Petrarch disparaged medical doctors in his *Invective contra medicum* (*Invectives against a Physician*) in 1353,[24] pointing to a disconnect between their (scholastic) way of thinking and their (generally empirical) practices,[25] subsequent scholars, both humanists and physicians, would increasingly be interested in the fruitful meeting points between humanistic, medical and scientific knowledge.

In his *Invective*, Petrarch perpetuated an old debate between the status of the liberal arts, as superior arts addressing the spirit, and mechanical arts, like medicine, as those addressing the body. His scholarly descendants, however, would cultivate a set of 'humanist habits' – to borrow Brian Ogilvie's memorable turn of phrase – that tested this dichotomy.[26] As Ogilvie, Nancy Siraisi and Chiara Crisciani have shown (following the pioneering work of Paul Oskar Kristeller and Eugenio Garin), the disciplines of medicine and humanism were not mutually exclusive during the Middle Ages and Early Modern period and, in fact, shared interests particularly closely at universities in northern Italy.[27] Simply put, many humanists were medically educated, and many physicians were humanistically trained. For instance, as students in the schools of arts and medicine, future physicians at the University of Padua counted natural philosophy, logic, astrology and rhetoric among their university studies.[28]

These scholars did not have the sense of disciplinary separation we so often see today. Instead, they exchanged ideas from complementary fields of inquiry. For example, in their writings, humanists and physicians shared interests in the genre of biography, the role of faith in healing, antiquarianism and the wonders of nature.[29] Physicians borrowed humanists' rhetorical tools for use in oratory, and, later in the fifteenth and sixteenth centuries, both communities would enrich each other's disciplines – philological and medical – through their shared translation efforts (especially of original Greek medical treatises). Of particular relevance to this discussion, fifteenth-century physicians increasingly applied traditional humanistic values associated with the study of history and rhetoric to genres of medical writing (such as case histories and health regimens) and to the study of nature more broadly.[30]

For humanistically trained scholars and physicians across the fifteenth century, the study of nature, in which medicine played a large role, carried with it moral overtones more commonly associated with the study of civil history and rhetoric (which humanists from Petrarch onward taught through the lens of ethics).[31] Humanist teachers pillaged Greek and Roman histories and poetry, especially, in search of accounts or details that provided moral *exempla* or that could be interpreted according to contemporary moral codes for their students.[32] While initially confined to 'preuniversity studies', these long-established practices increasingly were integrated into university curricula, especially during the second half of the fifteenth century – an integration that would birth what to modern eyes appear as disciplinary hybrids, like medical humanism and medical philology.[33] Scholars began to internalise the ethical study of human history and to map it onto their study of nature and its particular details.[34] Knowledge about the natural world, then, was not simply a form of erudition or a foundation for a community of scholars or physicians. It connoted the moral health of individuals and their communities.

While the ethical conceits accompanying the study of nature would truly blossom in the sixteenth century with the growth of natural history as a discipline, they were nascent at the time of the *Carrara Herbal*'s creation. In the late fourteenth century, humanist teachers began to encourage the study of nature and medicine in conjunction with the study of other branches of knowledge.[35] So, for instance, in his early fifteenth-century treatise describing the ideal education for young men and future leaders, *De ingenuis moribus et liberalibus adulescentiae studiis* (*The Character and Studies Befitting a Free-Born Youth*), Pier Paolo Vergerio (ca. 1369–1444) noted that[36]

> Indeed, knowledge about nature [*scientia de natura*] is especially appropriate to and in conformity with the human intellect, for through this knowledge we understand the principles and processes of natural things, both animate and inanimate, as well as the causes and effects of the motions and transformations of those which are contained in heaven and on earth, and we are able to explain many things that generally seem miraculous to the vulgar. There is nothing that is not pleasant to understand, but it is especially pleasant to concern ourselves with those things which cause sensible effects in the air and round about the earth.

Furthermore, Vergerio goes on to praise the study of medicine as very fine (*pulcherissima*) and useful (*commodissima*) to know – although he discouraged its practice as unbefitting for his elite students.[37]

Vergerio borrowed Petrarch's (and, long before him, Horace's) approach to the study of history and applied it to the study of nature and medicine as well: he associated these studies with pleasure (*iucundissimum est*) and utility (*commodissima*).[38] In their growing tendency to include natural philosophy and medicine as part of a liberal education, Vergerio and his fellow humanists complicated Petrarch's condemnation of the study of nature and medicine as useless.[39] It was from these seeds in 'pleasant and useful' study of nature and medicine that the *Carrara Herbal* grew.

Vergerio wrote *De ingenuis moribus* for Ubertino 'Fiorentino' da Carrara (1390–1407), Francesco Novello's youngest son.[40] So, the humanist's ideas about education were in circulation in the same milieu that generated the *Carrara Herbal*. In its form and content, the *Carrara Herbal* translated the rhetoric of moral health (associated with the humanistic study of civil history and the practice of contemplative reading) into the rhetoric of physical health (associated with the study and practice of medicine). The frontispiece of the *Carrara Herbal* shows the careful tension between these avenues of interpretation. It prominently displays the prince's initials and his personal and familial shields of arms set amid colourful, swirling acanthus-like leaves accented in gold (Plate 1).

The Carrara family's heraldic arms, the red *carro* (or 'cart', a play on the family name) on a black background, is represented three times on the frontispiece to the *Herbal* (f. 4r), which begins the section of the manuscript dedicated to medicines derived from plants. In addition, the *carro* is represented twice on the title page of the subsequent, unillustrated section dedicated to medicines derived from animals (f. 267r).[41] On the principal frontispiece, two large, gold 'Fs' set in quatrefoil frames complement the heraldic arms from the upper right and left corners. These initials identify the book as Francesco Novello's possession while they also may honour his father and namesake, Francesco I 'il Vecchio' (1325–1393, r. 1350–1388),[42] from whom he inherited his shield of arms or crest (*cimiero*).[43]

Francesco il Vecchio's crest, which he appropriated from Ubertino (d. 1345), the third Carrara lord of Padua (r. 1338–1345), is portrayed in the lower left corner.[44] Francesco Novello inherited this crest, which portrays a winged, golden-horned black figure – identified as a 'Moor' or 'Saracen' in contemporary Paduan chronicles – robed in red and gold and perched atop a black helmet. The helmet in turn rests upon the familial heraldic arms (*stemma*): the black shield bearing the *carro*. Another shield of arms mirrors the intergenerational family shield from the lower exterior margin. This crest is Francesco Novello's personal addition to the family heraldry. Set against a red background, the crest shows a helmet crowned with two wings – one black and the other white – atop the black shield bearing the representation of the *carro*.[45] Along with two of Francesco Novello's personal devices, these two shields frame the depiction of *citron* (*Citrus medica*, L., citron tree, f. 4r, Plate 1), and, with the other Carrara symbols, encircle the opening illustration of the *Herbal*.[46] Through this imagery, Francesco claimed the book for himself and his ancestral family. Further, these ornate identifiers position the *Herbal* in the Carrara tradition of book collection and its attendant sets of moral associations with the humanist educational enterprise. Moreover, by surrounding the Serapion text on citron trees and its accompanying illustration, the heraldic border reinforces Francesco Novello's commitment to medical study and the aesthetic beauty of nature.[47]

The frontispiece imagery anticipates the role of the codex itself as a vehicle that bridges visual and textual rhetorics associated with different avenues of patronage and elements of Paduan civic identity. By association with Serapion's text, the book conflates patterns of knowledge transmission and pharmacological innovation (ideas affiliated with the medical community and the University of Padua) with status and humanistic notions of moral and physical health (ideas affiliated with the collection and reading of illustrated books and with the experience of cultivated nature, or nature shaped by human invention).

The late medieval *fortuna* of an Arabic herbal

The textual content of the *Carrara Herbal* directly tied Francesco Novello to trends in the development of curriculum at the medical school of the University of Padua. Shifting currents in university medicine in the Latin West – beginning with efforts to translate Arabic and Greek medical texts in the late eleventh century at Salerno – would redefine how medicine and pharmacology were taught at universities across Italy.[48] The translation of Serapion's treatise into Latin contributed to these efforts. Its growing popularity – along with that of other medical texts originally composed in Arabic – among apothecaries and physicians across the Italian peninsula, and particularly at the University of Padua, likely contributed to Francesco Novello's interest in Serapion's work.[49] Owning the *Carrara Herbal*, the *signore* brought the advances in medicine and pharmacology emerging in the new curriculum into the purview of the court, where he claimed them as attributes of his imagined identity as prince of Padua.

The *Carrara Herbal* is an early example of a northern Italian illustrated translation of an Arabic book of *materia medica*. It was preceded by the slightly earlier production of illuminated manuscripts of the *Taqwīm al-Ṣiḥḥa*, translated into Latin as the *Tacuinum Sanitatis*, the 'Table of Health'; but the *Taqwīm* is not a book of *materia medica* in the strictest sense. Originally composed by the Christian physician Ibn Buṭlān of Baghdad (d. ca. 1063),[50] the *Tacuinum* includes information other than the therapeutics of *materia medica* found in pharmacopoeias. Specifically, it includes prescriptions that address the so-called six 'non-naturals' – air, food and drink, exercise and rest, sleeping and waking, repletion and excretion, and emotions – considered central to the preservation of health (especially to the preservation of aristocrats' health).[51]

Francesco Novello's commission of an illustrated version of Serapion's text responds, in part, to the illustrated *Tacuinum*, which was popular at the court of the Carrara rivals – the Visconti of Milan. However, Serapion's work, rather than Ibn Buṭlān's, was the more appropriate choice for the prince of Padua. The *Liber Serapionis aggregatus in medicinis simplicibus* held specific, local significance due to its association with the growing prestige of Arabic medicine in the medical school at the University of Padua (and, perhaps, its use in curricula as well).[52]

During the late medieval and Early Modern eras, Serapion's work was counted among the influential texts of the medical canon.[53] Over 50 extant manuscript copies and 11 printed editions of Serapion's treatise – dating from the thirteenth through sixteenth centuries – attest to its popularity in the Latin West.[54] It was a central text for pharmacists and physicians well into the sixteenth century, especially across the Italian peninsula. In the fifteenth century, distinguished scholars and physicians urged their students to study Serapion. For example, Saladino da Ascoli (fl. 1448–1463), the court physician to the Prince of Taranto, Giovanni Antonio Orsini del Balzo (ca. 1393–1463), described Serapion's treatise as one of only six essential readings for aspiring apothecaries in Part I of his *Compendium aromatariorum* (*The Book of the Pharmacists*, ca. 1450).[55] Even Niccolò Leoniceno (1428–1524), himself no friend of Arabic medicine, owned a copy of the Latin translation of Serapion's treatise (it was the only Arabic medical text that he owned) and noted that all students of pharmacy were essentially students of Serapion.[56] Of course, when Frater Jacobus penned his translation onto the pages of the *Carrara Herbal*, Serapion's treatise was just beginning its ascent to fame in the West.

Serapion's work gained such popularity and spread widely across Europe, in part, because of its compilatory form. For Francesco and the medical students, apothecaries and professors who would study Serapion's work, the treatise represented a synthesis of the pharmacological tradition from across the Mediterranean.[57] As a synthesis, Serapion's work was emblematic of the entire medieval

Pan-Mediterranean medical tradition. In the case of the *Carrara Herbal*, this synthesis of vast medical knowledge was housed in an ornate, illustrated book belonging to the Carrara lord. Regardless of how popular Serapion's treatise was among medical doctors, the quality of the materials and the illustrative apparatus in the *Carrara Herbal* distinguish it from its unillustrated counterparts and anchor it to wider trends of book collection, particularly among patricians in northern Italy, and to the history of Carrara family patronage.

Patterns of Carrara patronage

In 1390, when Francesco Novello regained Padua from Giangaleazzo Visconti (1351–1402), the *signore* of Milan, the Carrara lord helped secure his rule by appropriating his family's traditional avenues of patronage into his own. This patronage choice followed a distinctive pattern in which the Carrara princes practiced a type of imitation as emulation to demonstrate the continuity of the dynasty. Each Carrara *signore* built upon the identifiable patronage strategies of his predecessor, creating a visual continuity in their successive rules and simultaneously asserting an individual character for each ruler. Following his father, Francesco il Vecchio, in particular, Francesco Novello's principal avenues of patronage were the acquisition and circulation of books and the support of the University of Padua. Owning the *Carrara Herbal* allowed Francesco to participate in both avenues at once. It identified him as a member of a long line of patrons (from physicians to patricians) who commissioned and collected illustrated books, while its content connected the lord to the field of medicine, taught at the university and practiced at court.

Similar patronage strategies were used to good effect by Francesco Novello's father and his grandfather, Giacomo II (d. 1350, r. 1345–1350),[58] both of whom celebrated the university and fostered a culture of knowledge in Padua that they visualised in their libraries and in decorative cycles adorning their halls of state. When Giangaleazzo Visconti seized Padua in 1388, the *signore* of Milan took the contents of the elder Francesco's library as *spolia*. Francesco Novello's efforts to rebuild the Carrara library show his desire to remedy this loss and are evidence of the importance of book collection, not only to the younger Francesco, but also to his family heritage. While these efforts indicate that the elder Francesco's patronage influenced his son's vision of self as ruler of Padua, the contents of the younger Francesco's book collection diverged dramatically from his father's. Francesco il Vecchio's library connected the lord to patterns in his own father's patronage and centred around their mutual friendship with the poet Petrarch. The contents of the elder Francesco's library attested to his living relationship with the poet and so was characterised by the works Petrarch wrote and by those he read, while the younger Francesco's library – created after Petrarch's death – adopted a different focus.

Both Francesco il Vecchio and his father, Giacomo II, entreated Petrarch to settle in Padua. The poet accepted the invitations of father and son, both of whom welcomed him into their inner court circles. Petrarch's correspondence from his time in Padua shows that he admired the Carrara lords and considered his role at court as that of a teacher and mentor.[59] Defining the trajectory of humanist peda-gogy, Petrarch taught a moralised version of Roman history and used its heroic protagonists as examples to instruct the *signori* on the proper character and rule of a good and moral prince. He described his method of teaching in his letter to Niccolò Acciaiuoli (1310–1365), the Grand Seneschal to the new King of Naples, Louis of Taranto (1320–1362), in 1352.[60] In his letter, Petrarch urged Acciaiuoli to educate the king using examples drawn from the lives of virtuous men of history. Petrarch wrote:[61]

> Let [the King] borrow this quality, discipline, from that great leader, and additional ones from other men, so that by culling from all of them he may fashion a truly distinctive man. However many outstanding men preceded him, let him consider them all his teachers of life, his leaders toward glory. Examples enkindle noble minds no less than rewards, nor do words less than statues. It is of benefit to compare oneself to exemplary men who are highly praised, for beautiful is that imitation inspired by virtue.

Petrarch taught an imitative practice for contemporary rulers that involved study-ing and – more importantly – emulating the (moralised) lives of ancient leaders.

Perhaps the strongest literary expression of his teaching practice is *De viris illustribus* (*On Famous Men*),[62] which the poet dedicated to Francesco il Vecchio in 1367. According to Petrarch, the heroes of (primarily) Roman history, the *viri illustres* or illustrious men, provide a template for the development of a good and just modern ruler, and their personal and professional characters were the poet's blueprints for the return of good government to a corrupted Italy. Petrarch upheld each illustrious man as *magistra vitae* – a teacher or guide of life – and urged the Carrara lord to see these men as *exempla* to follow in his own life. Petrarch's understanding of this practice derived from the *Speculum principis* (*Mirror of Princes*) literary tradition, a tradition indebted to Seneca's first-century moral theory on monarchical rule expressed in *De clementia* (*On Mercy*),[63] in which the philosopher couched his political advice to the emperor, Nero (37–68 CE), in medical metaphors.[64]

In *De clementia*, Seneca (4–65 CE) sought to provide an education on proper ethical and political behaviour for the emperor.[65] The first sentence of Seneca's treatise specifically indicates that his argument is meant to serve as a 'mirror' for its reader.[66] He wrote: 'I have undertaken, Nero Caesar, to write on the subject of mercy, in order to serve in a way the purpose of a mirror, and thus reveal you to yourself'.[67] Here, Seneca used the mirror as a metaphor to relate the prince's person to intangible moral characteristics. Furthermore, in a technique that Petrarch would adopt, Seneca used the body of the ruler as a metaphor for his territories and his citizens. If the ruler did not conduct himself well and care for his (civic) body, his people's (and his city's) health would suffer. For example, Seneca wrote:[68]

For if – and this is what thus far [my essay] is establishing – you are the soul of the state and the state your body, you see, I think, how requisite is mercy; for you are merciful to yourself when you are seemingly merciful to another. And so even reprobate citizens should have mercy as being the weak members of the body, and if there should ever be need to let blood, the hand must be held under control to keep it from cutting deeper than may be necessary.

Seneca considered the relationship between the state and the ruler to be like that between the soul and the body, and he used the idea of careful surgery or phlebotomy as a metaphor to suggest how the emperor ought to control his unruly citizens.

Petrarch revitalised this metaphor in his discussion of the *viri illustres*. The poet and his followers used similar corporeal metaphors related to the health of the prince's body to illustrate an ideal prince's moral leadership. Petrarch argued that a leader would ensure the health of his civic body by patterning his life on Rome's great men. The resulting teaching practice influenced the artistic commissions of both Francesco Novello's father and grandfather. In different ways, Francesco il Vecchio and Giacomo II incorporated Petrarch's view of Roman history and its leaders into their artistic commissions. Through it, they sought to project images of themselves as the successors to Rome's great leaders and as proper vessels for the (moral) health of Padua and its people.

By collecting books inspired by his friendship with Petrarch, Francesco il Vecchio presented himself not just as the successor of Giacomo II – who was greatly admired by the poet – but also as a new *vir illustris*, a noble man in the tradition of Petrarch's heroes. Following Petrarch's example, the elder Francesco claimed books as signs of the contemplative life that the poet deemed requisite for an illustrious leader, signs Giacomo II also incorporated into his self-image. Building on his father's artistic patronage and commissions for the Reggia Carrarese, the family palace, Francesco il Vecchio adorned a new great hall, the *Sala virorum illustrium* (*Hall of Famous Men*), with portraits of Petrarch's heroes to remind his visitors of the poet's connection to Padua and to the city's lords.[69] Guided by Petrarch's teachings in the *Speculum principis* tradition, the elder Francesco commissioned the portrait frieze and collected books to help connect him to the ideal of healthy (moral) governance of Padua in the tradition of healthy (moral) governance of a Christianised Roman past.

Conversely, as Francesco Zago's list of books tells us, the younger Francesco clearly preferred contemporary medical treatises and books of *materia medica*. The only Petrarchan text on Zago's inventory is *De remediis utriusque fortunae* (*On the Remedies for Different Fortunes*),[70] in which Petrarch uses medical metaphors to convey his moralistic advice. He assumes the persona of a physician and 'prescribes' his advice as though it was a medicine.[71] Including this Petrarchan work, the subject matters chosen for Francesco Novello's library – and the way in which those subjects were conveyed in ornate illustrated manuscripts – projected an image of the prince as learned in contemporary medicine (metaphorical and literal) and in local history rather than in the histories of Petrarch's *viri illustres*. Through his illustrated book collection, Francesco Novello remade Petrarch's concept of the *viri illustres*, as they were understood by his father, into a new image. He accomplished this task, in part, by inverting Petrarch's use of medical metaphor. If Petrarch and his fellow humanists conveyed moral advice in the guise of medical practice, could not the actual practice of medicine be a guise for humanist moral advice?

The new *viri illustres*, as they were understood by Francesco Novello, were the most recognisable and lauded citizens of his present-day Padua (next to the Carrara lords, of course): medical doctors and humanist chronicler-historians. Possessing books about medicine and about local history affiliated Francesco with these two influential communities of educated men. Through his association with these communities, Francesco invested his self-image as the new ruler of Padua with their respective knowledge of medicine, history and the qualities of morality and health associated with these disciplines. In doing so, Francesco restructured his father's use of Petrarch's *viri illustres* as metaphors for his own personal qualities as the new Carrara leader.

Yet whether the admirable personal qualities of the lords' self-images were associated with men from ancient Rome or from fourteenth-century Padua, these qualities needed a Carrara body in which to manifest and upon which to play out the relationship between medical practice and medical metaphor. Francesco Novello's father and grandfather used figural portraiture as a heuristic device, mobilising allusions to the Roman *viri illustres* as their alternative selves. Francesco Novello, conversely, did not focus his commissions on figural portraits of himself. Rather, to consolidate his role as leader and to give a renewed vision to Petrarch's *viri illustres*, he brought his ancestors' use of portraiture into his illustrated book collection. Francesco had portraits and family heraldic devices originally commissioned by his predecessors directly translated into his new books, which explicitly connected Francesco to his ancestors and to their artistic patronages. In doing so, Francesco collapsed the hermeneutic apparatus on which the metaphorical association between the Carrara princes and Petrarch's *viri illustres* depended into a physical object associated with Francesco himself. Through its connection to medicine and so to medicine's use as a metaphor in humanists' rhetoric of exemplarity, the *Carrara Herbal* played a key role within Francesco's collection, one that helped him to assume his forefathers' strengths, as emphasised in their portraits, into himself.

*

The following chapters explore the creation, value and meaning of the *Carrara Herbal* primarily within the three traditional avenues of Carrara family patronage: book collection, support of the University of Padua (*Studium*), and family portraiture. Chapter 1 situates the content and imagery of the *Carrara Herbal* in the long history of collection of illustrated books of *materia medica* – from the sixth century to the thirteenth, from Byzantium to the Arabic Empire and into the Latin West. This chapter considers how the genre of illustrated books of *materia medica* could be used to convey messages about their owners' morality, health and status by creating specific reading experiences that alluded to privileged knowledge sets.

Chapter 2 focuses on the experience and benefits of reading the *Carrara Herbal* in particular. This chapter examines the *Herbal* and its imagery within popular medical and humanistic ideals in circulation at the Carrara court.

Chapter 3 considers how Francesco Novello used the *Carrara Herbal* to engage and modify the humanistic rhetoric of exemplarity, established in his father's book collection, and to refocus it onto the rising fame of Padua's *Studium* and its physicians. By commissioning the *Herbal*, Francesco Novello appropriated into his self-image the family's historic use of the University of Padua's successes as measures of its leadership and good governance. Such appropriation enabled Francesco to portray himself as a new type of heroic ruler – the 'physician prince' of Padua. To understand the complementary relationship between the self-images and patronage strategies of Francesco and his ancestors, Chapter 4 explores the artistic and civic commissions of Francesco's father and grandfather in more detail, especially their use of monumental portraiture to effect a positive, public view of the lords and their family.

Chapters 5 focuses on how Francesco Novello assumed the ideals about the Carrara family, established in his ancestors' use of portraiture and heraldry, and placed them into conversation with his own self-image. In particular, this chapter argues that the study and practice of physiognomy by Paduan physicians, artists and humanists provided Francesco Novello with a vector through which to appropriate his ancestors' self-imagery into his patronage and so into his view of self as the new prince of Padua. Chapter 6 analyses how Francesco Novello accomplished this appropriation. By translating historic portraits of the *signori* and their heraldry into his books, Francesco mobilised diverse physiognomic associations to advance an image of himself as heir and successor to the Carrara dynasty.

The representations of the Carrara lords and their heraldry in Francesco Novello's other books become a type of key – a paradigmatic instrument – with which to interpret the representations of plants and their accompanying textual content in the *Carrara Herbal*. The manuscript mediated between historic ideals of the prince's ancestors (as shown in their portraits and patterns of patronage) and Francesco's own self-representation as prince of Padua. As an attribute of the *signore*, it blended knowledge and tradition from medical and humanistic study in order to position Francesco as an ideal 'physician prince' who orchestrated the moral and physical health of his community. As a physical object, it actualised Francesco's image: like Francesco himself, the visual and textual rhetoric in the *Carrara Herbal* internalised past traditions and transformed them into tools capable of ensuring a 'healthy' future for the city of Padua and its citizens.

Notes

1 Brooks (2008: 19).
2 For a brief introduction to Francesco II da Carrara, see Ganguzza Billanovich (1977a).
3 Lazzarini (1901–1902: 26), and Bettini (1974: 55). In the successive months, priests named Cristoforo and Brussano brought forward four more volumes, which were added to the list. The inventory was part of a *consegna*, a note of consignment or delivery, acquired at the end of the eighteenth century by the Biblioteca Nazionale Marciana as

part of a register of letters that once belonged to Dondi dall'Orologio, a late seventeenth-century Paduan historian. Pélissier (1899: 6.177–80) published a transcription of the *consegna*. For a description of the larger contents of the *consegna* included with the inventory (Venice, Biblioteca Nazionale Marciana, lat. XIV, 93 [coll. 4530]), see Valentinelli (1870: 3.95–6). For the definition of *massaro*, see Kohl's glossary (1998: 422). For Zago's complete list, see Appendix.

4 On Francesco Novello's education, see Kohl (1998: 133). From a young age, perhaps as young as 4, the prince studied languages and literature (along with the art of war).

5 Few of the manuscripts on Zago's list have been identified with certainty because the former Carrara collection was fragmented and scattered even before the end of the Carrara dynasty. Shortly before his capture on 18 November 1405, Francesco Novello allegedly sent his most luxurious codices to Florence for safekeeping, along with the young Carrara children, money, jewels and silverware (Lazzarini 1901–1902: 29, and Bettini 1974: 55). The details and whereabouts of this family patrimony are unknown. Furthermore, in January and September of 1406, the chancellors of Padua gave many unnamed codices to Venice's 'Council of Ten', along with other documents from various Carrara governmental offices (Lazzarini 1901–1902: 27–8).

6 On the closing folio (289v), the scribe wrote: 'Frat Jacob Phyllipus de Pađ ordīs hēx scripsit' ('Frat[er] Jacob[us] Phyllipus de Pad[ua], ord[in]is he[remitarum] scripsit').

7 The primacy of plant materials in this genre of book accounts for the somewhat misleading name 'herbal'.

8 Whenever possible, for the spelling of ancient Arabic names I have followed the usage in the *Encyclopaedia of Islam*, 2nd edn. Ibn Sarābī is not included in *EI2*. For a brief introduction to Ibn Sarābī, see Harvey (2008).

9 Generally, scholars now date the treatise to between 1242 and 1248, in accord with Ullmann's careful analysis of the sources cited by Serapion (1970). Ullmann notes that Serapion cited al-Rāzī (Rhazes, ca. 854–925 or 935, see Richter-Bernburg 2006) and Ibn Wāfid (Abenguefit, 1008–1075, see Hopkins 1971), sources that provide a firm *terminus post quem* of the late eleventh century. However, Serapion also cites the lapidary written by al-Tīfāshī (d. 1253, see Ruska and Kahl 2000), which dates to 1242, locating the creation of Serapion's work to after the mid-thirteenth century (Ullmann 1970: 283–4, and Dilg 1999: 226). Serapion's work, in turn, is cited by the botanist Ibn al-Bayṭār in his pharmacopeia, *Kitāb Al-jāmi' li-mufradāt al-adwiya wa al-aghdhiya* (*Compendium on Simple Medicaments and Foods*). Al-Bayṭār died in 1248, providing a potential *terminus ante quem* (Ullmann 1970: 280–3). On al-Bayṭār, see Vernet (1971). While no Arabic version of his work remains extant, Serapion is believed to have been an Arabic-speaking author because he repeats errors found in Arabic texts of Dioscorides (first century CE) and Galen (129–ca. 216–17 CE). Furthermore, Serapion lists the drugs included in the second part of his treatise according to the Arabic *abjad* alphabet (Dilg 1999: 224). That Serapion lived and worked in al-Andalus is suggested in a chapter on the medicinal properties of cherries. He observed that the cherries grown 'in Oriente' (in the East) are different from those known 'apud nos' (among us) (Dilg 1999: 227). Citing Ibn Wāfid, a physician and pharmacologist working in Toledo, also suggests that Ibn Sarābī lived and worked in al-Andalus. On al-Andalus, see Delfina Serrano Ruano (2006).

10 Simon was papal curia chaplain and physician at the court of Nicolas IV, pope from 1288 to 1292 (Touwaide 2013b: 48). There is no extant Arabic version of Serapion's text preceding the translation into Latin – the entire transmission of Serapion's work rests on this single translation (Dilg 1999: 226). Simon finished his *Clavis sanationis* (a multilingual lexicon of *materia medica*) in 1290. Since Simon cites Serapion in the *Clavis*, he may have translated Serapion's book around this time or earlier (Dilg 1999: 226).

11 For his content, Serapion draws especially on Dioscorides' *De materia medica* (*On Therapeutic Substance*) and on Galen's *De simplicium medicamentorum temperamentis*

ac facultatibus (*On the Mixtures and Properties of Simple Medicines*) (Dilg 1999: 228). The Greek physician Galen of Pergamum theorised that each drug possessed a dominant 'element' which related it to the cosmic elements – earth, fire, water and air – found in the body (according to an Aristotelian concept of the physical world). Following the tenets of Hippocratic medicine, Galen considered disease a result of an imbalance of the four humours or fluids (blood, yellow bile, black bile and phlegm) within the body, which he correlated with the four elements and their qualities (hot, cold, wet and dry). While, broadly speaking, Hippocratic medicine (especially Galen's interpretation of it) focusses on the ability of the body to heal itself and rebalance its humours with the help of proper diet, good air, rest and hygiene, Galen added a complementary theory on the curative use of drugs, the properties of which were recorded in books of *materia medica*. Serapion's work integrates Dioscorides' knowledge of medical properties with Galen's organisational system. For a detailed discussion of the theories and practices of Dioscorides, Galen and other ancient physicians, see Nutton (2013). For an introduction to Galen and Galenic medicine, in particular, see Nutton (2004 and 2013: 222–53).

12 Dilg (1999: 228), and Harvey (2008: 1118).

13 The cycle of illustration remains incomplete, likely cut short by the expensive conflict with Venice that preceded the extermination of the Carrara family in 1406. On the final conflict between Venice and the Carrara, see Kohl (1998: 303–38).

14 For detailed descriptions of the four distinct genera of plant imagery in the *Herbal* and their relationship to the text, see Chapter 1, pp. 24–8. The illustrations for the sections of Serapion's treatise dedicated to medicines derived from other, nonbotanical sources were not completed. The existing illustrations are scattered throughout the codex and often cluster in small groups in the entries near the beginning of their respective chapters.

15 When discussing the *Carrara Herbal*, art historians have tended to isolate its imagery from its text and to focus on its realistic plant imagery as part of a progressive stylistic development toward the more realistic figural and nature imagery associated with the idea of Renaissance. Pächt established this reading of the *Herbal*'s imagery over half a century ago. For Pächt (1950), the plant images in the *Carrara Herbal* were part of a progression toward an increasingly illusionistic portrayal of nature drawn from direct observation, a progression that culminated in monumental, individualised landscape painting in Northern Europe and later in Italy. Several generations of art historical scholarship have challenged Pächt's view of Renaissance, in which verisimilitude assumes metahistoric value; yet his interpretation of the *Carrara Herbal* has remained influential. He posited that the imagery in the *Herbal* expanded upon that in a *Tractatus de herbis*, a treatise on medicinal plants, likely produced in Salerno, ca. 1280–1317 (London, British Library, Egerton 747). For Pächt, this *Tractatus* was the archetype for a new genre of illustrated herbal that strove to record lifelike observations of nature. As such, it began the return to a supposed veristic Late Antique aesthetic that heralded Renaissance. Pächt argued that the plant imagery in herbals had deteriorated into schematic and decorative illustrations worthless for identification of the plants, which he considered the purpose of these books. Similarly, in the sole study dedicated to the *Carrara Herbal*, Baumann (1974) followed Pächt and situated the *Herbal*'s imagery within what he perceived as a stylistic arc, a rise and fall of early pictorial naturalism, in the *Tractatus de herbis* manuscripts. He classified the images as 'Schema' (schematic portraiture), 'beginnendes Naturstudium' (early nature study), 'Naturbeobachtung' (portraiture derived from direct observation of nature), 'gepreβtes Herbarexemplar' (portraiture based on pressed specimens), and finally as 'Reduktionsformen' (simplification of form due to the copying process). More recently, Collins (2000) discussed the *Herbal* in her chronological survey of the development of botanical imagery. While valuable as the culmination of the sort of formal analysis Pächt undertook and the development of a stylistic chronology across the genre, Collins' argument remains

tethered to Pächt's conclusions. Like Pächt, Collins suggests that the reappearance of illusionistic plant imagery in the Egerton 747 and the *Carrara Herbal* is evidence of the illustrators' consultation of Antique examples of plant representations that sparked a fashion for empirical observation in late medieval natural philosophy. She concludes that by the fifteenth century, when their accompanying texts had become increasingly abbreviated and distanced from their original medical content, illustrated herbal manuscripts became simply 'picture books' for aristocratic bibliophiles (Collins 2000: 310). For an alternative interpretation of fifteenth-century herbals, especially the *Tractatus de herbis* now held at the British Library under the shelfmark Sloane 4016, see Touwaide (2013b).

16   Ineichen (1962–1966). My understanding of the content and medical terminology used in the *Carrara Herbal* is deeply indebted to Ineichen's comprehensive study of the text.

17   To my knowledge, Mariani Canova (1994 and 1999) is the sole scholar specifically to consider, albeit briefly, the *Carrara Herbal* within the patronage practices – in this case, illustrated book collection – of the Carrara family. The entries on books produced for the Carrara and members of their court in the catalogue for an exhibition of Paduan illuminated manuscripts, which Mariani Canova co-edited (1999), were especially useful to me in establishing a more comprehensive view of the Carrara libraries. Otherwise, although a rich tradition of scholarship exists on the Carrara family and their patronage, it has remained mostly silent concerning the *Carrara Herbal*. Historians Hyde (1966b and 1993) and Kohl (especially 1989 and 1998) have discussed the political and military realities of communal and seigniorial Padua in detail. Kohl's work, in particular, has been indispensable to my understanding of the network of political and social relationships that the Carrara cultivated and how the family's artistic commissions functioned to buttress these relationships. Yet neither Hyde nor Kohl addressed the significance of the Carrara manuscript commissions. Over a century ago, Lazzarini (1901–1902) published Zago's partial inventory of Francesco Novello's books, identified the *Carrara Herbal* as the 'Serapiom in volgare', and noted the prevalence of medical texts within the collection. However, he did not address the significance of the *Herbal* or the collection to Francesco Novello's patronage or sense of princely identity, either. More recently, art historians Plant (1981 and 1987), Saalman (1987), Norman (1995b), Warr (1996) and Derbes (2013) all have discussed aspects of the artistic patrimony of the Carrara family; however, none of them has considered the *Herbal* either as evidence of the trajectory of Carrara family patronage or as a record of its values.

18   The *Carrara Herbal* does not contain the first book of Serapion's treatise, which is dedicated to his theory of medicine (also an amalgamation of Greek and Arabic learning). While Serapion's work is independent of any accompanying medical treatises in the *Herbal*, in many of the extant copies produced during the height of the work's transmission, Serapion's treatise is bound with that of a ninth-century physician who bears a similar name, Yūḥannā b. Sarābiyūn. Ibn Sarābiyūn is known in the Latin West as Johannes Serapionis or Serapion the Elder. On the elder Serapion and his relationship to the younger, see Harvey (2008: 1118). The confusion between the two Serapions caused a lengthy debate over the dating of Serapion the Younger's treatise. The elder Serapion practiced in Damascus and wrote two treatises on diet and medicine in Syriac, which subsequently were translated into Arabic. Gerard of Cremona (ca. 1114–1187, see Burnett 2005) translated one of these texts – the so-called *Small Kunnāsh* (*Small Compendium*) – from Arabic into Latin, as *Practica Joannis Serapionis dicta Breviarium* (*Serapion's Practica, called Breviarium*), and this text often is found together with the *Liber Serapionis aggregatus* (as, for example, in the fourteenth-century medical miscellany, now London, British Library, Harley 3745). Of course, the confusion of these two physicians may have been a deliberate strategy: the younger Serapion could have adopted the name of the older physician specifically to conflate his identity with that of

a more established medical authority. If this is indeed the case, Serapion the Younger's *Kitāb al-Adwiya al-mufrada* is pseudepigraphic (Dilg 1999: 222–3).

19 For example, the first book contains entries for plants deemed 'temperate', while the second book contains entries for plants considered 'hot and dry' (elemental constitution) in the first degree. Galen's analysis of a drug's degree of intensity and its relationship to a patient's physical condition is complex. For a brief introduction, see Nutton (2013: 251). Serapion does not fully replicate this complexity in his treatise, perhaps because Galen himself did not do so in his categorisation of simple drugs and their properties. Galen gave detailed grades of intensity for only 161 of 475 plant simples (Nutton 2013: 251).

20 Since many of these variations of image/text placement occur toward the beginning of the codex, Baumann (1974: 26–7) suggests that the scribe and artist went through a number of alternative settings for image and text before settling on the dominant pattern. I think that this interpretation does not grant the artist or scribe enough credit in designing the reading experience.

21 See Chapter 2.

22 During the second half of the fourteenth century, the University of Padua surpassed even the prestigious University of Bologna due to the efforts of the Carrara family to entice great teachers to Padua. See Kibre (1962: 63–6), and Siraisi (1973: 29).

23 In general, practitioners of the scholastic medicine taught at universities in the Middle Ages, which privileged Aristotelian deduction of principles and causes (disputed in *quaestiones*), were rethinking the value of sense experiences (empirical, observation-based knowledge) to the field of medicine. Experience had always played a role in the study and – especially – in the practice of medicine; however, this type of knowledge lacked the cachet – the status of *scientia* – associated with the Aristotelian disputations. The literature on the study and practice of medieval medicine is vast. For a summary of the question and an introduction to the place of empiricism in late medieval medicine, see Crisciani (1990 and 2005: 297–9). For more in-depth analyses, see Riddle (1974); Kibre (1984); Siraisi (1990 and 2007); Nutton (1995a); and Givens et al. (2006).

24 Ed. and tr. Marsh (2003: 2–179).

25 On this dynamic, see Struever (1993).

26 Struever (1993: 661), and Ogilvie (2006: 141).

27 Garin (1961 and 1965); Kristeller (1978 and 1979: especially 21–32); Siraisi (2003 and 2004); Crisciani (2005); and Ogilvie (2005).

28 Grendler (2002: 24). The list of subjects is drawn from the first surviving roll of professors and the subjects they taught at the University of Padua, dated 10 November 1422, now Padua, Archivio Antico dell'Università di Padova, F. 648, ff. 35r–36v.

29 Siraisi (2001a: 2–3 and 2004: 192–3).

30 Siraisi (1987b [repr. 2001b] and 2007: especially 23–133).

31 Ogilvie (2005: 82). The connection between a construction of the moral self and the process of knowledge-building was established by the fifteenth century in educational treatises written by Pier Paolo Vergerio (ca. 1370–1445), Leonardo Bruni (ca. 1369–1444) and Battista Guarino (ca. 1434–1513). These teachers advocated a pedagogy in which their students were encouraged not only to learn about history and the natural world but also to emulate the great men of history, particularly of Roman history. This idea ultimately stemmed from Petrarch's veneration of ancient heroes in his *De viris illustribus* (*On Famous Men*), which Lombardo della Seta (d. 1390) – Petrarch's assistant and executor – completed in the last quarter of the fourteenth century. See Pier Paolo Vergerio, *De ingenuis moribus et liberalibus adulescentiae studiis* (*The Character and Studies Befitting a Free-Born Youth*) (ed. and tr. Kallendorf 2002: 2–91); Leonardo Bruni, *De studiis et litteris liber* (*The Study of Literature*) (ed. and tr. Kallendorf 2002: 92–125); and Battista Guarino, *De ordine docendi et studendi* (*A Program of Teaching and Learning*) (ed. and tr. Kallendorf 2002: 260–320). However, merging the values of

historical exemplars with the development of a more codified study of natural history truly became popular during the sixteenth century.

32 The literature on humanists' didactic interpretation of history and their teaching methods is extensive. As a starting point, see Kallendorf's introduction to his translations of four early humanists' treatises on education (2002: vii–xvi). See also the classic scholarship of Trinkaus (1970), and Kristeller (1979 and 1988), and the work of Greene (1982 and 1989); Grafton and Jardine (1986); Hampton (1990); and Bushnell (1996). On Paduan humanism, in particular, see Bolland (1996).

33 Grendler discusses the transition of humanist teachers from what he calls 'preuniversity' studies to the university (2002: especially 199–229). On medical humanism, see Reeds (1976); Siraisi (1990 and 2007); Nutton (1997); and Ogilvie (2006: 11–12 and 121). On the development of medical philology, in particular, see Nutton (1985a, 1985b, 1988 and 1995b). The humanistically trained scholars of the fifteenth and sixteenth centuries analysed, transcribed, translated, interpreted and glossed materials from all fields of inquiry in their attempt to recapture the knowledge of the past (and its languages) in the 'purest' form, an effort that (like all education) came with moral implications. Good scholarship correlated with good morals – knowledge had 'moral and aesthetic benefits', as Ogilvie puts it (2006: 92). Moreover, such knowledge was useful across many disciplines. The work of comparing and translating Greek medical treatises, for instance, was valuable to physicians and philologists alike, especially as the Greek texts became more available in the later fifteenth century. Such developments would inform the seventeenth-century studies of natural history, which Ogilvie (2006) defines as the 'science of describing' and cataloguing the particulars of nature, its properties and its uses. Because of their shared use of sources and philological interests, the boundaries between disciplines were much less codified in sixteenth-century universities than they are today (on curriculum at the Renaissance university, see Grendler 2002). A physician writing about history or a humanist writing about medicine was not unusual (Siraisi 1987b [repr. 2001b], 2001a and 2007: especially 63–105).

34 Ogilvie (2005 and 2006: especially 87–138).

35 Second- and third-generation humanists, like Vergerio, associated knowledge of nature with meticulous descriptions of the natural world, its objects and its properties. By emphasising the value of truthful recording of nature's particularities (their 'histories'), these late-fourteenth and early fifteenth-century humanists began to transform medieval conceptions of nature (which used natural objects and events as vehicles for ethical or theological commentary) into what would become the *naturalis historia* of the sixteenth and seventeenth centuries. On medieval bestiaries and spiritual exegesis, see Daston and Park (2001: 21–66), and Ogilvie (2006: 97–106). On the development of *naturalis historia*, see Grafton and Siraisi (1999). For a survey of humanists, authors and historians working at the Carrara court, in particular, see Capo (1976).

36 'Maxime vero scientia de natura intellectui humano consona atque conformis est, per quam naturalium rerum animatarum inanimatarumve principia passionesque et eorum quae caelo et mundo continentur motuum ac transmutationum causas effectusque cognoscimus, ac multorum quidem possumus causas reddere quae vulgo miranda videri soleant. Quae cum omnia iucundum est intellegere, tum maxime negotiari circa eas quae in aere et circa terram fiunt impressiones iucundissimum est' (Vergerio, *De ingenuis moribus*, 'Excellens studium tractat, armorum scilicet et litterarum', §44 [ed. and tr. Kallendorf 2002: 54–5]). Discussed and cited in different translation by Ogilvie (2005: 76).

37 Vergerio perpetuates the long-established association between natural philosophy and medical theory. He writes, 'Medicine is a very fine thing to know about and very useful for bodily health, but its practice contains very little that is suitable for the noble mind. Skill in the law is useful, both to the community and to the individual, and is held in great honour everywhere; indeed, it is derived from moral philosophy, just as medicine is from natural philosophy' ('Medicina igitur est cognitu pulcherrima et ad salutem corporum commodissima, verum exercitium habet minime liberale. Legum peritia

publice privatimque utilis est et magno ubique honori habetur, et ipsa quidem a morali philosophia derivata est, quemadmodum a naturali, medicina') (Vergerio, *De ingenuis moribus*, 'Excellens studium tractat, armorum scilicet et litterarum', §45 [ed. and tr. Kallendorf 2002: 54–5]).

38 The pleasure to which Vergerio refers is not the sense of pleasure as 'fun'; rather, it is the pleasure found in living well, in caring for the body and the soul, and in cultivating a likeminded community – all pleasures with useful physical and spiritual ends. On pleasure, utility and care of the soul (*anima cura*) for Petrarch, see Kohl (1974); Kahn (1989); Barbour (2004); and Zak (2010). On pleasure (of the mind) in the Renaissance *studiolo*, see Campbell (2004: especially 27–58). On pleasure and utility as understood by the fifteenth-century court physician Michele Savonarola (1385–1468), see Zuccolin (2012: 881).

39 Petrarch disavowed the study of the natural world, believing it vain and, ultimately, a distraction from more important philosophical and theological issues. See *De sui ipsius et multorum aliorum ignorantia* (*On His Own Ignorance and That of Many Others*) (ed. and tr. Marsh 2003: 222–363). Ogilvie (2006: 103–4) also discusses Petrarch's view of nature and natural philosophy.

40 The boy was named Ubertino 'Fiorentino' because he was born in Florence during the Carrara family's exile there (Kohl 1998: 257).

41 The artist centred the *carro* in the upper and interior margins of the title page of the bestiary section. The exterior marginal decoration is less ornate than that adorning the title page of the herbal section of the manuscript.

42 For a brief introduction to Francesco I da Carrara, see Kohl (1977).

43 Mariani Canova (1999: 154). For heraldry terminology, I have followed Boulton's (1990) descriptions of the three types of heraldry used by Italian princes: 1) the heraldic arms (*lo stemma* in Italian) is a design that covers the whole surface of a shield. Often, the design is a simple, geometrical motif portrayed in a contrasting colour to the shield; 2) the shield of arms (*il cimiero* in Italian) is a helm with a crest at its apex. These designs can allude to the heraldic arms, but often they do not, and they can be more whimsical in their form than the heraldic arms; 3) 'badges' or 'devices' are symbolic designs adopted by an individual. They are usually plants or animals whose significance is explained by a motto represented next to the badge. Boulton terms badges 'paraheraldic' because they are less formal and their use is less stable than the other forms.

44 Francesco il Vecchio assumed this personal crest rather than the shield of arms of his assassinated father, Giacomo II da Carrara (lord of Padua, 1345–1350, see Ganguzza Billanovich 1977d), which displays a hydra atop the helm and *carro*. Instead, Francesco il Vecchio resurrected the crest of his father's cousin, Ubertino da Carrara (d. 1345, r. 1338–1345; see Ganguzza Billanovich 1977i).

45 This crest is described in the *Cronaca Carrarese* (*The Chronicle of the Carrara*), a chronicle of the Carrara rule of Padua written by Galeazzo Gatari (1344–1405), a Carrara diplomat and historian, and his sons Andrea (ca. 1370–d. after 1454) and Bartolomeo (1380–1439). Gatari noted that Francesco Novello gave a pennant bearing this crest to Piero da Cortaruollo (fl. late fourteenth century) to carry into battle. He describes the pennant as 'ch'erra tuta rossa col cimiero da l'alla e con la targha dal carro' ('[the pennant] that was all-over red with the *cimiero* of the wing and with the *carro* shield') (Gatari, *Cronaca Carrarese*, 15 agosto 1404 [eds Medin and Tolomei 1931: 536; my translation]).

46 Two of Francesco's personal devices (badges), at least one which he may have based upon or borrowed from that of his father (Saccocci 2014: 193–5), rest between the shields of arms on the lower margin. In the device closest to Francesco il Vecchio's shield of arms, a hand holding an armillary sphere stretches out of a bell-shaped sleeve set against a dark blue background framed in gold. The device closest to Francesco Novello's personal shield of arms shows a 'comet': a gold cross set against a white background is encircled by a blue band inscribed with gold text, which, in turn, radiates

golden rays across a white background framed in gold. While damage to this second device makes the text difficult to decipher on the frontispiece to the herbal section (f. 4r), a similar device represented on the bestiary section's frontispiece (f. 267r) reveals the text more clearly. The band encircling the cross and containing the gold text in the representation of the comet device on the bestiary page is white rather than blue, increasing the legibility of the text, which reads: 'pour moy auxi' ('for me also'), one of Francesco Novello's mottos (Baumann 1974: 95–7). While Saccocci (2014: 195) mistakenly inverts the placement of the two devices in the *Carrara Herbal*, locating the blue-banded version on the bestiary frontispiece, and overlooks the text within the blue band, his point highlighting the differences between these representations of the comet device is convincing. Saccocci argues that the differences suggest Francesco il Vecchio also used this device, a point he corroborates through an analysis of a coin likely produced during the elder Francesco's rule. Such an exchange of devices between the elder and younger Francesco would be consistent with the other examples of Francesco Novello's imitation and appropriation of heraldry and his use of the initial 'F' in his artistic commissions. The armillary sphere device and the comet device also appear on coins and medals minted during Francesco Novello's seigniory (Mariani Canova 1999: 154; Gorini 2005; and Saccocci 2014: 189). Further, in the same passage describing the war pennants, Gatari recorded that one of Francesco Novello's standards depicted celestial worlds ('mondi d'oro') (*Cronaca*, 15 agosto 1404 [eds Medin and Tolomei 1931: 536]). Lazzarini (1901–1902: 29n2) suggested that the devices represented between the familial crests may be those described by Gatari.

47 See Chapter 3 for a more detailed analysis of the frontispiece imagery and its connection to courtly codices and university textbooks.

48 The literature on the transmission of Arabic medicine into the Latin West is diverse and extensive. As a starting point, see Siraisi (1973: especially 143–71); Kibre (1984); Reeds (1991: especially 3–38); Jacquart (1996); Dilg (1999); and Riva (2001), along with their relevant bibliographies.

49 Segre Rutz (2002: 196) notes the presence of the *Carrara Herbal* and many other medical texts originally composed in Arabic in Francesco Novello's book collection. She attributes Francesco's interest in Serapion's work to the importance of the *Liber Serapionis aggregatus in medicinis simplicibus* to late medieval pharmacology in Padua, in particular.

50 On Ibn Buṭlān, see Arnaldez (1997).

51 On the *Tacuinum sanitatis*, see, most recently, Collins (2000: 279); Bertiz (2003); Hoeniger (2006); and Touwaide (2009c–f). For a more extensive bibliography of the scholarly literature on the *Tacuinum*, see Chapter 2, p. 86n58. Although he does not use the term 'non-naturals', preferring instead 'necessary causes', these factors are central to Galen's theory of medicine (Galen, *Ars medica* [*The Art of Medicine*], 23 [ed. and Latin tr. Kühn 1821–1833: 1.367–9; English tr. Singer 1997: 374–5]). On the non-naturals and their role in Galenic medicine more generally, see Nutton (2013: 242 and 246–8).

52 Despite this connection to the university, it bears noting that both the *Tacuinum* and the *Liber Serapionis aggregatus* were available in luxury, illustrated versions in the northern courts of Italy. Together, they attest to a growing fashion for Arabic works outside of university settings and to their use in competition for status among *signori*.

53 Ineichen (1962–1966: 1.x), the philologist responsible for an extensive study of the translation of Serapion's text included in the *Carrara Herbal*, points to the primacy of Serapion's work in late-medieval medicine, as does Dilg (1999: 222).

54 For descriptions of the extant medieval and Early Modern manuscript copies of Serapion's treatise, see Thorndike and Kibre (1963: cols 751, 862 and 1077), and Dilg (1999).

55 Saladino da Ascoli, *Compendium*, I, 'Libri necessarii ipsi Aromatario', Benedictus Hectoris, 1488, ff. 1v (col. 2)–2r (col. 1). Also, see Dilg (1999: 221). For a discussion of the six works Saladino recommended, see Huguet-Termes (2008: 230–1).

56 Ogilvie (2006: 32). For a brief introduction to Leoniceno, see Touwaide (2008a). On Leoniceno's comments regarding Serapion, see Dilg (1999: 221).

57 The practice of synthesis was not unusual either before the advent of Serapion's text in the Latin West (as the popularity of the *Tractatus de herbis* tradition attests) or after it (as the imitative works of pharmacologists from the fourteenth to sixteenth centuries attest). For an introduction to the *Tractatus*, see Chapter 1, pp. 46–7. For a more detailed discussion of the *Tractatus*, see Ventura (2009), and Touwaide (2013b). Notably, the compendium of sources found in the *Tractatus* combines both the non-Classical Latin works and translations of Greek (Classical) and Arabic authorities. For a discussion of other authors practicing synthesis of medical sources in the Early Modern era (for instance, Gentile da Foligno [d. 1348], Matthaeus Silvaticus [ca. 1280–ca. 1342], Saladino da Ascoli, Quiricus de Augustis [fl. late fifteenth century] and the authors of the *Ricettario Fiorentino*), see Dilg (1999: 229).

58 For an introduction to Giacomo II, see Ganguzza Billanovich (1977d).

59 See Chapter 4.

60 Petrarch, *Rerum familiarium*, XII.2 (eds Rossi and Bosco 1933–1942: 3.5–17).

61 'Hoc ab illo, alia sumat ab aliis, e quibus omnibus perficiat clarum virum; quotque insignia nomina precesserunt, tot sibi magistros vite, tot duces ad gloriam datos sciat; non minus interdum accendunt generosos animos exempla quam premia, nec minus verba quam statue; iuvat laudatis se se conferre nominibus et pulcra emulatio est que de virtute suscipitur' (Petrarch, *Rerum familiarium*, XII.2, ll. 264–70 [eds Rossi and Bosco 1933–1942: 3.15; tr. Bernardo 2005: 2.139, with slight revisions to Bernardo's translation]). Petrarch continued on to describe King Robert (1277–1343), former King of Naples, as a 'suitable exemplar' (exemplar ydoneum [l. 273]). He urged Acciaiuoli to instruct Louis to 'contemplate that great man [and] . . . conform to his pattern of life; let him look upon [Robert] as though he were seeing him in a flawless mirror. He was wise, he was kind, he was high-minded and gentle, he was the king of kings' ('. . . Illum intueatur; ad illius regulam se conformet; in illo se nitidissimo speculo contempletur; ille sapiens, ille magnanimus, ille mitis, ille rex regum erat') (XII.2, ll. 275–8 [eds Rossi and Bosco 1933–1942: 3.16]).

62 For modern critical editions of *De viris illustribus*, see ed. Martellotti (1964); and eds and tr. Ferrone, Malta and de Capua (2006–2012).

63 Ed. Hosius (1914); tr. Basore (1928–1935: 1.357–447).

64 Seneca's *De clementia* is the oldest example of a *Speculum principis* in Latin (Stacey 2007: 4–5). Petrarch's use of the *Speculum* combines characteristics drawn from Seneca's treatise with his own Christian (Augustinian) values. For instance, in his letter to Niccolò Acciaiuoli (*Rerum familiarium* XII.2), Petrarch seems to criticise Seneca's dismissal of *misericordia* (pity) as a princely virtue and instead argues that pity is a better virtue for a prince than those praised by Seneca, namely *magnanimitas* (magnanimity) and *humanitas* (humanity) (Stacey 2007: 139).

65 Part of Seneca's project was to appropriate Cicero's discussion of civic virtue and moral duty, described in *De officiis* (ed. and tr. Miller 1913), into a new social order where the prince embodies the *civis*. In what Stacey (2007: 9) describes as a process of 'ideological re-characterization' after the Roman revolution, Seneca helped to transform republican values into imperial ones. Stacey's argument for Seneca's primacy in the *Speculum principis* tradition counters that of Quentin Skinner. Skinner (2002: 124–5) argues that Cicero's influence is most visible in the early humanists' contributions to the *Speculum principis* tradition, especially in Petrarch's. Previously, Skinner (1978: 117–19) expressed a similar idea about the debt to Cicero of the later, fifteenth-century *Speculum principis* tradition.

66 Stacey (2007: 4–5).

67 'Scribere de clementia, Nero Caesar, institui, ut quodam modo speculi vice fungerer et te tibi ostenderem perventurum ad voluptatem maximam omnium' (Seneca *De clementia*, I.I, l.1 [ed. Hosius 1914: 210; tr. Basore 1928–1935: 1.356–7]).

68 'Nam si, quod adhuc colligit, tu animus rei publicae tuae es, illa corpus tuum, vides, ut puto, quam necessaria sit clementia; tibi enim parcis, cum videris alteri parcere. Parcendum itaque est etiam improbandis civibus non aliter quam membris languentibus, et, si quando misso sanguine opus est, sustinenda est manus, ne ultra, quam necesse sit, incidat' (Seneca *De clementia* I.V, ll.1–2 [ed. Hosius 1914: 217; tr. Basore 1928–1935: 1.370–1]). This passage is discussed in greater depth by Stacey (2007: 152).

69 See Chapter 4 for a discussion and comparison of these commissions.

70 Ed. Fenzi (2009); tr. Rawski (1991).

71 On the role of Petrarch's *De remediis* in Francesco Novello's library, see Kyle (2015).

1 The *Carrara Herbal* and the traditions of illustrated books of *materia medica*

When Francesco Novello commissioned the *Carrara Herbal* in the 1390s, he commissioned a book that participated in two distinct traditions. On the one hand, the book participates in the long history of collection and production of illustrated books of *materia medica*. This history is separate from – yet runs parallel to – the history of collection and production of their unillustrated counterparts. On the other hand, the illustrations in the *Carrara Herbal*, while they reflect the composite nature of Serapion's treatise, also reflect the complex heterogeneous illustrative sets visible across the genre's history. Illustrated books of *materia medica* appealed to diverse readers, and neither their readership nor their illustrative traditions were static.

Physicians and pharmacists acquired and studied illustrated books of *materia medica*, and in this context the books' illustrations were not necessarily used for identification of plants in the field or even as part of medical pedagogy.[1] Rather, at different times in their history, such books served other purposes for these readers, perhaps as indices for finding therapeutic information, as mnemonic devices to assist in study, as methods of communicating medical knowledge irrespective of linguistic barriers or as ways to mitigate the risk of dangerous translation errors.[2] Paralleling these aspects of their collection, however, illustrated books of *materia medica* also appealed to wealthy collectors, often those with political authority and without much knowledge of medicine and its practice.[3] Among other purposes, such collectors used these books – together with other, complementary aspects of their patronage – to advance a certain vision of their identities, histories and cultural heritage. Generally, but not always, the quality of the manuscripts and their illustrations distinguish the commissions of powerful and wealthy patrons from their more practical or academic counterparts.

The *Carrara Herbal* brings together elements not only from the genre's diverse illustrative traditions but also from its diverse history of collection – a remarkable and new role for an illustrated book of *materia medica*. It connects to the collection and use of this type of book both by the medical community and by erudite collectors with a specific image to construct or uphold.

The illustrative apparatus and content of the *Carrara Herbal* – with its ties to advances in medicine and curricula at the university – locate Francesco as a patron and reader with one foot in the medical community and the other in the political one.

To establish the place of the *Carrara Herbal* within particular pictorial and textual traditions, I begin this chapter by describing its variety of imagery. Then, to understand its possible personal and political functions, I examine select examples of illustrated books of *materia medica* from across the genre's history that show the wide variety of uses, illustrative sets and collection-histories of these books. In particular, I consider the book given to Anicia Juliana (ca. 462–528), daughter of Byzantine Emperor Flavius Anicius Olybrius (d. ca. 472), as an example of how illustrated books of *materia medica* may have been amalgamated into strategies of self-representation through contact with different visual rhetorics associated with the owner's other forms of patronage.

Turning to the Arabic tradition, I consider illustrated copies of Dioscorides' *De materia medica* (*On Therapeutic Substance*) specifically produced for prominent physicians or high-ranking members of the courts at Baghdad and Cordova as examples of how these books could serve both professional and political purposes, which were not necessarily mutually exclusive. Lastly, turning to the Latin and vernacular traditions, I consider the illustrated books of *materia medica* produced for Holy Roman Emperor Frederick II Hohenstaufen (1194–1250) and those produced for patrons of more regional significance – the physician Manfred de Monte Imperiale (fl. ca. 1330–1340), the *signore* of Milan, Giangaleazzo Visconti (1351–1402), and perhaps Francesco Novello's father as well.[4] These examples further illuminate the hermeneutical flexibility of the genre and point to its varied uses across social and political lines.

Botanical illustration in the *Carrara Herbal*

In the *Carrara Herbal*, many of the plant images are remarkable for their precise attention to the defining visual characteristics of a particular species, not a generic example of it, a characteristic that is unique in fourteenth-century herbal manuscript illumination in the West. Yet many also retain elements of older illustrative traditions in which artists portrayed the plants as schemata, rather than as specific, individual specimens. These illustrations tend to depict the general shape of the plant and its significant parts but avoid the more precise details that convey a sense of illusionistic realness and individuality.[5] Furthermore, the artist hybridised aspects of these techniques, creating a completely new type of plant representation. Regardless of the style of their execution, however, the illustrations engage with the pages' surface area and its text in a variety of ways, all of which arrest the readers' progress through the text and steal their attention away from Serapion's words.[6]

The artist's representations of *malbavisco* (*Althaea officinalis* L. and *Lavatera thuringiaca* L., genera of marshmallow, f. 52v, Figure 1.1) are characteristic of a

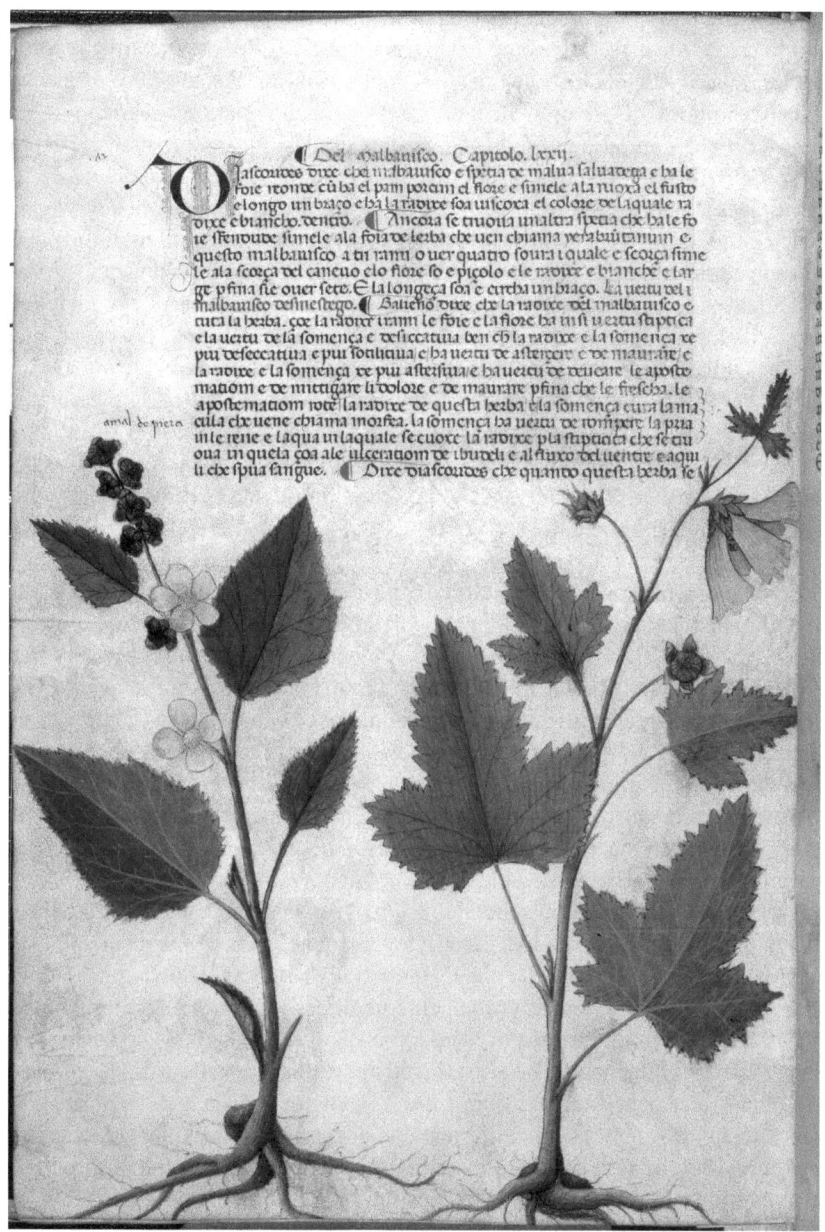

Figure 1.1 Malbavisco (*Althaea officinalis* L. and *Lavatera thuringiaca* L., genera of marshmallow)

Carrara Herbal
London, British Library, Egerton 2020, f. 52v
35 × 24 cm, gouache on vellum, Padua, ca. 1390–1400

style in which observation of single plant specimens played a large role.[7] With the goal to create the effect of seeing a particular species of plant, the artist recorded specific identifying details (such as the plant's fruit and its structure of growth) using techniques of pictorial illusionism like tonal variation, overlapping and *chiaroscuro* (the variation of light and shadow used by an artist to indicate depth). In the *malbavisco* representation at the right of the folio (*Lavatera thuringiaca* L.), for instance, the artist showed the funnel-shaped profile of the plant's flower and depicted the characteristic three to five sepals that frame the bottom of the petals. He showed the alternate pattern of leaf growth and depicted the underside of one of the leaves to reveal its prominent white veining. The artist also rendered the plant's distinct pumpkin-shaped fruits three-dimensionally. He portrayed them both frontally and in profile so that the viewer may observe how the bracts characteristically curl over the fruit.[8] Since the plant usually completes flowering and goes to seed in October, the artist likely observed and recorded it in late summer or early fall. The second type of *malbavisco* (*Althaea officinalis* L.), portrayed on the left side of the folio, shows a similar attention to detail, allowing the viewer to see the similarities and differences between the two genera of marshmallow.

The image of *meliloto* (*Lotus corniculatus* L., bird's foot trefoil, f. 15r, Plate 2) shows a more playful use of pictorial illusionism. Rather than illustrating the three-dimensional aspects of a living plant, as he did in the *malbavisco* representations, the artist showed the *meliloto* as a specimen pressed into this very book for preservation and study.[9] In his illustration, the artist pushed the plant toward the interior margin, leaving much of the vellum page exposed. This compositional gesture alerts the viewer to the strange positioning of the plant and its parts. The secondary stem, furthest to the left, bends awkwardly back in on itself, and the flowers that branch from the main stem appear squeezed against the page, their petals sandwiched together in a disorderly fashion, their peduncles (which link the flowers to the stem) bent dramatically.[10]

Although constructing the general illusion of a pressed specimen, the artist continued to articulate the principal identifying characteristics of the plant. He chose a composition that revealed the plant's underlying structure, showing its alternate arrangement of sessile leaves (which emerge directly from the stem), its flowers and its fruit (the long, disorderly, 'bird's foot-like' seedpods) isolated against the blank expanse of the page. The artist tinged the withering, yellow flowers – which resemble sweet peas (*Lathyrus odoratus* L.) – with a deep red, suggesting the plant's age.[11] Through his technical and compositional choices, the artist added a new dimension of visual play to his representation, a dimension that through its very playfulness draws the viewers' attention back to the role of the image in this particular book and to their role as readers.

In another type of image, the artist did not use verisimilar techniques. Instead, he used schematic ones. For instance, he depicted the *sponga marina* (*Euspongia officinalis* L., marine sponge, f. 14r, Figure 1.2), which Serapion included among plant *materia medica*, as a distinctly two-dimensional, asymmetrical ovoid mass covered with many small, pointed scales.[12] Without the modelling and shading of the more realistic plant images, the marine sponge appears flat on the page. The uniform ivory-grey

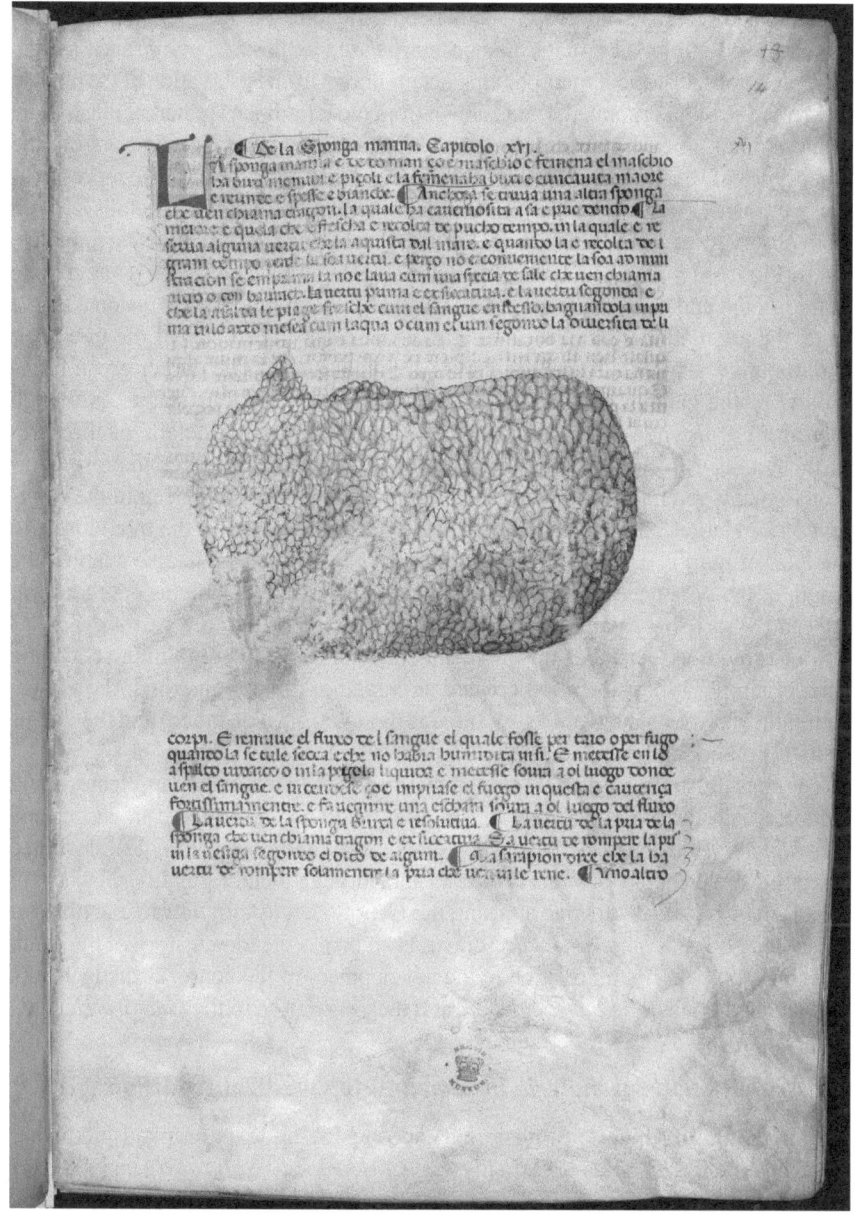

Figure 1.2 Sponga marina (*Euspongia officinalis* L., marine sponge)

Carrara Herbal
London, British Library, Egerton 2020, f. 14r
35 × 24 cm, gouache on vellum, Padua, ca. 1390–1400

colouration discourages the perception of depth or texture. For the *sponga* illustration, the artist used a different visual language than he used for the *malbavisco* and *meliloto* representations. Instead of incorporating details drawn from observation of the plant in nature, the artist incorporated details drawn from older traditions of herbal illustration.

In his final type of plant imagery, the artist amalgamated techniques from the other types of illustration within the *Herbal* to create hybrids. In these representations, the artist blended details derived from historical models with details derived from observation. In his illustration of *pino* (*Pinus pinea* L., Italian stone pine tree, f. 41r, Figure 1.3), for example, the artist presented his viewer with an aggregate of traditional and new representational types.[13] To depict the entire tree on a single page, the artist adapted the tree's overall proportions. The body of the tree itself is diminutive, while its fruits and leaves are magnified.[14] The darker green background of the canopy conveys the treetop's common bulbous shape, as though seen from a distance. Simultaneously, the artist emphasised details of the bark, as though seen from up close, showing the characteristic fissures that are common to many genera of pine trees and are particularly large and deep in the *Pinus pinea* L.[15] Harvested for their *pignóli*, the pinecones shown on the tree closest to the interior margin are given visual prominence by the artist. He also adapted the length of the pine needles, portraying them in large, pale green clusters that form fan- and whorl-shapes against the darker green mass of the tree's canopy, a pattern of growth associated with this genus of pine tree. By combining schematic and verisimilar types, the artist created an image of the tree in which the viewer simultaneously sees its overall structure (as though from a distance) and the details of its fruit, bark and needles (as though from up-close).

The four illustrative types employed by the artist alternatively participate in and compete with the heterogeneous illustrative traditions encountered in earlier and contemporary illustrated herbals. They distinguish the book from other illustrated and unillustrated books of *materia medica* and, through their originality, they help to establish the book's distinctive and singular identity. Let us turn now to examples of illustrated books of *materia medica* drawn from across the long history of the genre and consider them first in relation to the development of the genre, as distinct from unillustrated books of *materia medica*, and then in relation to the *Carrara Herbal*.

Illustrated books of *materia medica* and the medical tradition

The first author to mention illustrations accompanying texts on plant medicines was Pliny the Elder (23/24–79). In his *Naturalis historia* (*Natural History*),[16] Pliny noted that these images, while 'very attractive' (*blandissima*), have the potential to 'mislead' (*fallax est*) and so to corrupt the body of medical knowledge.[17] He believed that one of the goals of the illustrations was to imitate and record nature. While a pictorial representation of a plant could – and perhaps did, in some cases – serve as a guide to study, Pliny emphasised that a single picture was incapable of accurately capturing the diversity of forms a plant assumes during its lifecycle, and he cautioned against their use in books of *materia medica*. At best, Pliny argued, to be comprehensible, an image could only capture the plant at a single moment

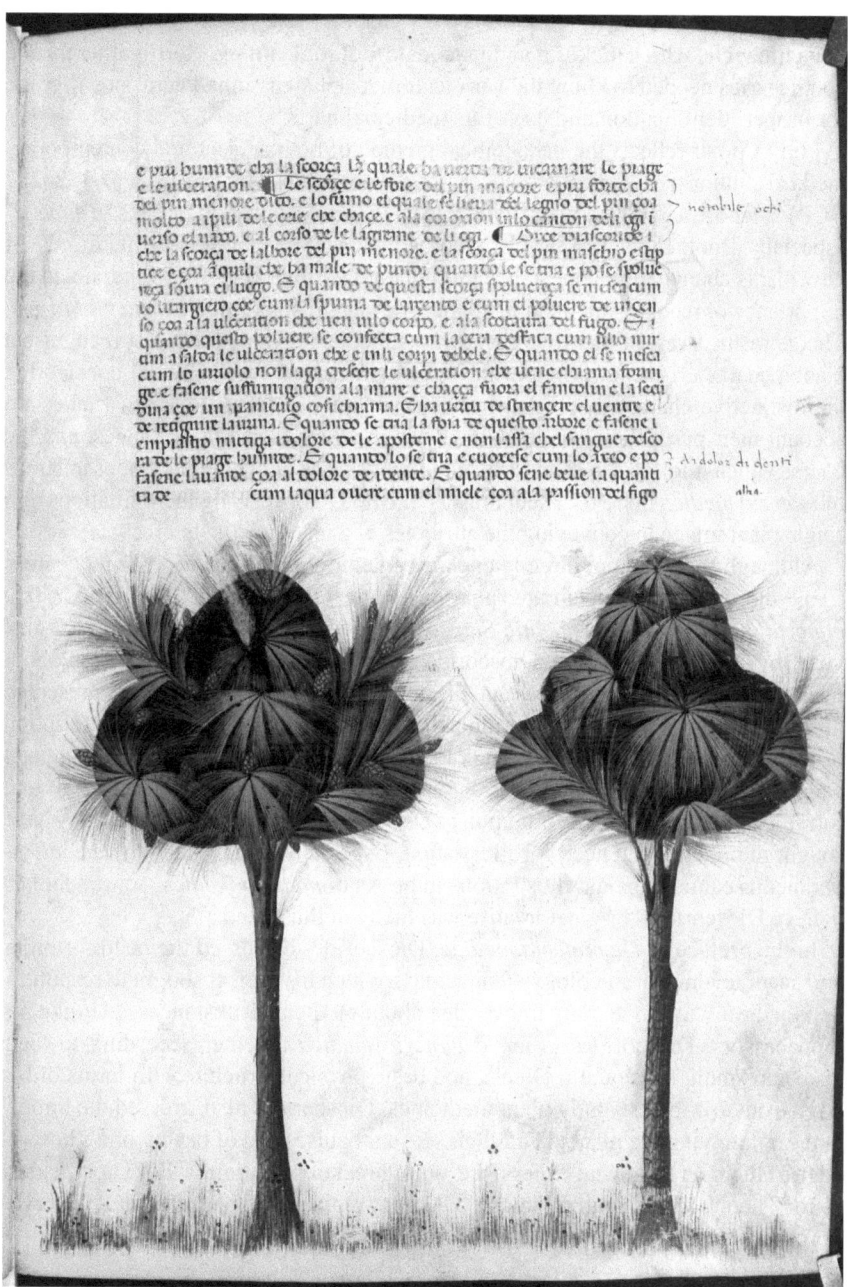

Figure 1.3 Pino (*Pinus pinea* L., Italian stone pine tree)

Carrara Herbal
London, British Library, Egerton 2020, f. 41r
35 × 24 cm, gouache on vellum, Padua, ca. 1390–1400

in its lifecycle, which makes it an inadequate tool for learning. Herb-gatherers and apothecaries needed to know the various forms a plant assumed across its lifetime for proper identification and use of its medicinal parts.

Pliny's point reflects the pedagogical method of both ancient and contemporary medical authorities. Aristotle's successor, Theophrastus of Eresus (ca. 372–287 BCE),[18] whose Περὶ φυτῶν ἱστορία (*Historia plantarum*; *Enquiry into Plants*),[19] especially Book IX, is the earliest recorded account of plant medicine, discussed how plants change their appearance throughout their lifecycle. He further noted the importance of recognising them in all their variety. In book I of *Historia plantarum*, Theophrastus stressed that to understand its medicinal value one must recognise a plant's characteristics at different times of its life. He wrote, '[when] considering the distinctive characters of plants and their nature generally one must take into account their parts, their qualities, the ways in which their life originates, and the course which it follows in each case'.[20] Pliny's critique of plant illustrations in books of *materia medica* upholds Theophrastus' method, emphasising the limitations of a single plant image in conveying the attributes of a plant across its lifecycle.

Although Pliny did not directly cite his contemporary, Dioscorides (first century CE),[21] the author of the celebrated pharmacological treatise Περὶ ὕλης ἰατρικῆς (*De materia medica*; *On Therapeutic Substance*),[22] Dioscorides shared Theophrastus' view. In *De materia medica*, Dioscorides recorded identifying information about over 1,000 medicinal substances and discussed their therapeutic uses. He presented this information according to a formula that included a detailed physical description of the substance, notes on the correct identification of its medicinally useful parts and instructions for their preparation and uses.[23] With his attention to detail and formulaic presentation of information in *De materia medica*, Dioscorides may have sought to preclude the need for illustration. Especially in light of Pliny's contemporaneous caution against illustrations in books of *materia medica*, some scholars believe Dioscorides' original treatise was likely unillustrated.[24]

In the preface to *De materia medica*, Dioscorides discussed the need for order and accuracy in pharmacology – concerns to which his project sought to respond – and the best ways to acquire knowledge about medicinal substances.[25] Unlike his predecessors, Dioscorides grouped *materia medica* together according to their taste and smell, therapeutic effects, and basic physical structure.[26] In terms of his advice on how to best study plant medicines, Dioscorides also stressed the importance of knowing the plants in all their seasonal guises and of basing one's knowledge of them on 'practical experience' and 'direct observation'.[27] For Dioscorides, as for Theophrastus, a single image could not replace the role of careful observation over the lifecycle of a plant.[28] Dioscorides wrote:[29]

> Anyone wanting experience in these matters [understanding botanical *materia medica*] must encounter the plants as shoots, newly emerged from the earth, plants in their prime, and plants in their decline. For someone who has come across the shoot alone cannot know the mature plant, nor if he has seen only the ripened plants can he recognize the young shoot as well. Great error is occasionally committed by those who have not made an appropriate

inspection, as a result of the changes in the form of the leaves, the varying sizes of stems, flowers and fruits, and some other characteristics. . . . But anyone who has seen these plants often and in many places will gain a particularly precise knowledge of them.

While Dioscorides' treatise is not the oldest recorded pharmacopeia and likely derives, at least in part, from older Alexandrian sources (as does much of Pliny's commentary on medicinal plants, for that matter), the transmission and diffusion of Dioscorides' work was unprecedented.[30] From its inception, possibly in the second half of the first century, Dioscorides' treatise was copied and revised, in both illustrated and unillustrated versions, across the Byzantine Empire, through Baghdad, the Arabic Empire (including Al-Andalus), and the Latin West. Not including its prolific print editions, Dioscorides' treatise is preserved in over 150 extant manuscripts from across the Mediterranean.[31] It is safe to say that his views on how to acquire and disseminate knowledge about plant medicines spread just as widely as his pharmacology.

Perhaps following the guidelines implicit in the pedagogical methods of Dioscorides and Theophrastus, Pliny considered illustrations of plants in books of *materia medica* as inadequate educational tools for herb-gathers or physicians. Yet the production and collection of illustrated and unillustrated books of *materia medica*, and especially those dedicated to plant medicines, grew concurrently across the Mediterranean region – particularly (if ironically) in books containing versions of Dioscorides' *De materia medica*.[32] The persistent collection of these books demonstrates that illustrated pharmacopoeias were desired, despite any limitations they might impose on learning about the lifecycles of medicinal plants. These books served other purposes for their owners, one of which Pliny alluded to when he labelled the illustrations of plants as 'most attractive'. By focussing on the attractive qualities of the illustrations, illustrated books of plant *materia medica*, especially, can become as much about facilitating memorable and pleasurable viewing and reading as about understanding and using plant drugs. Doing so, they participate in another knowledge set, one dedicated to understanding the value of pleasure to moral and physical health – a point to which I will return in the next chapter.

For now, consider the following examples drawn from the long history of illustrated versions of Dioscorides' *De materia medica*. In its many copies and revisions, the number of substances and the ways in which they are organised vary. This fluctuation of substances was likely a result of the necessarily open nature of discourse on medicinal plants and their uses, which depended on the changing ecosystems and medical practices of the locales where the books circulated. New *materia medica* were introduced, either as they were discovered or to incorporate local medicinal plants and healing traditions, while others were abandoned, either as impractical or as unattainable.[33] The illustrations also reflect this natural coming-and-going of medicinal substances. However, whether old or new, local or foreign, the illustrations that accompany *materia medica* range from schematic to realistic and can be grouped into general sets according to textual recensions.[34] Arguments about which type of representation was original to the first illustrated copy of

Dioscorides' treatise are ongoing.[35] But regardless of the types of illustrations in these codices, their very presence points to the continued and cross-cultural value of illustrated books of *materia medica* as distinct from their unillustrated counterparts. While these few examples cannot adequately convey the diversity within each textual and illustrative tradition, they reveal certain aesthetic and epistemological values that potentially connect these books and their collectors across geographical and temporal arenas.[36]

The illustrative tradition in the Greek Dioscorides

In the Greek tradition alone, there are over thirty extant illustrated copies of Dioscorides' treatise.[37] The oldest illustrated copy is known in modern scholarship as the *Vienna Dioscorides*.[38] It contains over 300 illustrations of plants and an opening series of frontispieces, which includes what is considered the earliest surviving portrait miniature of a real person, Anicia Juliana (ca. 462–528), the daughter of Emperor Flavius Anicius Olybrius (d. ca. 472) and descendant of the Theodosian dynasty, to whom the book is dedicated.[39] According to an inscription on the dedication page of the codex, the book was a gift for Juliana from the citizens of the Honorata district of Constantinople in gratitude for the Christian church built there, a church Juliana financed.[40]

In his *Chronographia*, Theophanes the Confessor (ca. 750–818) described a church of the Theotokos (Θεοτόκος) built in Honoratai in his account of the year 512.[41] Since the frontispiece of Juliana's book identified the location of the church (Honoratai), Theophanes' chronicle, which names the church and gives a date of construction coinciding with Juliana's lifetime, seemed to confirm the date of the codex's creation. Scholars have traditionally dated the codex to 512 because of these two sources, but recently this date has come under scrutiny. Ernst Gamillscheg, Byzantinist and palaeographer with the Österreichische Nationalbibliothek, current home of the *Vienna Dioscorides*, pointed out that the first quire, which includes the portrait with the inscriptions along with several other opening frontispieces, postdates the illustrations in the remainder of the codex.[42] Also, upon revisiting the textual sources, Byzantinist Andreas E. Müller concluded that the reference in Theophanes is unreliable and, consequently, the frontispieces can be – at best – tentatively dated to ca. 512/513 CE.[43]

Despite the confusion surrounding the codex's exact date of production, Juliana's Dioscorides remains a widely known and celebrated early example from the Greek tradition of illustrated books of *materia medica*. The large codex – weighing 14 pounds – contains a variety of texts and illustrations, including a shortened, alphabetised version of *De materia medica*[44] and five other abridged, annotated and illustrated medical treatises by other Greek authors.[45] The *Vienna Dioscorides*, then, is a compilation of illustrated Greek medical texts – despite the misleading name by which it is now known.

In the Dioscorides section, the unknown artist(s) – with few exceptions – represented each plant on its own page.[46] The full-page illustrations face a page of text that describes the plant's properties and medicinal usage according to Dioscorides' formulaic presentation of information. This section includes 383 illustrations of plants, while the other sections include many illustrations of insects, lizards, snakes and birds. Across the codex's many texts, and including within the Dioscorides itself, the illustrations range in type from realistic representation to schematic sketch, further suggesting that the separate treatises within the book were not completed at the same time or by the same hand.

Regardless of their origin, however, many of the illustrations in the Dioscorides section are indeed very beautiful – for instance, the detailed representation of blackberry (*Rubus fruticosus* L., f. 83r), which rambles across the page, or the understated bulb onion (*Allium cepa* L., f. 185r) with its fan of overlapping blue-green leaves.[47] Yet, especially in the other treatises that accompany the Dioscorides, many illustrations – as John Scarborough memorably describes them – prompt the viewer to growl at their dreadfulness.[48] The snakes and lizards, in particular, are repetitive and unimaginative. The inconsistent style and quality of the illustrations in the *Vienna Dioscorides* suggest that the codex was likely not produced specifically for Juliana and not at the imperial scriptorium either. Instead, the citizens of Honorata may have purchased the book on the market as a 'ready-made' compilation of earlier illustrated Greek medical treatises bound together into a single volume and then commissioned only the opening frontispieces with which to 'wrap' their gift.[49] The frontispieces, then, were likely produced distinct from- and later than the illustrations in the treatises, but in their visual language they attempt to bring together the codex's pharmacological texts and to align them with attributes of Juliana's status and learning – flattering her as the recipient of this gift.[50]

The frontispieces provide evidence for how this assortment of older illustrated medical treatises could be transformed to demonstrate the gift-givers' support for Anicia Juliana and so to advance her public image. They lay out a way of reading the texts and their illustrations in relation to Juliana as a learned *patrikia*, especially one from a ruling family (albeit one in decline). The series begins with the image of a peacock (f. 1v), an ambiguous symbol that could refer to paradise and immortality (as is often seen in the context of mosaics in medieval and Byzantine Christian churches) or to the attribute of Hera (Juno) – a bird befitting an empress.[51] The following four frontispieces portray legendary and historical physicians in conversation with each other (or with their students). The first of these physician portraits shows the fabled centaur, Chiron, with several of his most-esteemed pupils (f. 2v).[52] The next portrait is also a group portrait, which shows seven physicians identified as Galen (129–ca. 216/17 CE, in the central position), Dioscorides (first century CE), Crateuas (120–63 BCE), Nicander (fl. second century BCE), Rufus of Ephesus (fl. first century CE), Andreas of Carystos (d. ca. 217 BCE) and Apollonius (fl. first century BCE to first century CE) (f. 3v).[53]

Two separate frontispieces follow, which show legendary scenes from Dioscorides' life. These scenes are pivotal to reframing the medical content of the book into a vocabulary perhaps more suited to the advancement of Juliana's public persona. They transition the readers' attention from the historical medical authorities to personifications of ideals associated with learning, discovery and leadership, personifications that prepare the reader to interpret the dedicatory portrait and the book's content in relation to Anicia Juliana. The first of these legendary scenes portrays a personification of *Heuresis* (discovery/invention) giving Dioscorides the mandrake root – a powerful narcotic (f. 4v).[54] The second shows an artist painting an image of the mandrake in the company of Dioscorides, who is writing his description of the root, and a personification of *Epinoia* (knowledge), who watches over the physician (f. 5v, Figure 1.4).[55] The final, culminating frontispiece contains

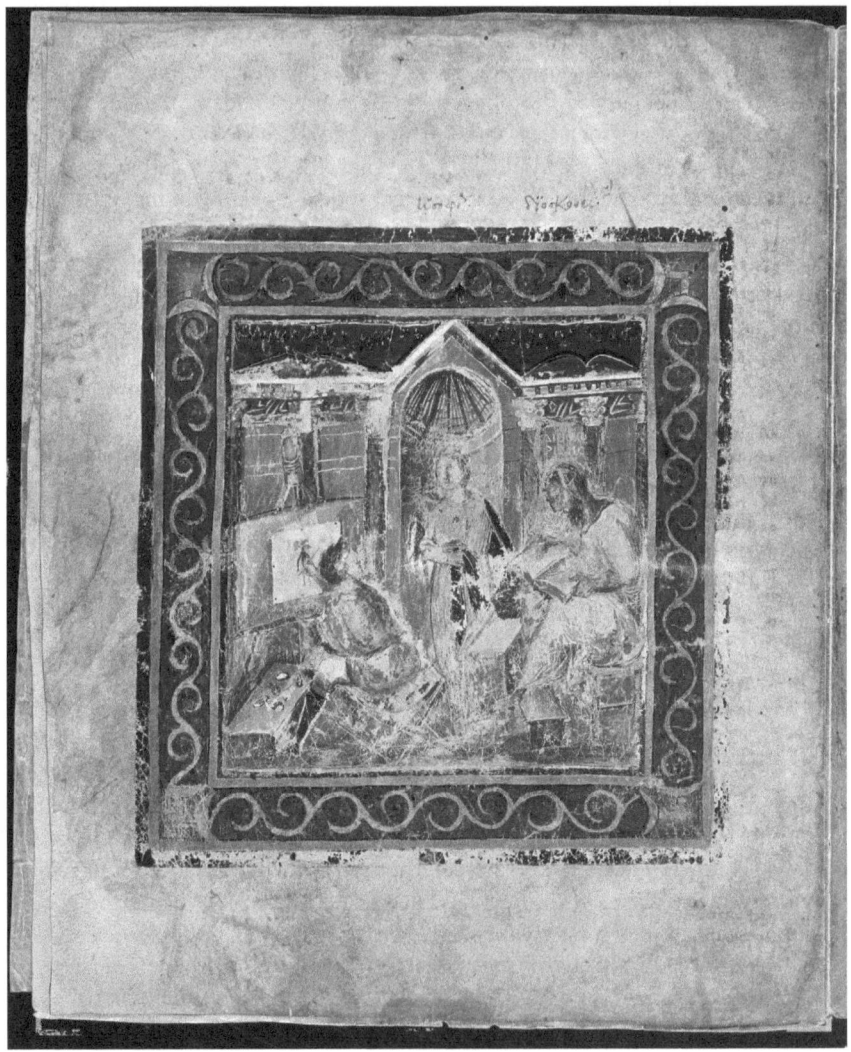

Figure 1.4 Portraits of *Epinoia* (Knowledge), Dioscorides and Painter

De materia medica
Vienna, Österreichische Nationalbibliothek, *medicus graecus* 1, f. 5v
37.6 × 31.2 cm, Constantinople, ca. 512/13 CE

Source: ÖNB

the dedication miniature and the inscription that identifies Juliana as the recipient of this book (f. 6v).

Set within an elaborate frame in the shape of an eight-pointed star (each point containing a letter of her name, ΙΟΥΛΙΑΝΑ), the dedication frontispiece shows Juliana enthroned, with a codex in her left hand and coins falling from her right. She wears a white tunic and purple and gold dalmatic, and a bejewelled diadem or headdress rests on her brow. Juliana is flanked by two female personifications (identified by inscriptions): on Juliana's left, *Phronesis* (intelligence/practical wisdom) points to a book balanced on her knee, while on Juliana's right, *Megalo-psychia* (magnanimity/greatness of soul) carries gold coins in the folds of her dress. A smaller female personification of *[Eu]cha[r]istia [ton] technon* (gratitude, especially of the arts) kisses Juliana's feet (*proskynesis*), beside a putto labelled *Pothos tes philoktistou* (love of building) that hands Juliana an open codex bound in red – in all likelihood, a representation of the *Vienna Dioscorides* itself.[56] The personifications that accompany Juliana tie her to rhetoric associated with virtuous rulers.[57] Bente Kiilerich argues that the sum of these personifications and the portrait of Juliana results in a merging of her role as *patrikia* and as an embodiment of *Sophia* – wisdom.[58] An inscription in a later hand identified the portrait of Juliana specifically as *Sophia* (σοφία). This presentation of Juliana partially corresponds to the manner in which she describes herself in the running frieze of the interior of Saint Polyeuktos, a church she commissioned in part to resecure her power in an environment increasingly less supportive of the Anicii and their heirs.[59]

Magnanimity, wisdom and prudence – these are all virtues prized in rulers and praised in Classical sources (in Aristotle's *Ethica ad Nicomachum* [*Nicomachean Ethics*] and Seneca's *De clementia* [*On Mercy*], especially). The later medieval and Renaissance literary traditions that partially derive from the Classical texts, such as books of secrets and so-called 'mirrors' for princes, also praised these virtues.[60] The many representations of books in the frontispieces of the *Vienna Dioscorides* – in the physician portraits and in the dedication page – point to their importance as conduits for ideas and knowledge and as signs for a set of learned virtues connected with the ideal ruler, those virtues personified alongside Juliana.[61] This aspect of the iconography of Juliana's book is important to the understanding of later illustrated books of *materia medica* commissioned by or given to patrons of political importance. In later commissions, including the *Carrara Herbal*, we also see the ideological associations of the book object used to support a view of the patron as learned and virtuous.

While scholars debate the reasons why the citizens of Honorata would chose an illustrated book of *materia medica* as a gift for their benefactor, the nature of the book object and its attendant meanings likely informed their choice.[62] The codex contains diverse Greek medical sources, illustrated in memorable – if not always beautiful – ways. The frontispieces promise the reader an experience in which he or she learns the wonders of nature and the keys to health from the likes of Chiron, Dioscorides and Galen. The dedication miniature, however, not only honours the book's dedicatee, but it also shows any other reader exactly who, by virtue of her generosity, orchestrated not just the building of a church but this reading experience as well: the *patrikia*, Anicia Juliana.

Juliana would not have been the book's only reader. Within households and among other readers of similar social standing, books circulated.[63] The way Juliana is presented in the frontispiece not only honoured her, it also presented a particular (albeit sometimes ambiguous) image of her to the book's other readers.[64] Like *Heuresis* giving Dioscorides the mandrake, Juliana instigates the reader's own *heuresis*. Whatever discoveries or delights the readers take from their encounter with the texts and images in the codex Juliana enabled through the greatness of her patronage (which, of course, is also an image of Juliana meant to be part of the readers' *heuresis*). Like *Epinoia*, who witnesses Dioscorides recording his discoveries for the benefit of future readers, the enthroned Juliana gives access to and witnesses the readers' own study, an act associated – by way of the accompanying personifications – with the cultivation of a good leader's virtues. These qualities of the illustrated book of *materia medica* – as an instrument of valuable knowledge conveyed in a form that can suggest the restricted or privileged nature of this knowledge and the potential rewards of such access – are visible in other examples across the history of collection of such books.

The illustrative tradition in the Arabic Dioscorides

Like its Greek versions, the Arabic translations of Dioscorides' *De materia medica* and their accompanying illustrative traditions have a long and varied history of production and collection.[65] The Nestorians translated Dioscorides' text into Syriac in the sixth century, but the ninth-century translation efforts in Baghdad to assume Greek knowledge into an Arabic context account for its wider dissemination outside of the Greek world. Iṣṭifan b. Basīl (known in the Latin West as Stephanos, fl. 847–861)[66] and Ḥunayn b. Isḥāk al-ʿIbādī (known as Johannitius, 808–873, a Christian physician and translator working in Baghdad) translated the work of Dioscorides and other Greek medical authorities from Greek into Arabic.[67] The Arabic text was revised and translated again in the tenth century in both the eastern and western (Cordova) Islamic world, and the Syriac version was retranslated in the twelfth century as well.[68] All versions appear to have circulated widely, as attested by the many Arabic commentaries.[69]

Twelve illustrated Arabic Dioscorides manuscripts remain extant.[70] The type of imagery in the illustrated copies varies across these versions, as does the quality of Arabic.[71] For my purposes here, the history of two manuscripts in the Islamic world, in particular, demonstrate the connections between the collection of illustrated books of *materia medica* and status (political and professional), pleasure, and the acquisition of medical knowledge. The history of a lost Greek copy of Dioscorides' *De materia medica* given to ʿAbd al-Raḥmān III (891–961), emir and subsequently caliph of Cordova (912–961), points to a continuous connection between political status, knowledge and gift-giving associated with these manuscripts. Likewise, the illustrations in an Arabic copy of Dioscorides created in Baghdad before the city's fall to the Mongols in 1258 and now held at the Süleymaniye Kütüphanesi in Istanbul under the shelfmark

Ayasofia 3703 (dated 1224) suggest the role pleasure played in the privileged experience of reading of these codices.[72]

In the tenth century – a century after its more widespread introduction to the Arabic world – an illustrated Greek Dioscorides served as a gift for an emperor, much as it did for the Byzantine Emperor's daughter, Anicia Juliana, four centuries earlier. The tenth-century codex was a gift from the then-Byzantine Emperor (likely Armanios, identified as Romanus II [fl. 948], co-regent of Constantine VII Porphyrogenitus [905–959]) to the court of ʿAbd al-Raḥmān III in Cordova.[73] In his dictionary of physicians, *Uyūn al-anbāʾ fī ṭabaqāt al-aṭibbā* (*Lives of the Physicians*), produced in the 1240s, the historian and biographer Ibn Abī Uṣaybiʿa (ca. 1203–1270) noted the presence of a beautifully illustrated Greek Dioscorides in the library of ʿAbd al-Raḥmān III. Abī Uṣaybiʿa also noted both the caliph's request for a translator from the Byzantine emperor and the concurrent circulation of Stephanos' ninth-century Arabic translation of Dioscorides in the court at Cordova.[74]

The request for an expert and the use of an earlier translation of Dioscorides' work attest to the importance of access to the information in the text and to the drive to amend or build upon it.[75] The Byzantine emperor did send an expert eventually; a monk named Nicholas arrived in 951–952. While Nicholas' work with the Greek codex likely contributed to or prompted efforts at collaborative translations to replace or modify Stephanos' older one, these efforts did not produce an official new translation.[76] Despite the absence of a new translation, however, the caliph's effort to further integrate the Greek text into the community – where an earlier version of that text's translation was already in use – points to the text's practical and ideological value in Al-Andalus. D. Fairchild Ruggles describes this event eloquently: 'the Byzantine gift was not simply a beautiful *objet d'art* but a treasure of information'.[77] Like a physical treasure, this 'treasure of information' had currency in the community, which reinforced the appropriateness of a distinguished version of this book as a possession of al-Raḥmān. The caliph's request for a translator not only brought together a group of Arabic, Latin, Greek and Hebrew-speaking scholars to interpret the Greek Dioscorides, but it also publicised the book's presence at court and connected al-Raḥmān to the transmission of prized and useful knowledge.

The significance of illustrated books of *materia medica* to privileged and influential members of society – as vectors for self-making or as means to knit their social or political identities together with community needs and values – is shown in a different context in the unique set of illustrations that accompany Dioscorides' treatise in the manuscript now known as Ayasofia 3703. These large illustrations almost completely cover the page and combine representations of plants with figural scenes and landscapes drawn from illustrative traditions associated with mosaics and with different literary genres favoured by educated audiences.[78] As Richard Ettinghausen and Alain Touwaide have pointed out, all aspects of this manuscript – from its large images to its beautiful *naskhi* script – are of the finest possible quality, which suggests that a wealthy physician, patron or member of the court (likely in Baghdad) commissioned the codex.[79] Illustrations dominate the book's pages and, before it was dismantled in the late nineteenth century, every other folio contained two full-page illustrations that faced each other.[80] Further, on the pages with text and imagery, the scribe confined the accompanying text to an 'airy' thirteen lines per page (to borrow Touwaide's description).[81] These characteristics immediately point to the cost, quality and exclusivity of the manuscript while simultaneously emphasising its literary and illustrative contents.

An artist named 'Abdallâh ibn al-Fadl (fl. first half thirteenth-century) completed the illustrations. He modelled many of the plant drawings on those found in a contemporaneous Arabic Dioscorides, also now held at the Süleymaniye Kütüphanesi, Ayasofia 3702.[82] The illustrations in this manuscript, in particular, evoke those in a ninth-century Greek Dioscorides produced in Syria, Palestine or Southern Italy,[83] which may have taken as its model the oldest type of illustration to accompany Dioscorides' treatise.[84] While certainly indebted to Ayasofia 3702, and so to *graecus* 2179, al-Fadl made the imagery in Ayasofia 3703 unique by altering his source imagery and adding to it in a way that evoked other illustrations and imagery enjoyed by privileged readers, which in turn connoted different sets of knowledge and values.[85]

In particular, al-Fadl looked to illustrative traditions in the anonymous *Kalīla Wa-Dimna* (*Kalīlah and Dimnah*)[86] and the *Makāmāt* (*Assemblies*) by al-Harīrī of Basra (1054–1122) – texts that belong to humanistic rather than medical discourse.[87] The *Kalīla* is a collection of animal fables with a long history of translation and transmission from India, through Persia, the eastern and western Arabic Empire, Spain, Italy, and – in printed editions – across the rest of Europe.[88] The scenes in Ayasofia 3703 depicting plants flanked by animals are reminiscent of scenes in these fables (Figure 1.5).[89] The text of the *Kalīla* was originally composed in Sanskrit (likely in the third century CE) and subsequently translated into Persian in the sixth century by a physician named Burzoy. The physician-translator added five stories to the original five in the Sanskrit, although one of his stories often is excluded from subsequent translations.[90] In the mid-eighth century, Ibn al-Mukaffa' (724–759) translated the text into Arabic from Pahlavi (Middle Persian) and added five more stories, while his contemporary, Abān al-Lāhiķī (ca. 750–816), versified the tales.[91] The stories originating in the Sanskrit and Persian versions of the compilation often present negative exemplars and focus on amoral behaviour, while those added in the Arabic translations focus on positive exemplars and just behaviour.[92] The eponymous characters are two jackals from the longest of the stories, 'The Lion and the Bull', who represent the poles of good and bad judgement.[93]

In its Arabic version, the *Kalīla* often includes a preface by al-Mukaffa' that specifically names the audience and the purpose of the text. He wrote:[94]

> He who peruses this book should know that its intention is fourfold. Firstly, it was put into the mouths of dumb animals so that light-hearted youths might flock to read it and their hearts be captivated by the rare uses of animals. Secondly, it was intended to show the images of the animals in varieties of paints and colours so as to delight the hearts of princes, increase their pleasure, and

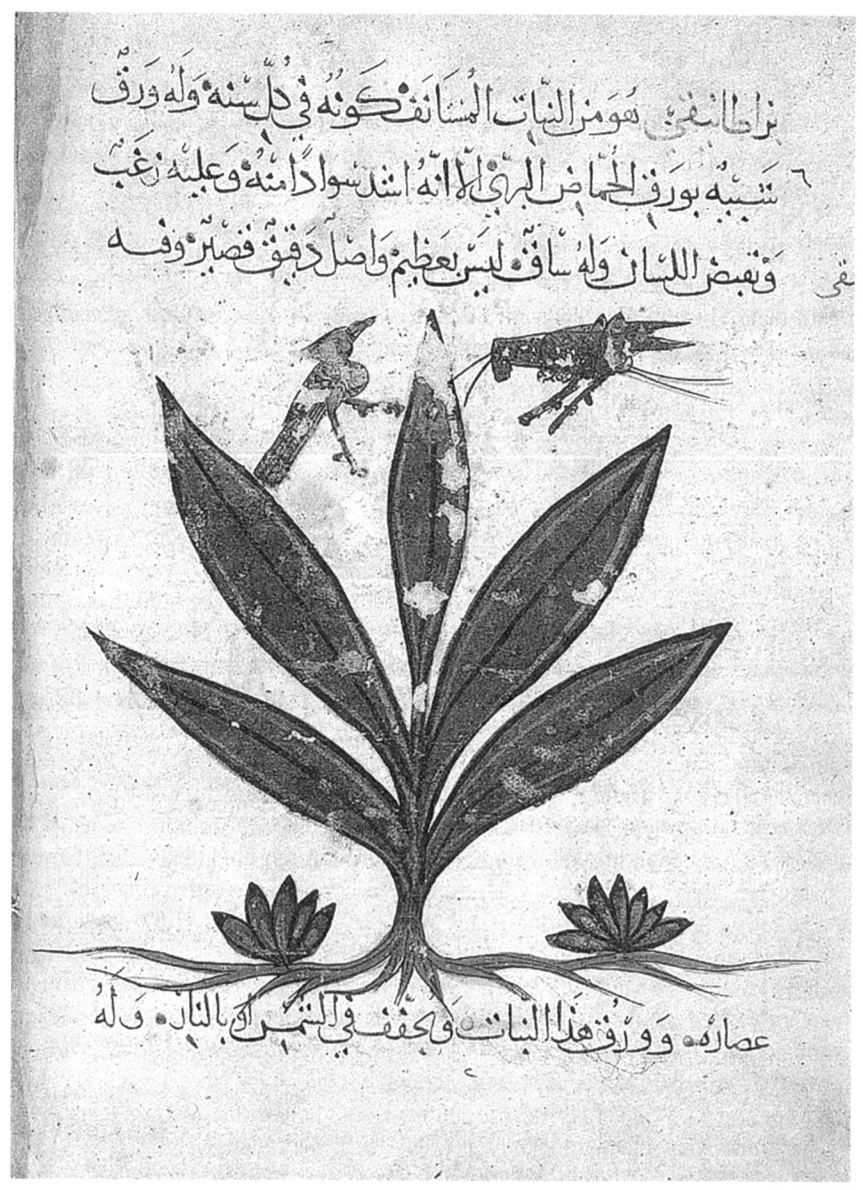

Figure 1.5 Bird and grasshopper with water dock (?) (*Rumex aquaticus* L.)

'Abdallâh ibn al-Fadl, *De materia medica*
Istanbul, Süleymaniye Kütüphanesi, Ayasofia 3703, f. 3b
33 × 24 cm, Baghdad (?), 1224

Source: Süleymaniye Kütüphanesi

also the degree of care which they would bestow on the work. Thirdly, it was intended that the book should be such that both kings and common folk should not cease to acquire it; that it might be repeatedly copied and re-created in the course of time thus giving work to the painter and copyist. The fourth purpose of the work concerns the philosophers in particular (i.e. the apologues put into the mouths of animals).

In its Arabic version, then, the text had didactic (and economic) purposes, but it also sought to delight. Furthermore, as al-Muḳaffaʿ tells us, its illustrations were instrumental to fulfilling these purposes, especially for princes. This principle of didactic delight applies readily to other Arabic illustrated books produced for a privileged audience, as demonstrated in the illustrations in the *Makāmāt al-Ḥarīrī* – one of al-Fadl's other illustrative sources for Ayasofia 3703.

In the *Makāmāt al-Ḥarīrī*, both the textual content and its illustrations share the purposeful delight invoked by al-Muḳaffaʿ in his preface to the *Kalīla*. Al-Fadl borrowed architectural and environmental settings from the *Makāmāt* as well as scenes of figures speaking or encircling plants.[95] The work is a late eleventh- or early twelfth-century fictional account of the adventures of the wandering hero, Abū Zayd. Like the much-later escapades of another picaresque hero, Don Quixote, Abū Zayd's adventures were immediately popular; over 200 manuscript copies from the twelfth and thirteenth centuries remain extant.[96] The *Makāmāt* is celebrated not only for its illustrations but also for its beautiful and witty use of Arabic. The author plays with the language, creating sophisticated puns – sometimes double and triple puns – to accompany Abū Zayd's exploits.[97] In certain recensions, the illustrations accompanying the text echo this linguistic play.

Like the illustrated Dioscorides and the *Kalīla*, the illustrations paired with al-Ḥarīrī's text range in type from highly stylised to more realistic. Oleg Grabar categorises the types of imagery as 'literal', 'descriptive' or 'interpretative'.[98] He specifically points to the wittiness and often-satirical qualities of the 'interpretative' illustrations (which create a 'mood' rather than simply attempt to record the action of the stories) and the scenes or environments portrayed in the 'descriptive' imagery (which physically locate the stories in cityscapes relevant to the lives of contemporary readers). In his discussion of the 'interpretative' and 'descriptive' imagery in an ornate thirteenth-century copy,[99] Grabar argues that the artist, Yaḥyā ibn Maḥmūd al-Wāsiṭī (fl. thirteenth century), sought to further delight the viewer by accompanying the wittiness of the text with playfulness and charm in the imagery. Al-Wāsiṭī's illustrations provide what Grabar terms 'psychological and intellectual' interpretations of the textual content.[100] A high degree of facility with the language was necessary to access the interplay between image and text in the *Makāmāt* and its linguistic humour. Such facility only came with a high degree of education, which points to the intended audience of this manuscript in particular: it was the purview of an elite, literate class.[101]

In the illustrated Dioscorides of Ayasofia 3703, al-Fadl borrowed the figural scenes from the *Makāmāt al-Ḥarīrī* tradition, keeping some of the playfulness and pleasure associated with their original context: for instance, al-Fadl's illustrations of physicians interacting echoes scenes of al-Ḥarīrī and Abū Zayd speaking.[102] The scenes of physicians preparing medicines in Ayasofia 3703, like many scenes in the *Maḳāmāt al-Ḥarīrī*, are highly decorative and full of repeating patterns and motifs (Figure 1.6). Like an ornate textile or mosaic, they catch the reader's eye and invite him or her to linger on their delicate details and intricate beauty.[103] Although not

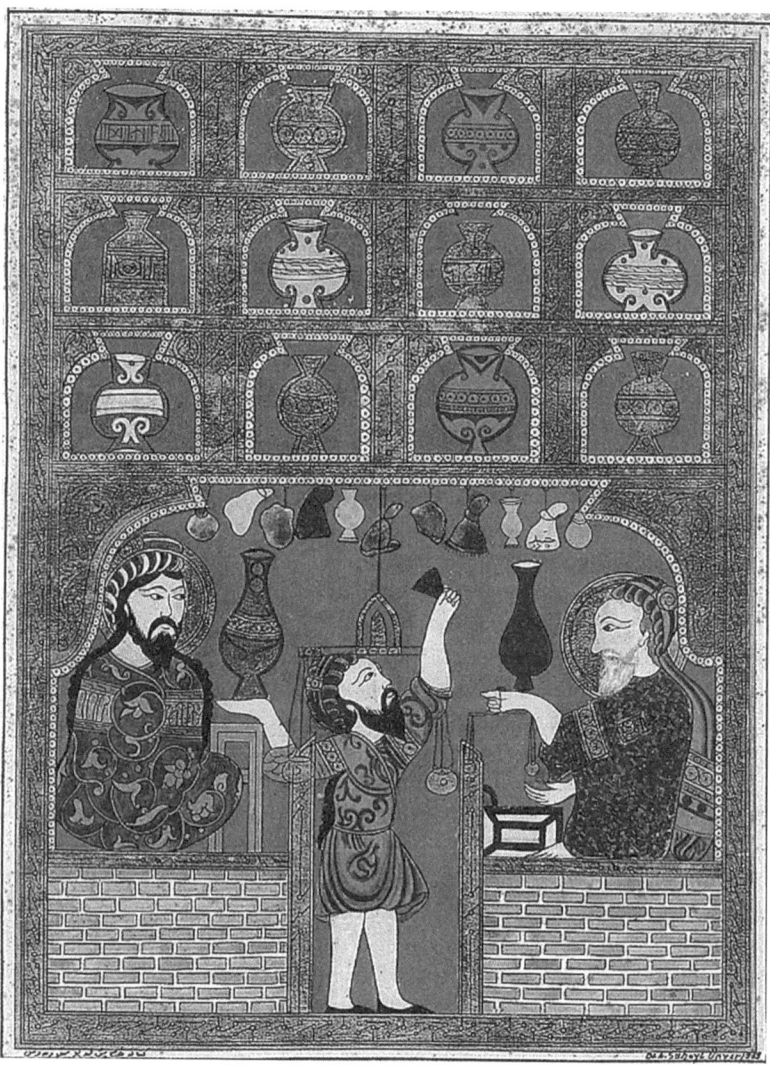

Figure 1.6 Physicians preparing medicine

ʿAbdallâh ibn al-Fadl, *De materia medica*
Istanbul, Süleymaniye Kütüphanesi, Ayasofia 3703, f. 2b
33 × 24 cm, Baghdad (?), 1224

Source: Süleymaniye Kütüphanesi

all illustrated Arabic recensions of Dioscorides' *De materia medica* incorporate imagery from other literary genres, the diverse imagery in Ayasofia 3703 shows a connection between humanistic and scientific texts established by the merging of their respective illustrative traditions.[104]

These two examples from the Arabic tradition of the illustrated Dioscorides affirm a continuity in the role of such books in collections of the social and political elite and suggest the valued role physicians and their knowledge of medicine could play in those strata of society. The books contain respected knowledge, and the object that presents this knowledge ensured its association with the highest echelons of educated society.

The illustrative traditions of materia medica in the Latin West

Turning to the Latin West, we see both a change in the transmission of medical knowledge and a continuity in the roles played by illustrated books of *materia medica* in patterns of exchange, gift giving and identity building as established in the Greek and Arabic traditions. Furthermore, select illustrative traditions that accompany medical treatises in the Latin West echo the synthesis of imagery drawn from humanistic, scientific and even architectural contexts in al-Fadl's illustrations for Ayasofia 3703.

The Latin books of *materia medica* produced around the same time as Ayasofia 3703, while neither reproducing Dioscorides' text in its entirety nor faithfully,[105] also contain illustrative cycles that demonstrate values shared by the books' patrons. The illustrations in these medical texts are diverse and include plant imagery (schematic and realistic), scenes of physicians interacting with patients and scenes drawn from Classical mythology. Like the previous traditions, the illustrated Latin books of *materia medica* vary widely in textual and visual content. The few examples explored here point to thematic and visual continuities with the earlier Greek and Arabic traditions, but they are not emblematic of the entirety of the Latin production, which is highly diverse.[106]

Dioscorides' complete treatise remained relatively unknown in Latin culture until its reintroduction in the eleventh-century Latin translations made at Salerno from Greek and Arabic copies.[107] From the sixth- through the thirteenth centuries, the *Herbarium Apuleii Platonici* (*The Herbal of Apuleius Platonicus*) remained the predominant treatise on *materia medica* in the Latin West.[108] The *Herbarium* is a fourth- or fifth-century compilation of medical information often found in combination with texts broadly derived from Dioscorides' *De materia medica* (especially the sixth-century Pseudo Dioscorides' *Ex herbis femininis* [*From Female Herbs*]).[109] The author of the *Herbarium* is unknown, although he is sometimes misidentified as Apuleius of Madaura (ca. 125–180), the author of the *Asinus aureus* (*The Golden Ass*).[110] The name Apuleius, however, may deliberately refer to Aesculapius's follower of the same name, an idea confirmed by incipits in some of the extant manuscripts. These incipits tell the reader that Chiron, the wise physician-centaur and teacher of heroes, and Aesculapius, the Greek god of healing, gave Apuleius this knowledge.[111] Certainly, Chiron and Aesculapius would be appropriate teachers (and so authorities) for the author to claim as his own.

Despite the mythical origins of his name, the information recorded by Apuleius derives from several identifiable fourth-century Greek and Latin sources, especially from the chapters on plant medicine in Pliny's *Naturalis historia* condensed into the Late Antique *Medicina Plinii* (*Medical Pliny*). Like the later *Tractatus de herbis* (*Treatise on Medicinal Plants*), the *Herbarium* tradition takes its name from the largest book in a relatively consistent compilation of medical texts.[112] It contains over 130 chapters, each one dedicated to a single plant that is illustrated and accompanied by a list of synonyms and a list of ailments – organised *a capite ad calcem*, from head to foot. Instructions follow on how to use the plant to address each symptom.

Two thirteenth-century examples of the illustrated *Herbarium* commissioned by Emperor Frederick II Hohenstaufen (1194–1250) point to the production and collection of illustrated books of *materia medica* by elite, political patrons during the Middle Ages in the Latin West.[113] Frederick commissioned these books to enjoy and consume – for their imagery and for the knowledge they contain – and to display his status and self-image to other readers.[114] In their form and content, the copies of the *Herbarium* reveal Frederick's chosen identity as a scholar-king and patron of the contemporary study of medicine. In Frederick's manuscripts, earlier textual and illustrative traditions were altered and edited to form a new variety of herbal, one that alluded to the progressive medicine taught at Salerno, which Frederick championed.[115]

It is well known that Frederick valued and promoted the physicians gathered at Salerno and the innovative scientific and medical knowledge established and taught there. Generally, in his manuscript commissions Frederick sought to amalgamate this new knowledge – drawn especially from Greek and Arabic medical texts – into older Latin sources, a technique that produced distinctive, personal reference books.[116] Similarly, the iconography of the illustrations in his herbals draws together into single codices specific elements from different copies of the *Herbarium* produced during the text's long history. In their comprehensive synthesis of the earlier visual and textual varieties of the *Herbarium*, Frederick's manuscripts are visual and textual records of the history of the genre itself.[117]

Like many illustrated copies of Dioscorides' *De materia medica*, Frederick's copies of the *Herbarium* include illustrations of individual plants, often flanked by synonyms of the plant's name and preceded by their textual descriptions. The illustrations dominate the surface of the page with both colourful botanical and figural representations.[118] In general, the schematic type of plant and animal illustration reproduced by Frederick's illustrators is characteristic of the three recensions of the *Herbarium* manuscripts, from the earliest sixth-century copies through to their twelfth-century successors. The mythological figures and illustrations of medical treatments in Frederick's codices, in particular, likely refer to ninth-century versions of the *Herbarium* produced in both Italy and the north. The anecdotal narrative scenes, such as the image of a man bitten by a rabid dog placed next to textual entries on the cures for such bites, drew on twelfth-century Italian versions (Figure 1.7). Conversely, the prefatory portraits of physicians and didactic scenes of preparation, collection and application of herbal remedies grew out of the northern twelfth-century renditions (Figure 1.8).

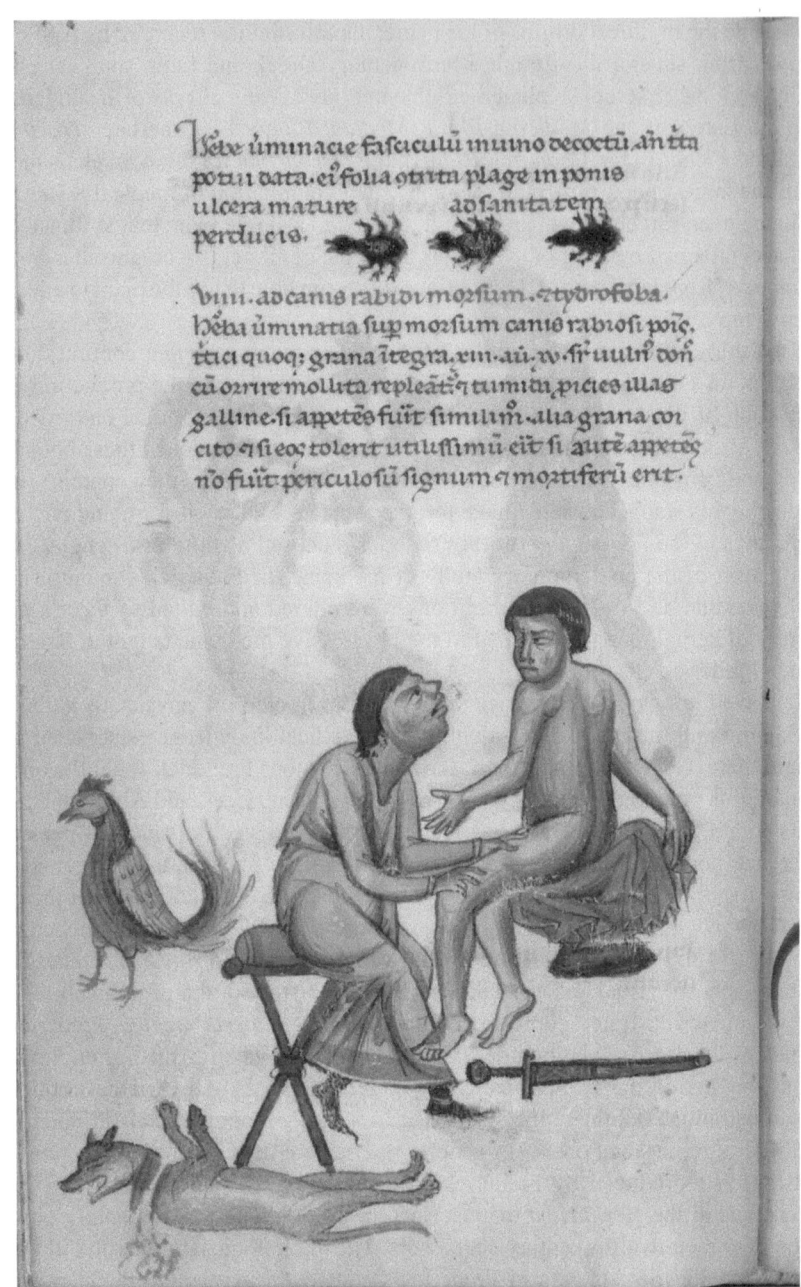

Figure 1.7 Verminatia (Verbena officinalis L., vervain) as treatment for rabid-dog bite

Herbarium Apuleii Platonici
Florence, Biblioteca Medicea Laurenziana, plut. 73.16, f. 34v
17.5 × 11.4 cm, Southern Italy, ca. 1220–1250

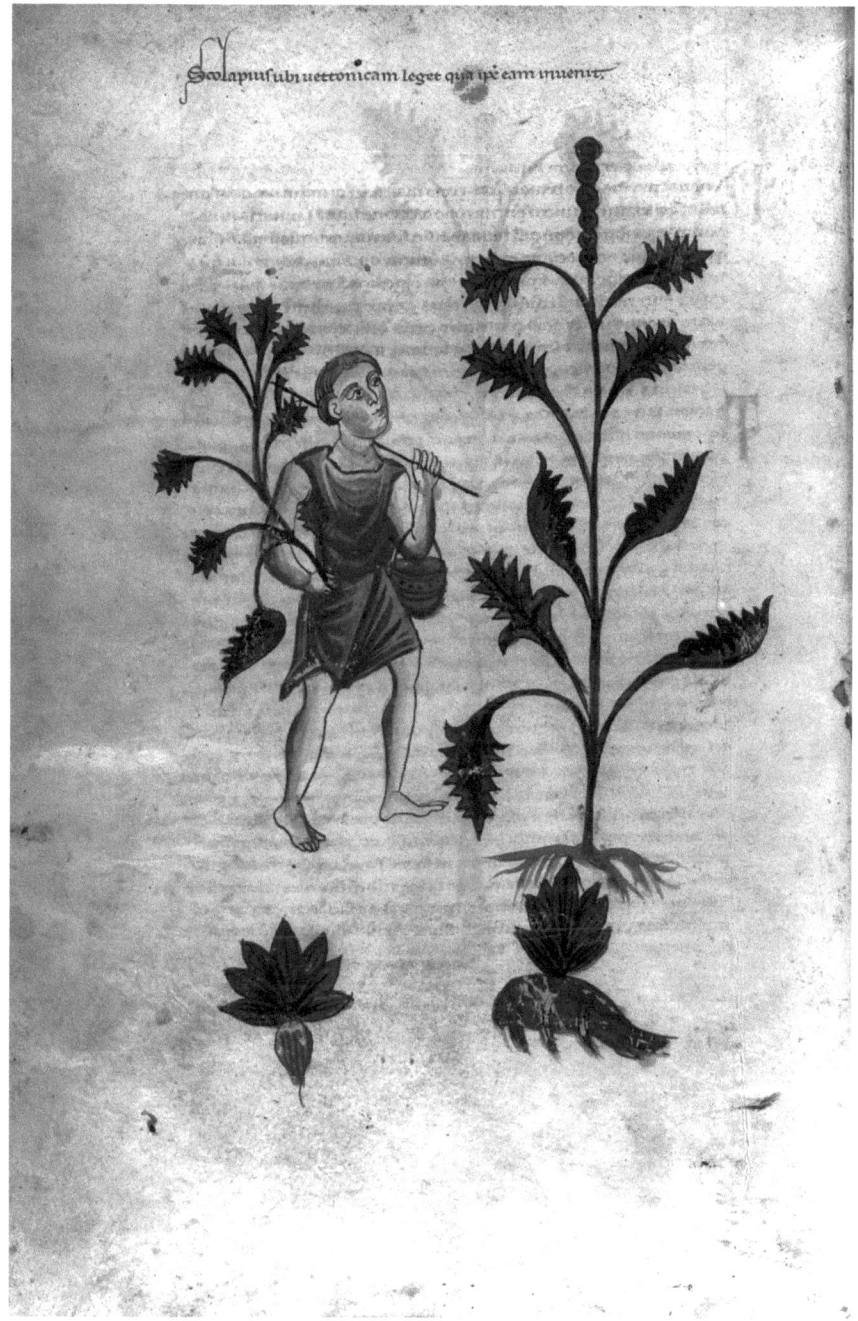

Figure 1.8 Portrait of Aesculapius with betony plant (*Stachys officinalis* L.)

Herbarium Apuleii Platonici
Vienna, Österreichische Nationalbibliothek, lat. 93, f. 5v
28 × 18.5 cm, Sicily, ca. 1220–1266

Source: ÖNB

Frederick's syncretical manuscripts point to the emperor's interest in the past (especially an imagined Classical past associated with Apuleius' text) and in the medical innovations occurring in Salerno during his rule. This interplay between old and new knowledge and the diversity of illustrations and illustrative traditions in Frederick's *Herbarium* manuscripts functions in a similar way to the playful cross-genre references in al-Fadl's illustrations of the Arabic Dioscorides, Ayasofia 3703. The illustrations create a rich and pleasurable reading experience infused with attributes of different textual and illustrative histories. To distinguish old sources from new ones and to recognise the different iconographies, however, the reader would need an education and exposure to pictorial and textual traditions accessible to select few. The combinations, then, invest the reading experience with exclusivity and promote a certain erudite image of the books' owner.

Through their amalgamation of textual and illustrative traditions, these manuscripts projected an image of Frederick as a progressive and scholarly leader whose knowledge bridged centuries of learning. In addition, as Giulia Orofino argues, Frederick's collection of these herbals may have emulated his ninth-century ancestors' commission and collection of this type of manuscript.[119] Allegedly, Frederick's ancestors associated books on plant medicine with Imperial Roman patronage, which they, in turn, strove to imitate.[120] Through their connection to Frederick's imperial genealogy and an imagined Classical past, the *Herbarium* manuscripts visually and textually advanced the emperor's sense of himself not only as a sophisticated leader but as an heir to empire as well.

The late thirteenth-century development of the *Tractatus de herbis* tradition also sought to synthesise all known knowledge of *materia medica*, whether from Greek, Arabic or Latin traditions, into a single volume.[121] This treatise was illustrated from its inception. Scholars tentatively attribute authorship of the *Tractatus* to the otherwise unknown Bartholomaeus Mini of Senis.[122] Bartholomaeus' work contains information on 524 plants and their medicinal properties. The author presented the plants in alphabetical order according to Latin plant name, beginning with aloe (*de aloe*) and ending with sugar (*de zuchara*).[123] Each entry, while variable in length, follows a consistent pattern that includes a description of the plant's characteristic features, its synonyms and instructions for its use.[124]

The earliest extant *Tractatus* (London, British Library, Egerton 747, ca. 1280–1317) includes the text from an unillustrated treatise known as the *Circa instans*, compiled by Salernitan physician Matthaeus Platearius (d. 1161).[125] The Egerton *Tractatus* also includes original textual content and information drawn from earlier Latin botanical treatises, especially from Apuleius' *Herbarium*, the versified book of *materia medica* known as *Macer Floridus* (*De viribus herbarum/On the Virtues of Herbs*) and an alphabetised, Latin version of Dioscorides *De materia medica*.[126] Furthermore, the author of the *Tractatus* fused these popular Western derivatives of Dioscorides' medicine with those preserved in Arabic treatises.[127] While the original patron and owner of the Egerton *Tractatus* remains unknown, the codex may have served as a reference book for the medical community at Salerno.[128]

An anonymous artist richly illustrated the book with both schematic and verisimilar representations of plants, a combination that produced imagery art historian Otto Pächt memorably termed 'half picture, half diagram'.[129] Much like the imagery in the earlier illustrated books of *materia medica* discussed previously, the diversity of representational styles in Egerton 747 delights readers as they learn about the accompanying plant medicines. The experience of reading the Egerton *Tractatus* is an even more layered one, perhaps, since in many instances the imagery quite literally overlaps the text, both challenging and charming the manuscript's readers (Figure 1.9). In addition to plant representations, the *Tractatus* also includes narrative and figural scenes, figured initials that enclose author portraits (on two incipit pages), and several formulaic images of scorpions and snakes.

For my purposes here, a manuscript indebted to Egerton 747 – the influential and widely copied *Tractatus liber de herbis et plantis*, also known as the *Herbal of Manfred de Monte Imperiale* – is more relevant to the cultural milieu that produced the *Carrara Herbal*.[130] Allegedly, a scholar-physician working in southern Italy in the first half of the fourteenth century, the eponymous Manfred, wrote and illustrated this herbal.[131] However, the book is a composite of information and imagery drawn from the Egerton *Tractatus*, among other sources, to which Manfred added his own reflections. Following a pattern we have seen in examples from other traditions of illustrated books of *materia medica*, Manfred altered his models to suit his purposes. He included an illustrated version of the *Liber medicinae ex animalibus* (*Book of the Medical Uses of Animals*), a fifth-century treatise on animal-derived drugs attributed to the unknown author Placitus Papyriensis. He also included an augmented version of the *Clavis sanationis* (ca. 1290), the glossary of Greek, Arabic and Latin medical terminology compiled by Simon of Genoa (fl. late thirteenth century) around the same time he translated Serapion's work into Latin. The glossary gives Manfred's codex a *terminus post quem*: Simon likely compiled his 'key' while serving as the papal curia chaplain and physician to Pope Nicolas IV (1288–1292).[132]

Manfred's herbal is important to the study of illustrated books of *materia medica* and their dissemination and collection in northern Italy, especially. It shows the developing connection of these books both to the personal collections of erudite readers and to the university community in the late fourteenth century. In its long history of transmission, Manfred's book also affirms the relationship between acquiring knowledge of nature's medicines and delighting in their visual representations. Although the cause or person responsible for the book's northern migration remains unknown, several illustrated herbals produced in the Veneto and Lombardy regions likely take Manfred's book as a model and so attest to its presence in northern Italy in the second half of the fourteenth century (none of them is a direct copy, however).[133] Furthermore, the earliest extant *consignatio* (library inventory) of the Visconti-Sforza collection, taken in Pavia in 1426, records Manfred's book as part of the family's collection.[134] Since the Visconti claimed Francesco il Vecchio's books as spoils of war in 1388, it is possible that Manfred's book once belonged to the former Carrara lord. This possibility is strengthened when we consider that at least one of the illustrated books indebted to Manfred's herbal was likely produced in Padua (Paris, Bibliothèque de l'Ecole des Beaux-Arts, Masson 116).[135]

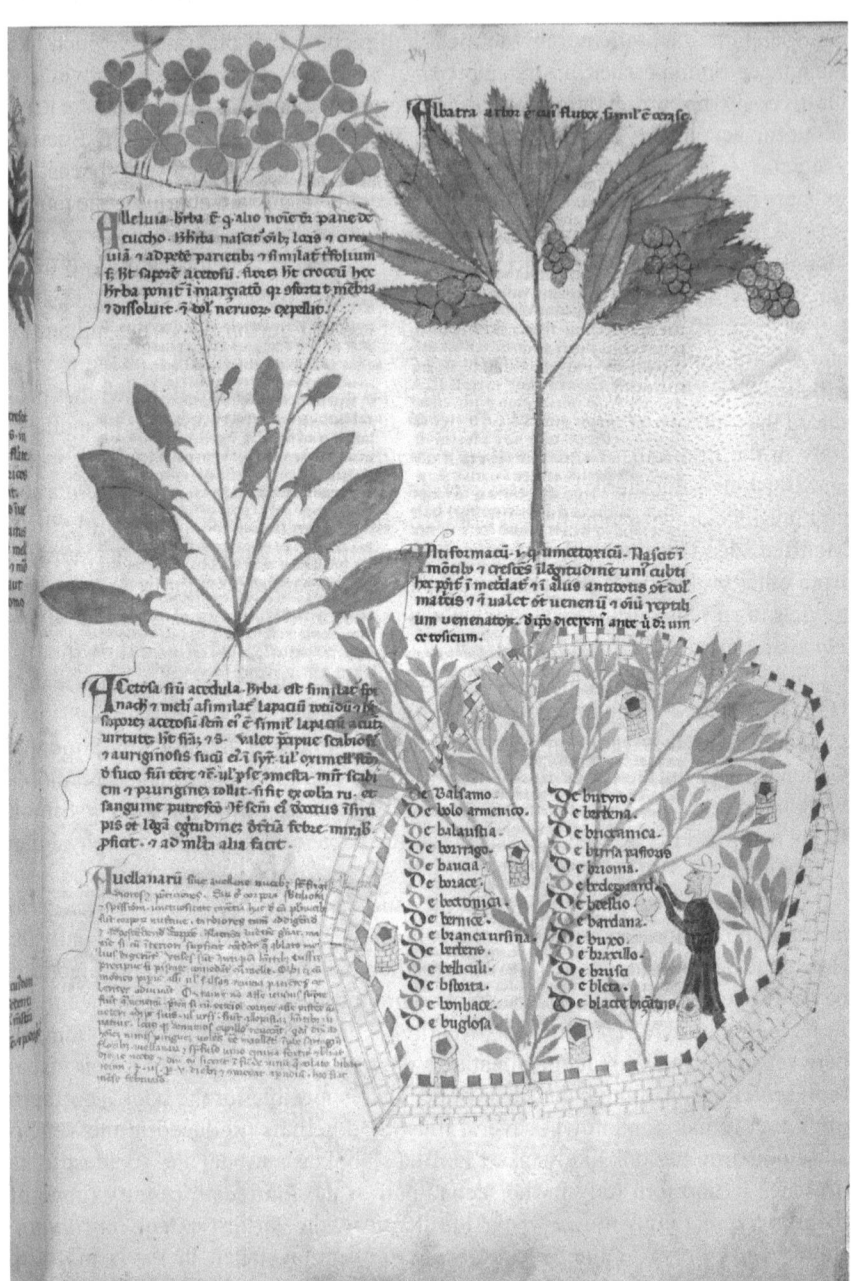

Figure 1.9 Allelulia (*Oxalis acetosella* L., wood sorrel), *acetosa* (*Rumex acetosa* L.,
sorrel), *albatra* (*Arbutus unedo* L., strawberry tree) and *balsamus* (*Commiphora
gileadensis* L., balsam)

Tractatus de herbis
London, British Library, Egerton 747, f. 12r
36 × 24.2 cm, Salerno (?), ca. 1280–1310

Art historian Felix Baumann dated the Masson *Tractatus* to 1370–1380 due to stylistic similarities he perceived between its figured scenes and those in contemporary illustrated romances, especially *Guiron le Courtois* (Paris, Bibliothèque nationale, nouv. acq. fr. 5243) and *Lancelot du Lac* (Paris, Bibliothèque nationale, fr. 343).[136] François Avril narrowed the date range to 1376–1379 and identified Padua as the site of production due to stylistic similarities between the manuscript's illustrations and the frescoes produced by Altichiero (1330–1390) or Jacopo Avanzo (ca. 1350–1416).[137] If this attribution and date-range are correct, they connect Manfred's herbal – as a model for Masson 116 – to Padua during Francesco il Vecchio's rule.

Even though illustrated books of *materia medica* were not the principal focus of his collection, Francesco il Vecchio likely possessed at least one in his extensive library.[138] Hypothetically, the initial migration north of Manfred's herbal may even have been the result of Francesco il Vecchio's continuation of his ancestors' efforts to recruit professors to the University of Padua from Bologna. The rise of these two medical schools and universities in northern Italy transferred the locus of medical knowledge and teaching from Salerno northward in the fourteenth century.[139] Moreover, the book's author and its history of use would have reinforced Francesco il Vecchio's desire to construct an image of himself as a contemplative scholar, book collector and as a patron of the growing medical schools at the University of Padua – three aspects of patronage upon which Francesco Novello would found his own self-image.

Although the original owner insignia in Manfred's herbal has been effaced, the resonance of its content and iconography with parts of Francesco il Vecchio's cultivated persona and its subsequent presence in the Visconti library after the conquest of Padua point to Carrara ownership. As part of Francesco il Vecchio's collection, Manfred's herbal becomes a potential model for the ideological significance of the *Carrara Herbal* as a book in Francesco Novello's library. While the books' illustrations share some formal similarities and their texts both address *materia medica*, it is the idea of Manfred's herbal as an illustrated book of plant medicines produced by and for a physician and subsequently acquired by an erudite bibliophile that the *Carrara Herbal* imitates.[140] By imitating an illustrated herbal from which other contemporaneous illustrated herbals derived, the *Carrara Herbal* firmly inserted itself into a hierarchical lineage of production and collection of illustrated herbals and emphasised the continuity of the Carrara family's efforts to create a prestigious book collection.

The opening series of portrait frontispieces in Manfred's herbal visually articulate another lineage that would have appealed to the Carrara *signori*, and especially to Francesco Novello.[141] In a way similar to the series of frontispieces in Anicia Juliana's Dioscorides (*Vienna Dioscorides*), the series in Manfred's book articulates the ideal image of the manuscript owner as a wise reader and a successor to the knowledge traditions encapsulated within the book. In Manfred's herbal, the opening author portrait – executed in pale-coloured pen and wash – shows Manfred seated with a large book cradled in the crook of his right arm (f. 1r, Plate 3). He raises his left hand in a gesture of speech to a group of students, two of whom hold out plants – betony (*Stachys sylvatica* L.) and feverfew (*Tanacetum parthenium L.*) – for identification and analysis. Words stream from Manfred's mouth toward his students. Paraphrasing a Hippocratic adage, Manfred says, 'Prima et ultima medicina propter corpus et animam est abstinentia' ('Moderation, by means of body and soul, is the first and greatest medicine').

The portrait shows Manfred as a master of medicine in the act of teaching the next generation of physicians. Age lines Manfred's face, and his grey beard falls in waves across the front of his long, hooded robe. Conversely, his students show the glow of youth, their eager faces either clean-shaven or depicted with a short, neat beard. In the upper right corner of the page, the hand of God emerges from a series of concentric blue spheres in a gesture of blessing. Words stream downward from God's hand toward Manfred: 'Omnia probate quod bonum est tenete' ('Investigate all things, holding fast to what is good'). This quotation, from the first letter of Paul to the Thessalonians, 5:21, shows Manfred's practice and his teaching as divinely assisted and authorised. Moreover, following the medieval *Glossa Ordinaria* tradition, this verse and those immediately preceding it point to the importance of learning from elders who have 'tested' their knowledge and so determined what is good – a message Manfred, as a teacher, would value.[142]

The next two pages display eight portraits of medical authorities and their commentators whose works were central to the curriculum of the Neapolitan medical school and the medical community at Salerno. Four of the figures are named, and all are portrayed seated on benches in discussion with one another. To visualise the conversations and to identify the speakers, words excerpted from their most-recognisable works flow from the figures' mouths. The upper register of the first series of author portraits shows Hippocrates (ca. 460–ca. 371–350 BCE) citing the incipit from his *Prognostica* to the Arab translator Ḥunayn b. Isḥāk (Johannitius), who, in turn, speaks lines from his *Isagoge in Artem parvam Galeni* (f. 1v).[143] Beneath them, Hippocrates is portrayed again, now citing the incipit of his *Aphorismi* to Galen (Figure 1.10).[144]

On the following page the upper register shows an unknown doctor (perhaps Yuḥannā Ibn Māsawayh [777–857], known to the Latin West as Mesue) conversing with Bartolomeo of Salerno (fl. 1150–1180), a commentator on the texts of the authorities depicted on the preceding page.[145] Below them, the Aristotelian commentators Ibn Rushd (known to the Latin West as Averroes, 1126–1198) and Porphyry (?) (234–ca. 305) face one another in discussion (f. 2r).[146]

The medical treatises compiled in Manfred's herbal do not directly connect to the works of these authors. Instead, their portraits visually map the contents of Manfred's own knowledge and elevate him and his book as the ultimate, even divinely ordained, resource for medical learning. Within Manfred, the book's original reader, ancient medical authorities separated by vast stretches of time converse, merging their theories and practices into a new medicine embodied by Manfred himself. Pictured prior to the ancient doctors, Manfred's body is much larger and more individuated, highlighting his importance and authority. Manfred supersedes them and shows his status as the current master of medicine whose learning encompasses all of the previous knowledge of the ancient sources as well

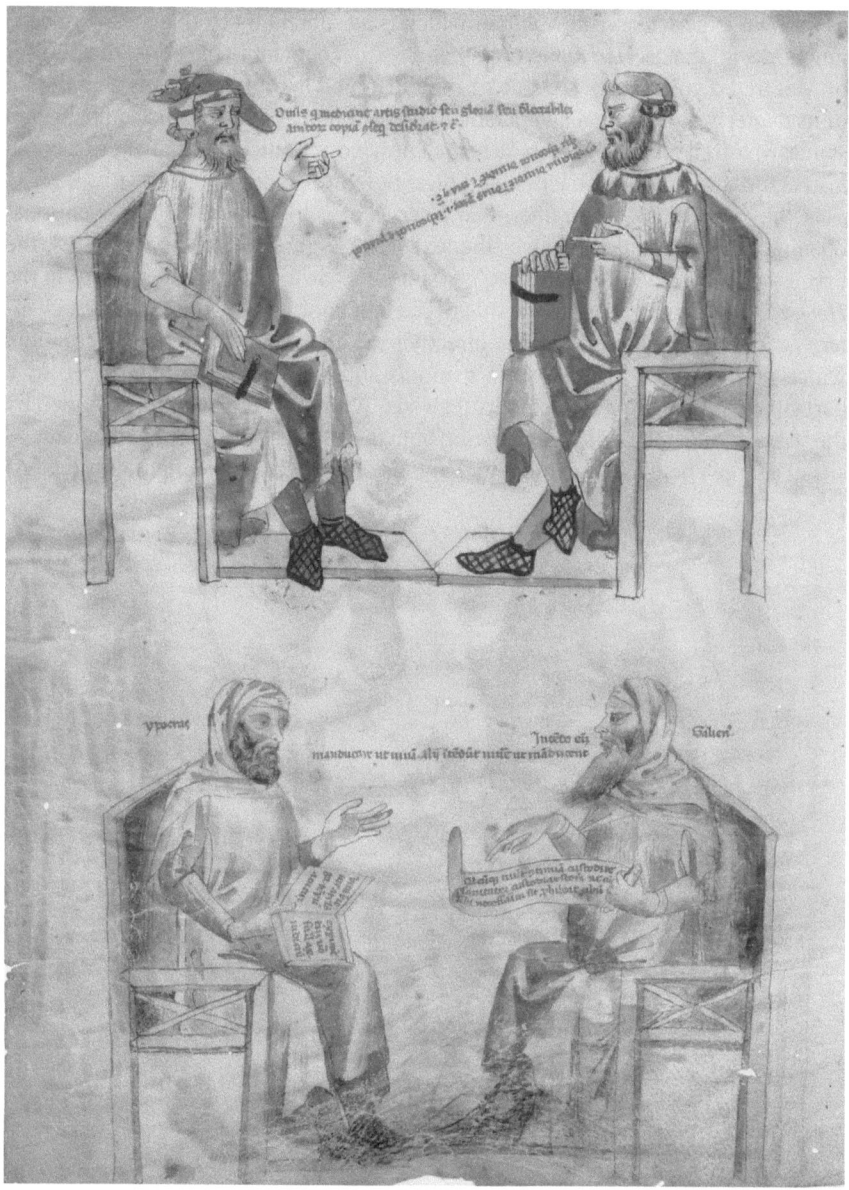

Figure 1.10 Portraits of Hippocrates and Johannitius (above), and Hippocrates and Galen
(below)

Lippo Vanni or Roberto d'Oderisio, *Tractatus de herbis*
Paris, Bibliothèque nationale de France, lat. 6823, f. 1v
34.5 × 24.7 cm, Southern Italy, ca. 1330–1340

Source: Bibliothèque nationale de France, Département des manuscrits, Latin 6823

as his own experiences (the value of which is attested to by God, no less). In conjunction with the diverse iconography and textual content in the book, the portrait of Manfred demonstrates the role of the illustrated herbal to serve as an emblem of its owner's professional and personal interests and as a sign of his authority and status. Manfred physically embodies the knowledge of different ancient authors in his person through the collection and digestion of their texts.

In the *Carrara Herbal*, rather than a series of author portraits, a conventional opening figured initial introduces the text (f. 4r, Figure 1.11). The initial 'E', the first letter in the title of the treatise's first book,[147] is the only figured initial in the *Herbal*. Along with the complete title of the first book and the title of its first chapter, 'del citron', the initial is placed directly beneath the upper marginal decoration, which portrays Francesco Novello's initials and family heraldry connected by a garland of flowing gold and colourful swirls. Within the architecture provided by the 'E', an unnamed figure – suggesting both the author, Serapion, and the reader – sits at a large enclosed desk modelled in black paint with white highlights against

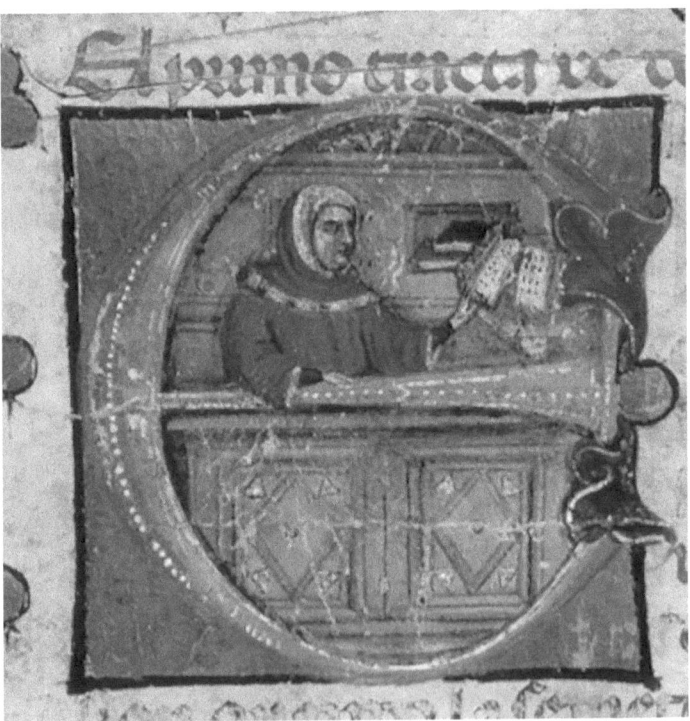

Figure 1.11 Frontispiece (detail of figured initial 'E')

Carrara Herbal
London, British Library, Egerton 2020, f. 4r
Gouache on vellum, Padua, ca. 1390–1400

© British Library Board, Egerton 2020

the initial's gold ground. The central horizontal axis of the 'E' provides the tabletop for the desk. Dressed in the familiar hooded robe of a scholar, the figure touches an open book perched on a bookstand, denoting the object of his attention. Per visual convention, two books on a shelf beside the figure and another on the bookstand further identify this space as a library or study (*studiolo*). The uniform, reflective gold background of the scene focusses the reader's attention on the scholar and his open book, prompting the reader to identify with the scholar who, like him or her, sits at a large desk contemplating this very book.

Considered as a portrait of the ideal reader, the initial is also a portrait of the patron, Francesco Novello. It visualises the action of reading and shows Francesco as a scholar in the active process of studying, of building his knowledge. Accompanied by Francesco's heraldry, the figured initial in the *Carrara Herbal* – like the author portrait of Manfred – connects this book to the collection of illustrated books of *materia medica* as avenues to promote or to corroborate a certain identity of their owners. Manfred augmented his book collection with his herbal to show himself as the new master of medicine. Likewise, as the next chapters will show, Francesco Novello augmented his book collection with the *Carrara Herbal* to show himself in a certain light: as a book collector from a family of book collectors, an ally of the university, and as a 'healer' of Padua.

Notes

1 On the illustrated *Tractatus de herbis* (now London, British Library, Egerton 747) as a physician's book, see Givens (2006). Also, consider the fate of the *Carrara Herbal* itself: around 1445, its images were copied by Andrea Amadio (fl. second half, fifteenth century) and included in the over 400 plant images he created for an illustrated herbal – its folios made of paper, not vellum – commissioned (and written) by the Venetian physician Niccolò Roccabonella (1386–1459) (now Venice, Biblioteca Nazionale Marciana, lat. VI, 59 [coll. 2548]). Later in the Quattrocento, Roccabonella's book appeared in an apothecary's shop in Venice where, perhaps until as late as the second half of the sixteenth century, it was displayed for the shop's clients (Ambrosoli 1992 [tr. 1997: 99]). On the *Roccabonella Herbal*, see Baumann (1974: 126–7); Mariani Canova (1988: 25–6); Paganelli and Cappelletti (1996); Collins (2000: 281); and Segre Rutz (2002: 195–8).
2 For these different interpretations of the function of illustrations across the long trajectory of illustrated books of *materia medica* and especially in books belonging to physicians, see Givens (2006; on indices and memory) and Touwaide (2013b; on transmission and translation).
3 Finely illuminated books were expensive commodities, regardless of their subject matter. They have long been associated with collections of luxuries possessed and displayed by the social and political elite to convey their affluence and status. Several scholars have discussed the relative costs of book production during the late medieval and Renaissance periods. Buettner (1992: 76) demonstrated the high cost of secular illuminated manuscripts in Burgundian France through comparison. She noted that books for princes' collections ranged from 100 to 600 francs, and compared this cost to that of the 'most expensive type of horse' at 100 francs. Also, Alexander (1994: 16–17) noted that Vespasiano da Bisticci (1421–1498), the book purveyor (*cartolaio*) for the Medici and other wealthy families, estimated the value of Federico da Montefeltro's (1422–1482) library at 30,000 ducats. Similarly, an inventory of the Aragonese manuscript collection taken in 1481 described 266 printed books and manuscripts put up as collateral to secure

loans worth 38,000 ducats (roughly 143 ducats per book) for a war against the Turks (Alexander 1994: 16–17).

4 On the Visconti and illustrated books of *materia medica* at their court in Pavia and at the courts of their allies, see Segre Rutz (2002: 11–13, 123–70 and 171–202); Collins and Raphael (2003: 22); and Hoeniger (2006).

5 Hoeniger (2006: 67).

6 The second book on hot and dry medicines in the first degree is an appropriate cross-section of the manuscript's characteristic illustrative techniques. This book contains the largest group of plant representations (27) within a single tract. I draw my examples from this book.

7 In the *malbavisco* illustration, the artist portrayed two species of the plant. Baumann (1974: 47) suggests a modern, Linnaean identification of the plants as *Althaea officinalis.* L. (left), common marshmallow, and *Lavatera thuringiaca* L. (right), tree mallow. For clarity, when citing plant names I have identified the plants according to the names given to them within the text under consideration, followed by their Linnaean identifications and their modern common names in parentheses. For plants in the *Carrara Herbal*, the identifications are based on my observations and those of Ineichen (1962–1966) and Baumann (1974).

8 Baumann considers the *malbavisco* images as examples of what he terms the 'Gepreβtes Herbarexemplar' category (pressed herb specimen) (1974: 47 and 91). I disagree. Unlike a pressed plant, the plants shown here retain the shapes of their flowers, as well as the three-dimensional quality of their fruits. The artist's use of an oblique light source (to the upper left of the plants) articulates the curved 'V' shape of the leaves: the left side of the leaves is in shadow, while the right side is lit. Also, the careful construction of the root systems to show the interweaving roots full of shadowy crevices provides yet another visual cue to depth. Baumann argues that the eight images sharing his pressed-plant categorisation attempt to show the vestiges of the plant's three-dimensionality to convey a sense of careful observation of the plant in nature. He points to the spread-out and flattened quality of the leaves in this category to illustrate his argument.

9 Baumann (1974: 36 and 90) considers *meliloto* an example of the 'Naturbeobachtung' category (nature study) rather than the 'pressed herb specimen' category. I disagree with his attribution of this plant to a category whose purpose was to create the illusion of a three-dimensional, living plant. As my observations point out, the *meliloto* image contains many visual cues to suggest its forced two-dimensionality due to pressing.

10 While not a literal, material-based *herbarium siccus* (plant catalogue comprised of dried specimens), the *Carrara Herbal* and its images of pressed plants evoke a tradition of preserving plants in books, but long before the earliest extant record of this practice (Baumann 1974: 91). In the 1540s, as the large botanical gardens were being established in Padua and Bologna, Luca Ghini (1490–1556), a professor of medicine and botanist at the University of Bologna (1534–1544), created his own *herbarium siccus* as a guide to the identification of plants. While no longer extant, many scholars consider Ghini's book as the first *herbarium siccus* (Arber 1912: 139, and Findlen 1994: 166, among others). Baumann (1974: 91) points to two slightly earlier examples of pressed plant specimens: the 1493–1494 correspondence between Pandolfo Collenuccio (1444–1504) (in Ferrara) and Angiolo Poliziano (1454–1494) (in Florence) shows that Collenuccio, while travelling through Tyrol, sent pressed botanical specimens to Poliziano. In his reply to Collenuccio, however, Poliziano notes that the scholars to whom he showed these specimens were sceptical of Collenuccio's method as a reliable form of scientific communication (*Politiani opera* 1533: 1.218). For a discussion of this letter, its possible date and its importance to Poliziano, see Godman 1998: 105–6. Baumann (1974: 91) also notes that a northern Italian herbal, now Brescia, Biblioteca Querini, B.V. 24 (ca. 1506), contains painted representations of plants next to the actual pressed specimens.

11 Like the *malbavisco*'s fruits, the red-tinged flowers of the *meliloto* suggest a late stage in the plant's growth. Pavord (2005: 130) notes many visual indicators in the verisimilar images in the *Carrara Herbal* that suggest the artist observed and recorded the plants in late summer or early autumn.

12 Similarly, Baumann (1974: 35) calls the *sponga marina* an example of 'Schema' (schematic portraiture).

13 Baumann (1974: 46) calls the *pino* illustration an example of 'Schema mit Naturbeobachtung' (schematic portraiture with some direct observation of nature).

14 The artist used this technique to focus attention on different aspects of the tree in several of his other tree illustrations. For examples, see Baumann (1974: 89).

15 Baumann (1974: 89) suggests that, in some of his tree images, the artist may have drawn on the representative techniques discussed by Cennino Cennini (1370–1440) in his late fourteenth-century *Il libro dell' arte* (*The Craftsman's Handbook*, chapter LXXXVI 'The Way to Paint Trees and Plants and Foliage, in Fresco and in Secco' [tr. Thompson 1969: 56]). Perhaps following Cennini's instructions, the *Carrara Herbal*'s artist primed the representation of the trunk and canopy of the *pino* with black paint, upon which he then layered the details of the tree, such as its needles – portrayed in different shades of green and highlighted with yellow – and its uneven bark. Cennini's method aimed to create a greater illusion of depth than that seen in older traditions of painting trees. In schematic representations of trees, the artist individually articulated the leaves and branches so that they stand out, starkly flat, against the page. The *Carrara Herbal* contains examples of both methods for depicting trees. Baumann (1974: 89) further suggests that the artist's use of Cennini's method may be evidence that he looked to illustrative sources outside of the herbal tradition for the *Carrara Herbal*'s illustrations, perhaps to the contemporaneous *Tacuinum Sanitatis* illustrative tradition. Baumann gives examples from a copy of the *Tacuinum Sanitatis* (now Vienna, Österreichische Nationalbibliothek, series nova, 2644) and the *Historia Plantarum* (now Rome, Biblioteca Casanatense, MS 459). I remain sceptical that the *Carrara Herbal*'s artist would have had access to these luxury codices associated with the Visconti court in Pavia.

16 For an introduction to the wide-ranging contents in Pliny's *Naturalis historia*, see the essays in Gibson and Morello (2011), and their relevant bibliographies. For an introduction to Pliny's views on nature, in particular, see Beagon (1992).

17 Pliny wrote: 'In addition to these [Latin authors], there are some Greek writers who have treated of this subject, and who have already been mentioned on the appropriate occasions. Among them, [the early Greek herbalists and rhizomists] Crateuas, Dionysios and Metrodoros, adopted a very attractive method of description, though one which has done little more than prove the remarkable difficulties which attended it. It was their plan to delineate the various plants in colours, and then to add in writing a description of the properties which they possessed. Pictures, however, are very apt to mislead, and more particularly where such a number of tints is required for the imitation of nature with any success; in addition to which, the diversity of copyists from the original paintings and their comparative degrees of skill, add very considerably to the chances of losing the necessary degree of resemblance to the originals. And then, besides, it is not sufficient to delineate a plant as it appears in one period only, as it presents a different appearance at each of the four seasons of the year [budding and foliation, blossoming, fructification, and fall of the leaf]' ('Praeter hos Graeci auctores prodidere, quos suis locis diximus, ex his Crateuas, Dionysius, Metrodorus ratione blandissima, sed qua nihil paene aliud quam difficultas rei intellegatur. Pinxere namque effigies herbarum atque ita subscripsere effectus. Verum et pictura fallax est coloribus tam numerosis, praesertim in aemulationem naturae, multumque degenerat transcribentium socordia. Praeterea parum est singulas earum aetates pingi, cum quadripertitis varietatibus anni faciem mutent') (Pliny, *Naturalis historia*, 25.4 [eds Jan and Mayhoff 1897: 4.118; tr. Bostock and Riley 1856: 5.80]). For a different translation and interpretation of this passage, see ed. and tr. Jones (1956: 7.140–1). On Crateuas the rhizomist, see Touwaide (2003).

18 The scholarly literature on Theophrastus is extensive and diverse, reflecting the philosopher's wide-ranging interests. For translations and introductions to his works, see Fortenbaugh (1992–1993). For an introduction to his views on botany and medicine, see Sharples (1995).

19 For original Greek and an English translation, see Theophrastus, *Historia plantarum* (ed. and tr. Hort 1916–1926).

20 Theophrastus, *Historia plantarum*, I.1 (ed. and tr. Hort 1916–1926: 1.2–3).

21 The scholarly literature on Dioscorides' life and work is vast. As a starting point, see Wellmann (1903); Riddle (1971, 1980 and 1986); Scarborough and Nutton (1982); Touwaide (1994 and 2007c); and Nutton (2013: especially 178–82).

22 Ed. Wellman (1906–1914), tr. Beck (2005).

23 Although Dioscorides provides data on substances from the three kingdoms of nature, about seventy percent of the substances in his pharmacopeia are plants. Dioscorides employed the following formula to organise his entries: 1) he records the most common name of the substance followed by any other names by which it might be known; 2) he gives a detailed description of the substance and any potential variations; 3) he identifies the parts of substances most medicinally useful; 4) he gives information on how to correctly prepare medicines from these parts; 5) he identifies the substance's therapeutic properties; 6) he provides other useful information, including notes on preparation, dosages and any other nonmedical or cosmetic uses for the substance (Touwaide 2014: 84–5).

24 Orofino (1991: 144–9).

25 In his preface, a dedicatory epistle to his benefactor and friend Areius, Dioscorides tells his readers that he aimed to provide accuracy, order and reliability to pharmacology and to reclaim it from what he considered the superstitious and spurious works of both earlier and contemporary physicians, several of whom he names. For biographies of the physicians Dioscorides criticises, see Scarborough and Nutton (1982: 202–6). In these prefatory remarks, Dioscorides also describes his treatise's organisational principle: 'For since I know, on the one hand, from personal observation in utmost detail most items, and, on the other hand, since I have a thorough understanding of the rest from accounts on which there has been unanimous agreement and previous examination in each case by natives, I shall try to use both a different arrangement [than my predecessors] and to list the materials according to the natural properties of each one of them' (*De materia medica*, Preface, §5 [tr. Beck 2005: 3]). Sadek (1983: 3–6) provides a slightly different translation of the dedicatory epistle, translating the preface that precedes Dioscorides' treatise in its Arabic version known as the *Leiden Dioscorides* (Leiden, University Library, cod. or. 289), dated 1083. In this version, Dioscorides describes his method as follows: 'I have taken the liberty of arranging these matters according to their kinds and species although it might disturb the alphabetical order of the names' (tr. Sadek 1983: 5). For the preface in its original Greek, see ed. Wellmann (1906–1914: 1.1–5).

26 The *materia medica* usually appear in five distinct volumes, which may represent therapeutic categories or, since the number of words in each volume are roughly equal, may refer to the original transmission of the text in five papyrus scrolls (Touwaide 2007a: 43). The five conventional volumes include: 1) aromatic oils, salves, trees and shrubs and their products; 2) animals, parts of animals, animal products, cereals, pot herbs and sharp herbs; 3) roots, juices, herbs and seeds; 4) roots and herbs not previously mentioned; and 5) wines and minerals (Riddle 1971: 120, and Scarborough and Nutton 1982: 191). Dioscorides also may have organised the substances according to their place on the *scala naturae* – the scale of natural properties (Touwaide 2007a: 43–4). The scale reflects attributions or connotations of positive and negative values associated with certain characteristics in the substances. For instance, the opening chapter in *De materia medica* begins with Iris, which is associated with light and warmth, while the final chapter closes with Soot, which is associated with darkness, humidity and cold (Touwaide 2007a: 43).

27 *De materia medica*, Preface, §5 (ed. Wellmann 1906–1914: 1.3; tr. Scarborough and Nutton 1982: 196).

28 Orofino (1991: 144–9) discusses Dioscorides' position on illustrations of plants in further detail, concluding that he would not have supported an illustrated version of his text.

29 *De materia medica*, Preface, §7–8 (ed. Wellmann 1906–1914: 1.4; tr. Scarborough and Nutton 1982: 196–7).

30 Compilations of medical materials drawn from the three kingdoms of nature – vegetal, animal and mineral – have a long history, dating back to ancient Egypt and Classical Greece. Their illustrated counterparts do, too (as Pliny pointed out). Dioscorides' *De materia medica*, however, dominated pharmacology across the Mediterranean (Touwaide 2006a: 117–18). On the connection to Alexandrian pharmacy, in particular, see Touwaide 2007a: 41–3.

31 For an overview of the transmission of *De materia medica*, see Riddle (1980). For a helpful overview of the historiography of the transmission of Dioscorides' text, see Touwaide (2014: 113n13, 114n16 and 115n24).

32 Pliny's comments confirm the existence of early examples of plant illustrations accompanying pharmacological texts, which suggests that this facet of the genre developed concurrently with its potentially more widely read textual counterpart (Brubaker 2002: 208).

33 On the ebb and flow of textual and illustrative entries in books of *materia medica*, see Touwaide (2013b: especially 103–28).

34 Touwaide (2014: 85).

35 On the primacy of schematic types of illustration, see Orofino (1991), and Touwaide (2008b: col. 935). On the primacy of realistic types of illustration, see Singer (1927); Pächt (1950); Blunt and Raphael (1979); Mariani Canova (1999); and Collins (2000).

36 On the many illustrative traditions that accompany the Greek, Arabic and Latin recensions of Dioscorides' *De materia medica* and other herbals, see Collins (2000). While I approach some of her conclusions and descriptions with reservations, Collins' book remains a beautiful and useful addition to the discussion on illustrated herbals.

37 On extant Greek manuscripts, see Touwaide (1988 and 2008b: 934).

38 Vienna, Österreichische Nationalbibliothek, *medicus graecus* 1 is considered the earliest extant illustrated version of the Greek Alphabetical Recension of *De materia medica*. This recension is a compilation of information extracted from the Greek original and put into alphabetical order (Touwaide 2006b: 35). It includes information drawn from Galenic theory and from the earlier pharmacopoeia of Crateuas, as well (Singer 1927: 5–7). In part because of its antiquity, the scholarship on this manuscript is extensive. For the foundational scholarship, see Premerstein (1903); Premerstein et al. (1906); Singer (1927); Buberl (1937); and the classic study by Gerstinger (1970) that includes commentary and facsimile. For more recent analyses, see Mazal (1981 and 1998, in which Mazal's commentary accompanies a small facsimile); and Collins (2000: 39–50).

39 Nathan (2010: 95).

40 In 1903, Premerstein deciphered the inscription (110). Kiilerich (2001: 171) transcribes an edited version of Premerstein's interpretation of the inscription in both the original Greek and English translation. It reads, 'Hail, oh princess, Honoratae extols and glorifies you with all fine praises; for Magnanimity (*Megalopsychia*) allows you to be mentioned over the entire world. You belong to the family of the Anicii, and you have built a temple of the Lord, raised high and beautiful'.

41 Kiilerich (2001: 171–2), and Brubaker (2002: 189). The reference to the church is found in Theophanes *Chronographia*, 512/13 CE (ed. de Boor 1883–1885: 1.157), which Brubaker further discusses (2002: 211).

42 Gamillscheg (2007).

43 Müller (2012: 109).
44 The *Vienna Dioscorides* contains the chapters on plants arranged in alphabetical order. The alphabetical reorganisation of Dioscorides' therapeutic substances may have begun as early as the late-second or early-third century, when they were assumed into the work of Galen, *De simplicium medicamentorum temperamentis et facultatibus* (*On the Mixtures and Properties of Simple Medicines*) (Touwaide 2014: 87). Galen divided Dioscorides' substances into categories according to the three kingdoms of nature and then alphabetised the individual chapters within each category. Alternatively, the reorganisation may date to the late-third or early-fourth century and may have been used by the Greek physician Oribasius (ca. 325–400) (Singer 1927: 24, and Touwaide 2006c: 190; on Oribasius' life and works, see Touwaide 2007b).
45 In addition to information derived from Dioscorides' *De materia medica*, the *Vienna Dioscorides* contains five other treatises on medicine: the *Carmen de viribus herbarum* (*Poem on the Virtues of Herbs*), a first- or second-century text that discusses plants with magical properties; Euteknios' (fl. between the third and fifth centuries) prose paraphrases of the *Theriaka* and *Alexipharmaka* (originally composed in verse by Nicander of Colophon [fl. second century BCE]); an anonymous paraphrase of Oppian's (fl. second century CE) *Halieutika* (*On Fishing*); and an anonymous paraphrase of *Ornithiaka*, a treatise on birds attributed to Dionysios Periegetes (fl. second century CE). The illustrations in these other texts play by different rules than those in the alphabetised Dioscorides – they often share space on the page with the text and, with the exception of the treatise on ornithology, are decidedly formulaic. See Brubaker (2002: 197–201), and Scarborough (2002: 180–2). On the bird illustrations, in particular, see Weitzmann (1959: 16), and Kádár (1978). Brubaker (2002: 206–7) also noted that within the version of Dioscorides' text contained in the codex, the 383 illustrations of plants fall into about a dozen categories of plant types, and many remain schematic and do not secure the plant's identification.
46 For a discussion of these exceptions, in which text and image are combined on one page, see Brubaker (2002: 191).
47 Scholars have long sought to connect such verisimilar imagery in the *Vienna Dioscorides* with a non-extant Hellenistic predecessor from which they assumed its tendency toward verisimilitude stemmed (Singer 1927: 6–7; Pächt 1950: 27; Pavord 2005: 85; and others). Conversely, Brubaker and Touwaide stress that there is little evidence to suggest an ancient precedent for the artist's sources. Brubaker (2002: 206) posits that the plant imagery may be original to the sixth century. Touwaide (2008b: 935) argues that the earliest imagery to accompany Dioscorides' text was likely schematically rendered. He suggests that the illustrations recorded in a ninth-century copy of *De materia medica* produced in Southern Italy or Syria – now Paris, Bibliothèque nationale de France, *graecus* 2179 – likely approximate the original imagery more closely. The reservations with which these scholars approach the verisimilar illustrations in the *Vienna Dioscorides* correspond in spirit with Pliny's criticism of illustrated herbals as 'unreliable' aids to plant identification. Given Pliny's concerns, it seems likely that at least some of the so-called Classical *exempla* would contain illustrations of questionable realism.
48 Scarborough (2002: 181).
49 With thanks to Alain Touwaide for the metaphor of the frontispieces as a type of 'wrapping paper' for the codex as a 'prefabricated' gift.
50 See Kiilerich (2001), and Gamillscheg (2007).
51 Kiilerich (2001: 183). Collins (2000: 42 and 98n76), following von Premerstein, notes that the peacock frontispiece may have been moved from its original position in the treatise on ornithology to the beginning of the codex during the manuscript's rebinding in 1406.
52 Brubaker (2002: 209) identifies these figures as Machaon (son of Aesculapius, god of healing), and the physicians Sextius Niger (fl. first century CE), Pamphilos (fl. first

century CE), Herakleides (fl. second century BCE), Xenocrates (fl. first century CE) and Manteos (fl. third century BCE). Brubaker's identifications follow Collins' (2000: 42).

53 Collins (2000: 42), and Brubaker (2002: 209).

54 On Mandrake's narcotic properties, see Scarborough (2002: 187). On identifications, in addition to Scarborough, see Collins (2000: 44), and Brubaker (2002: 207).

55 Collins (2000: 44), and Scarborough (2002: 186–7).

56 Kiilerich (2001: 172).

57 Kiilerich (2001: 178).

58 Kiilerich (2001: 172).

59 On the politics of Anicia Juliana's patronage, see Blair-Dixon (2004). For discussion of the inscription, see Mango and Ševčenko (1961); Brubaker (1997); Conner (1999); and Kiilerich (2001: 181–2).

60 On their relationship to Aristotle's *Ethica ad Nicomachum*, in particular, see Kiilerich (2001: 178–9).

61 Kiilerich (2001: 180–1) specifically points to the iconography of the kings praised in the Christian tradition – especially King Solomon.

62 These reasons range from the citizens' desire to flatter Juliana by portraying her as a compassionate and 'care-giving' leader to their desire to flatter her by portraying her imperial ambitions. Scarborough (2002: 182) suggests that the citizens of Honorata may have considered the knowledge contained in the book as necessary and valuable for the matron of a household of the highest status in the Byzantine Empire. Similarly, Brubaker (2002: 213) hazards that the choice of an elaborate herbal as a gift may reflect contemporary ideals of compassionate women who care for the sick. Kiilerich (2001: 189–90) and Nathan (2010: 95–102) point to the frontispiece imagery, in particular, as a flattering support for Juliana's imperial ambitions.

63 On the *Vienna Dioscorides* as a 'show book', see Nathan (2010: 96).

64 On the artist's perhaps deliberately opaque imperial references, see Nathan (2010: 101).

65 On the transmission and influence of Dioscorides in Arabic medicine, as a starting point, see Reeds (1991); Nutton (1995a and 2008); Touwaide (1995, 2005c, 2005d, 2009b and 2011); Jacquart (1996 and 2010); Jacquart and Paravicini Bagliani (2007); and Siraisi (2007), along with their bibliographies.

66 On Iṣṭifan b. Basīl, see Arnaldez (1978).

67 Ḥunayn b. Isḥāk al-ʿIbādī is also responsible for a translation of the Syriac Dioscorides into Arabic. For an overview of historiography on the transmission of *De materia medica* as well as a summary of the history of its transmission from the fifth-century transliterations into Latin, through the sixth-century translations from Greek into Syriac (made by the Jacobite monk Sergius of Res'aina), to the ninth-century translations into Arabic, revisions of the Latin transliteration, and up through the translation back into Greek, see Touwaide (2009b and 2011: 195–6). On Ḥunayn b. Isḥāk al-ʿIbādī ('Ḥunayn ibn Isḥāq'), see Iskandar (1997).

68 Touwaide (2006a: 117).

69 Touwaide (2006a: 117) notes especially the North African and Spanish commentators, Ibn al-Gazzâr (d. 980), al-Zahrāwī (936–1013), al-Ghāfiḳī (d. ca. 1165) and Ibn al-Bayṭār (1197–1248).

70 Sadek (1983: 13).

71 On the Arabic in the translations, see Sadek (1983). In addition, Sadek charts the range of illustrations in the earliest dated Arabic Dioscorides, the so-called *Leiden Dioscorides* (now Leiden, University Library, cod. or. 289), dated 1083 CE. Sadek notes that the plant images range in type from stylised representations, which he compares with tooled wrought-iron work (128), candelabra (130), and geometric motifs (134), to plants depicted with the suggestion of their local habitats or environments (132).

72 The manuscript is available in partial facsimile with commentary. See Touwaide (1992–1993).
73 Sadek (1983: 9). Touwaide (2011: 216) further suggests that, as the result of a diplomatic effort between Cordova and Constantinople, a letter containing a medical treatise in Arabic brought to Constantinople in the tenth century may have responded to the codex, or the codex may have responded to the letter. Regardless, an exchange of medical knowledge resulted in both the Greek to Arabic transmission in Cordova and the Arabic to Greek transmission in Constantinople. This exchange is further evidence that the transmission of medical knowledge was not one-way. Touwaide (2011: 216–20) argues that Byzantine appropriation of Arabic knowledge occurred in three phases. First, in the tenth century, Arabic knowledge was brought to Constantinople as part of the diplomatic exchange outlined earlier. Then, in the eleventh century, Arabic texts translated into Latin in Salerno and Sicily subsequently were translated into Greek and introduced into Byzantium. Lastly, the Greek appropriation of Arabic medical knowledge resulted from collaborations, likely in Constantinople after the fall of Baghdad in 1258, between native Greek and Arabic speakers who together produced lexica of plant names in different languages.
74 Sadek (1983: 203), and Ruggles (2000: 20).
75 Ruggles (2000: 20).
76 Sadek (1983: 12), and Touwaide (2005a: 97). Nicholas likely glossed the plant names from Greek into Latin, and Hasdāy ibn Shaprūt (915–970), al-Raḥmān III's Jewish physician, then translated the names from Latin into Arabic (Ruggles 2000: 20).
77 Ruggles (2000: 20).
78 Touwaide (2009a: 161–2).
79 Ettinghausen (1962: 87–90), and Touwaide (2009a: 159).
80 Over the course of the manuscript's long life, several of its full-page illustrations were cut out. Late in the nineteenth century, however, Friedrich R. Martin (1868–1933) sold many more pages on the antiquarian market in Istanbul. Touwaide (2009a: 159–60) reconstructs the manuscript 'virtually' and discusses the significance of its original, highly ornamented state.
81 Touwaide (2009a: 159).
82 Touwaide (2009a: 160).
83 This manuscript is now Paris, Bibliothèque nationale de France, *graecus* 2179.
84 Touwaide (2009a: 160). On Paris, *graecus* 2179, see Touwaide (1994).
85 Touwaide (2009a: 161) posits that al-Fadl may have had access to these other illustrated books, or model-books for these other genres, as a member of a workshop that produced luxury copies of several different genres of literature.
86 The *Kalīla* was translated into English as *The Fables of Bidpai* in the sixteenth century. For a brief introduction to the text and to its English translation, see Keith-Falconer (1885).
87 Touwaide (2009a: 161).
88 On the illustrated *Kalīla*, especially in Persia, see O'Kane (2003). On its translation and transmission, see Brockelmann (1927).
89 Touwaide (2009a: 161).
90 O'Kane (2003: 23).
91 Brockelman (1927: 4.695–6), and O'Kane (2003: 23).
92 O'Kane (2003: 23).
93 O'Kane (2003: 23).
94 Cited by O'Kane (2003: 23–4) from Rice's translation of Shaykhu's 1905 edition of the Arabic text, itself drawn from a manuscript dated 1338 (Rice 1959: 209). The preface is present in the earliest extant illustrated Arabic copy of the *Kalīla*, now Paris, Bibliothèque nationale de France, arabe 3465 (ca. 1225).
95 Touwaide (2009a: 161).
96 Grabar (2006: 189).

97 See Grabar's introduction to the facsimile edition of the *Maḵāmāt al-Ḥarīrī*, now Paris, Bibliothèque nationale de France, arabe 5847 (2003). Elsewhere, Grabar (2006: 189) memorably describes this linguistic play as 'verbal pyrotechnics'.

98 Although I do not entirely agree with Grabar's interpretation of 'visual systems' in the 13 illustrated versions of the *Maḵāmāt al-Ḥarīrī*, his comparison across iconographical groups is a useful way to organise the variety of illustrations in these manuscripts. Grabar (2006) compares the 'literal' illustrations in the *Maḵāmāt al-Ḥarīrī* (Paris, Bibliothèque nationale de France, arabe 3929) with the 'descriptive' (Leningrad, Academy of Sciences, MS 523) and 'interpretative' ones (Paris, Bibliothèque nationale de France, arabe 5847). To access the depth of the imagery, Grabar argues, readers needed knowledge of contemporary social values, knowledge that contributed to multiple levels of interpretation not only of the images, but of their relationship to the text as well. Further, Grabar (2006: 204) proposed that the illustrations, in part, served to prompt delight: 'we may consider them as metaphors, as parts of a system of visual signs parallel to the text, with its own set of rules, but which did not seek to illustrate so much as to provide pleasure, joy, or excitement as one read the book'. Although Grabar does not seek to analyse the significance of visual pleasure within the experience of reading the book, his point about the pleasure of the illustrations is an important one.

99 This manuscript is now Paris, Bibliothèque nationale de France, arabe 5847.

100 Grabar (2006: 200).

101 In his commentary on the manuscript now Paris, Bibliothèque nationale de France, arabe 5847, Grabar (2006: 189) notes that many of the extant copies of the *Maḵāmāt* were produced in centres in Egypt, Iraq and Syria known for their educated elite. He identifies the intended audience as 'highly literate Arabic-speaking bourgeoisie'.

102 Touwaide (2009a: 161).

103 Touwaide (2009a: 162) further notes the influence of late-Antique and Middle Eastern mosaics on al-Fadl, as well as scenes of philosophers speaking to each other found in illustrated Arabic copies of their works.

104 Touwaide (2009a: 161–2). Touwaide notes that Ayasofia 3703 was not unique in its illustrative strategy. He points to similar uses of illustration in Arabic copies of Galen's treatise on theriac, which also contains scenes of people interacting and portraits of physicians. See also, Balty-Guesdon (1996), and Kerner (2004).

105 Touwaide (2007c: 671).

106 The Latin illustrated books of *materia medica* contain several different texts and combinations of texts. Although a complete illustrated Latin translation of all five books of Dioscorides' *De materia medica* existed by the close of the tenth century, this treatise was not the work on *materia medica* most widely disseminated in the Latin West. That position was reserved for the *Herbarium Apuleii Platonici* and the later *Tractatus de herbis*, examples of which I discuss later. The singular illustrated translation of Dioscorides into Latin (the so-called *Old Latin Dioscorides*) – now Munich, Bayerische Staatsbibliothek, Clm 337 – dates to the late tenth century. Two text fragments of this recension remain extant as well. Both are held in Paris and are unillustrated: Paris, Bibliothèque nationale de France, lat. 9332 (eighth or early ninth century) and lat. 12995 (later ninth century). See Riddle (1980), and Collins (2000: 148–9).

107 In a translation no longer extant, Dioscorides' *De materia medica* first passed from Greek into Latin, possibly in the fifth or early sixth century. Yet this translation did not account for the text's greatest transmission into Latin culture, which happened much later. On the history of the Latin transmission of *De materia medica* and its relationship to the occupation of Constantinople (1204–1261), in particular, see Touwaide (2006b). Elsewhere, Touwaide (2011: 196–9) charts a history of translation efforts: among others, Constantine 'the African' (d. ca. 1078) at Salerno and Gerard of

Cremona (d. 1187) and Michel Scot (fl. twelfth–thirteenth century) at Toledo contributed to the translation of the Arabic Dioscorides into Latin. These efforts continued at Montpellier in late thirteenth and early fourteenth centuries in the work of Arnaud of Villanova (ca. 1240–1311). For relevant bibliography on each translator, see Touwaide (2011: 196n3 and 197n4). On Constantine 'the African', in particular, see Jacquart (1996). The translation of the Greek medical treatises directly into Latin occurred almost simultaneously at Salerno with the work of Alfanus (ca. 1015/20–1085) and was continued by Burgundio (ca. 1110–1193), a Pisan judge who translated several of Galen's treatises, and Pietro d'Abano (1257–ca. 1315), who continued Burgundio's work and commented on Dioscorides *De materia medica* as well (he also may have translated it) (Touwaide 2011: 198–9). Efforts at translation of the Galenic corpus, especially, continued at the Angevin court of Naples in the fourteenth century by Niccolò da Reggio (ca. 1280–ca. 1350) (Touwaide 2011: 198–9). Of course, as Jacquart (2010) and Touwaide (2011: 200) rightly note, the history of transmission of Greek medical knowledge into the Latin West is a complicated one. The trajectory of translation and transmission outlined here does not account for all manuscripts or orally transmitted knowledge and cannot provide a complete account of the influence of Greek medicine in the Latin world.

108 See Sigerist and Howald (1927).

109 Riddle (1981: 46–7).

110 On the rationale for adopting the name Apuleius, see Voigts (1978), and Maggiulli and Buffa Giolito (1996).

111 For example, the incipit for the *Herbarium* now Lucca, Biblioteca Statale, MS 196, reads: 'alium apulei platonici quem accepit a Chirone centauro et ab Aescolaphio'. On this incipit, see Collins (2000: 227n102).

112 For the texts included, see Sigerist and Howald (1927). For analysis of these texts, see Singer (1927: 47); Maggiulli and Buffa Giolito (1996: 68); and Collins (2000: 166).

113 These manuscripts are now Florence, Biblioteca Laurenziana, plut. 73.16, and Vienna Österreichische Nationalbibliothek, lat. 93.

114 Because there are no extant inventories of Frederick's collection, we cannot be certain that these codices were produced by Frederick's *scriptorium*. However, Orofino (1990) argues persuasively for the connection of both manuscripts to Frederick's court, as either a commission made by Frederick or his son Manfred (1232–1266), on account of the relationship between the manuscripts' iconography and content and Frederick's personal interests.

115 For analysis of the process of amalgamation, see Orofino (1990), and Collins (2000: 211–18).

116 Collins (2000: 219). The Hohenstaufen court valued the pursuit of knowledge and cultivated the perception of its progressiveness. Frederick is remembered for his many commissions of scientific texts on astronomy and medicine and for his own treatise on falconry, *De arte venandi cum avibus* (*The Art of Hunting with Birds*), in which he synthesised contemporary technical expertise with Classical hunting traditions and information from Arabic sources on hunting with birds. In addition, he is remembered for his emphatic support of the medical community at Salerno. This community was central to the diffusion of Greek and Arabic medical knowledge into the West. It flourished under Frederick's rule partly because he declared that physicians could practice in his kingdom only if they had studied at Salerno. On the role of Arabic medicine in the curriculum of the so-called Salerno school (the *Articella* textbook, especially), see McVaugh (1971), and Jacquart and Paravicini Bagliani (2007). For discussion of Frederick's interests and their relationship to his books, see Orofino (1990).

117 Frederick's *Herbarium* manuscripts combine the layout of text and image from the ninth-century southern Italian *Herbarium* tradition with the colouration of its ninth-century northern European counterparts. They also join the lavish character of the

Carolingian illustrative tradition – which depended on its ninth-century predecessors – with the careful revision of source texts characteristic of the twelfth-century manuscripts produced in southern Italy (Collins 2000: 209).

118 The following description of Frederick's *Herbarium* manuscripts and the iconographical blending in their illustrations follows Collins (2000: 183, 188 and 218).

119 Orofino (1990: 345).

120 Collins (2000: 219).

121 *Tractatus de herbis* is the title of a specific treatise within a larger compilation of diverse medical texts. The term was first applied to compilations of Latin translations of Arabic and Greek treatises on botanical medicine in an eighteenth-century catalogue for the Biblioteca Estense in Modena (Baumann 1974: 100n12). It remains, however, a convenient title to indicate the conventional group of texts within these thirteenth- and fourteenth-century codices, as well as to distinguish the text of the *Tractatus* itself from that of its predecessor, the *Circa instans*. Touwaide (2013b: 20) further defines the work as an ambitious attempt to synthesise all knowledge of *materia medica* from 'remembered classical' sources (the Greek originals) and contributions made by the Arabic physicians, plus a lexicon of plant names in other languages and any folkloric legends associated with those plants.

122 On the identity of the treatise's author/compiler, see Ventura (2009: 91).

123 Touwaide (2013b: 38–9).

124 Touwaide (2013b: 38–9) identifies this pattern: 1) therapeutic properties; 2) name of plant and its synonyms; 3) description of plant; 4) therapeutic uses of plant.

125 Dating to between 1280–1317, the Egerton *Tractatus* is the first extant, illustrated copy of a new version of the *Circa instans*, an earlier unillustrated treatise about simple medicines compiled by Platearius (see ed. Malandin 1986). The absence in Egerton 747 of the *Opus pandectarum medicinae* (*Encyclopedia of Medicines*), by physician Matthaeus Silvaticus (ca. 1280–ca. 1342), provides a potential *terminus ante quem*: Matthaeus' work was dedicated to Robert of Anjou in 1317 and, afterwards, was used extensively by the teaching community at Salerno. It would have been an obvious choice to include in a reference or teaching compilation of works like the *Tractatus* (Collins 2000: 286n39). For a summary of the scholarship on Egerton 747, see the introduction to the recent facsimile edition (Collins and Raphael 2003). As a starting point for more detailed study of Egerton 747, see Givens (2006); Ventura (2009); and Touwaide (2013b: 51–3), together with their bibliographies.

126 The three texts participate in the Latin illustrative and textual traditions of botanical and medical knowledge maintained in Europe prior to the wider reintroduction of Dioscorides' medicine in the fourteenth century. They contain both superstitious and mythical entries on plants, as well as fragmented information culled from Antique sources. Specifically, Egerton 747 contains the following works: the *Tractatus de herbis* (ff. 1–106v); plant illustrations without text (ff. 106v–9v); a lunar calendar and details on astrological forecasting (ff. 109v–11r); *Antidotarium Nicolai* (ff. 112v–24r); a work on dosages of medicines (ff. 124r–5r); a list of substitutions (ff. 125v–7v); three fragments describing weights and measurements used in the formulation of prescriptions (ff. 127v–8v); a list of synonyms for *materia medica* in other languages (ff. 128v–46r); and a supplement to the *Antidotarium* (ff. 146v–7v) (Touwaide 2013: 51–2).

127 Collins (2000: 244), and Collins and Raphael (2003: 6). The other texts appended to the illustrated *Tractatus* all originated in Salerno, which strongly suggests the codex's origin there. For a discussion of these additional texts and the glosses added to the text of the *Tractatus*, see Givens (2006).

128 The attribution to the Salerno community rests of several key identifiers: the manuscript's pattern of foliation follows that used at Salerno; two figured initials portray scholars (f. 1r and f. 122r) at the beginning of texts relevant to the curriculum at the medical school (*Circa instans* and *Antidotarium Nicolai*); and several of the texts

included in the manuscript were required reading in Salerno by around 1280 (Givens 2006: 116).

129   Pächt (1950: 30). Pächt further identified the book's illustrations as a fusion of first-hand observation of nature with lost Antique illustrative models. He proposed that the codex was the botanical equivalent of the animal model book, *Il taccuino di disegni* (*The Notebook of Drawings*), attributed to the workshop of Giovannino de' Grassi (now Bergamo, Biblioteca Civica 'A. Mai', Cassaforte 1.21). Pächt (1950: 31) argued that the model book and Egerton 747 were central to the dissemination of a renewed naturalistic style to other artists and workshops. His thesis was widely accepted, and his views significantly influenced the scholarship on this manuscript produced in the second half of the twentieth century.

130   Paris, Bibliothèque nationale de France, lat. 6823. Earlier scholarship on this manuscript debates its origin – as northern Italian (Milanese), Tuscan (Pisan or Bolognese), Salernitan or Neapolitan – and its potential relationship to Egerton 747. See Pächt (1950); Belloni et al. (1958); Degenhart and Schmitt (1968–1980); Baumann (1974); Opsomer-Halleux (1978); Avril (1984 and 1986); and Toresella (1990). Generally, on account of the attribution of the frontispieces' illustrations to Lippo Vanni (fl. mid-fourteenth century) or Roberto d'Oderisio (ca. 1320–1382), both working in Naples, a Neapolitan origin is now accepted (see p. 65n141 in this volume). For an introduction to the manuscript and its historiography, see Collins (2000: 268–73), and, most recently, Touwaide (2013b: 46–8).

131   Manfred describes himself as both author and illustrator in the incipit, which reads in part: 'Cum ego, Manfredus de Monte Imperiali, in artis speciarie semper optans scrire virtutes et cognoscere rerum proprietates, de simplicibus medicinis, ut recte cognate fuissent ab aliis et maxime a conficientibus medicinam, manu mea volui scribere librum et congregare omnes herbas et alia medicinalis secundum quod scripta inveni in multis libris autoribus; de quibus herbis quas cognovi et quorum nomina subtus subjecit, in libro hoc scripsi et per figuram demonstravi . . .' (f. 3r). For another analysis of the incipit, see Collins (2000: 291n102).

132   On the dating of Simon's *Clavis*, see Paravicini Bagliani (1991: 191–7 and 247–51), and, in relationship to Manfred's herbal, see Touwaide (2013b: 48).

133   Scholars have extensively debated the potential relationships between Manfred's herbal and illustrated versions of the *Tractatus de herbis* produced in northern Italy. See, for instance, Pächt (1950); Baumann (1974); Avril (1986); and Collins (2000). Most recently, Touwaide (2013b) has challenged aspects of these older interpretations and charted different and more nuanced familial relationships, especially between the *Tractatus* manuscripts now known as New York, Pierpont Morgan Library, M 873 (last quarter of fourteenth century); Paris, Bibliothèque de l'Ecole des Beaux-Arts, Masson 116 (ca. 1370–1380); London, British Library, Sloane 4016 (ca. 1440); and Rome, Biblioteca Apostolica Vaticana, Chigi F. VIII 158 (late fifteenth- or early sixteenth century). Scholars also have noted potential connections between Manfred's herbal and the illustrated herbal known as the *Historia Plantarum*, now Rome, Biblioteca Casanatense, MS 459 (ca. 1394–1395) (Pächt 1950: 34; Baumann 1974: 104–5 and 161–71; and Collins 2000: 273–8; on the *Historia Plantarum*, in particular, see Segre Rutz et al. 2002). Through comparative analysis with styles of costumes and figuration in other contemporary manuscripts, Baumann (1974: 105 and 161–71) and Avril (1986: 282) have suggested a northern Italian (Veneto) provenance for New York, Pierpont Morgan, M 873 and Paris, Beaux-Arts, Masson 116. On account of the stylistic affinity between Masson 116 and the works of Altichiero and Jacopo Avanzo – artists working in Padua in the late 1370s – Masson 116 is widely believed to have been produced in Padua (Avril 1986: 282n41; Collins 2000: 275; and Touwaide 2013b: 43).

134   Pellegrin (1955: 278–9).

135   In addition, one manuscript that borrowed Manfred's imagery, the *Historia Plantarum* (Rome, Biblioteca Casanatense, MS 459), is connected decisively to the Visconti court

and dates to after Giangaleazzo's conquest of the Carrara. This pattern of influence suggests that the manuscript was in the Padovano or Veneto during the last quarter of the fourteenth century and transferred to Lombardy by the end of the century, which further suggests the possibility that Manfred's herbal belonged to the Carrara. On the *Historia Plantarum*, see Segre Rutz et al. (2002).

136 Baumann (1974: 104–5 and figures on 131–54). On costuming and architecture in *Guiron le Courtois*, see Arslan (1963). Scholars debate the origins of the workshops that produced these manuscripts, and proposed sites of creation range from Milan to Padua, Venice, and Verona (see Avril 1984: 94–8, and Sutton 1991). On similar stylistic grounds, Masson 116 has also been compared to the illustrated *Tacuinum sanitatis* manuscripts (Cogliati Arano 1976, and Opsomer-Halleux 1991).

137 Avril (1986: 286n41) compared the verisimilar treatment of architecture, people, plants and animals, and the treatment of costume and colouration in Masson 116 to the work produced by Altichiero and Avanzo in Padua, particularly to the frescoes in the Chapel of San Felice (formerly San Giacomo) at the Basilica of Sant'Antonio. Collins' analysis and dating of the manuscript follows Avril's (2000: 275).

138 Francesco Novello's commission of the *Carrara Herbal* itself suggests that Francesco il Vecchio's library possessed this type of book. Francesco Novello intended to restore and exceed the greatness of his father's library. If he could not reclaim his father's books physically, he could reclaim them through imitation. Following this logic, the *Carrara Herbal* is the heir to a specific manuscript that once belonged to the elder Francesco and that was among the spoils taken from the Carrara library by Giangaleazzo Visconti in 1388.

139 See Siraisi (1973 and 2001a); and Grendler (2002).

140 The *Carrara Herbal* is not a direct copy of Manfred's book. The herbals share similar textual content as illustrated books of *materia medica*, and both books include formally similar examples of realistic and conventional imagery. For instance, the depictions of cucumber (*Cucumis sativus* L.) and watermelon (*Citrullus lanatus* [Thunb.] Matsum. & Nakai) in the *Carrara Herbal* (*del citron piçolo che fi chiamà citrollo*, f. 162v, and *de la anguria*, f. 163r) are remarkably similar to their corresponding representations in Manfred's herbal (*de cucurbita* and *de citrulis*, f. 42v). In both renditions, the illustrators show the characteristics of the plants' leaves, flowers and pattern of growth. Also, like the *Carrara Herbal*'s illustrator, Manfred (or his illustrator) incorporated into his work the schematic representational conventions found in the earlier herbals. For instance, he depicted *mandragore* (*Mandragora officinarum* L., mandrake, f. 89v) anthropomorphically. Mandrake has long been associated with the human body due to the tendency of its long, parsnip-like root to bifurcate or branch out into a shape that resembles legs, torso, and arms. Furthermore, Manfred juxtaposed verisimilar and schematic plant imagery. For instance, he portrayed *cottilidon sive cinbalaria vel unbillicus veneris* (*Cotyledon umbilicus* L., pennywort, left, f. 47r) schematically, while he portrayed its neighbour, *cepe* (*Allium cepa* L., onion, right, f. 47r), more realistically.

141 The series precedes the incipit page that identifies Manfred as both illustrator and author of the manuscript. The portraits, however, were not executed by Manfred himself. He likely commissioned them from either the Sienese artist Lippo Vanni, who was working in Naples ca. 1340–1344, or the Neapolitan artist Roberto d'Oderisio, also working in Naples during the 1340s and 1350s, whose frescoes at the Church of Santa Maria Incoronata show similar attention to costuming and individual facial features. On d'Oderisio's authorship, see Degenhart and Schmitt (1980: 351). On Vanni's authorship, see Avril (1984: 69).

142 The twelfth-century 'ordinary interpretation' of the Vulgate verses, attributed to Anselm of Laon (d. 1117) and his school, reads as follows: '[I. Thess. 5.19–21] *Extinguish not the spirit* because it is the will of God to do all these things, you older people who – through the Holy Spirit – have the gift of intelligence, do not conceal

it, because if you do that you too may lose it. Do not spurn their prophecies [of older, intelligent people] and substitute yourselves, but [on the other hand] do not accept all things [i.e., all prophecies] indiscriminately, but test [*probate*] them, i.e., break them down with reason, and hold on to whatever is found to be good' (*'Spiritum nolite. Quia voluntas Dei est facere haec Omnia, vos majors qui habetis per Spiritum sanctum, donum intelligentiae, nolite illud abscondere, quo merito et vos perderetis. Vos subditi prophetias illorum nolite spernere, tamen non Omnia indiscrete accipiatis, sed probate, id est ratione discutite et quod bonum invenitur tenete'*) (*Biblia Latina cum glossa ordinaria*, I. Thess. 5.19–21 [eds Migne and Hamman 1852: col. 620, unpublished tr. Margaret Musgrove; personal correspondence]). Until the mid-twentieth century, the *Glossa Ordinaria* was attributed to Walafrid Strabo (ca. 808–849). On the attribution of the *Glossa*, see Smalley (1941), and Matter (1997).

143 For identification of the physicians, see Collins (2000: 292n113), and Touwaide (2013b: 46–7). Johannitius, a Christian physician working in Baghdad, is credited with the first translation of Dioscorides from Greek into Syriac and Arabic (see Sadek 1983, and p. 36 in this volume). Touwaide (2013b: 46) suggests that the physician opposite Johannitius may be Constantine 'the African', another scholar-physician who translated Arabic treatises into Latin.

144 Galen returns the maxim 'Intendo enim manducare ut vivam, alii intendunt vivere ut manducent' ('Truly, I intend to eat so as to live; others live but to eat'). The maxim shows Galen as a student of Hippocratic medicine in which diet is integral to the preservation of health.

145 Bartolomeo speaks the incipit from his commentary, *Practica*. On the identification of the other physician as Mesue, see Touwaide (2013b: 46).

146 Collins (2000: 292n113).

147 'El prima tractà xè de le medexine temperè' – 'The first book on temperate medicine' (Serapion, ed. Ineichen 1962–1966: 1.3).

2 The healthy pleasures of reading the *Carrara Herbal*

In Chapter 1, we considered the history of production and collection of illustrated books of *materia medica* from across the Mediterranean world. These books appealed to readers from a variety of social, professional and political standings and for reasons just as various. Physicians and druggists acquired these books.[1] For this community, the books may have served as memory aids or indices, or as reference tools or instruments to facilitate cross-cultural communication.[2] However, for these readers and for others more distant from the medical professions, illustrated books of *materia medica* also could serve as vectors for the construction of self-images, which ranged from discerning readers and connoisseurs of valuable knowledge to political impresarios or even knowledge brokers.

The desire to possess a beautiful manuscript that provides a distinctive reading experience was certainly also part of the allure of illustrated books of *materia medica*, and perhaps especially so for Francesco Novello and for other patrons untrained in the medical arts or in pharmacology. Yet ideals of pleasure and beauty always circulate within specific social, aesthetic and historical contexts in which pleasure and utility are seldom mutually exclusive. The pleasure of reading illustrated books of *materia medica* came with attendant usefulness: it enhanced one's knowledge – and, depending on the books' readers, brought new ways of categorising, applying or displaying this knowledge. It enhanced one's status or image among other learned readers or collectors through possession of the knowledge itself and through the manner in which that knowledge was presented.

The *Carrara Herbal* participates in this history: the pleasure of reading the book draws together complementary categories of utility, enriching readers' status, knowledge and health. In this way, the function of the *Carrara Herbal* and other illustrated books of *materia medica* diverges from that of their unillustrated counterparts, in which pleasure's role – while likely still present for the avid reader – is less pronounced. On its surface, as a book full of elaborate scribal adornments and abundant illustrations, the *Herbal* cultivated a reading experience that can be associated with so-called courtly codices – smaller, illustrated books popular among the elite classes at the courts of northern Italy.[3] Through its association with such a pleasant – and often quite exclusive – reading experience, the *Herbal* provided a visible link not only to Francesco's status and his family's traditions of book collection but also to contemporaneous notions about the importance of pleasurable reading to the health of patricians and leaders. On a deeper level, the textual and visual content of the *Herbal* also connected it to intellectual currents outside of the court. In conjunction with the other books on medical theory and practice in his library, the *Herbal* served as an emblem of Francesco's specific scholarly interests, which, in turn, alluded to his support for the University of Padua's medical schools. In both contexts – by creating a privileged reading experience characterised by plea-sure and by emphasising his pursuit of the new medical knowledge at the schools in Padua – the *Herbal* consolidated Francesco's identity as a 'healthy' Carrara prince: it connected him to contemporaneous humanistic and medical discourses about pleasure, nature and social class in circulation at the university and at court.

The experience of reading the *Carrara Herbal*

To read the *Carrara Herbal* is both an aesthetic and academic act. It requires time, concentration, careful handling and a space structured to accommodate the book itself. The manuscript is bulky and awkward – approximately 35 × 24 × 8 cm – and was even larger before it was cropped (likely in the eighteenth century).[4] It was not a *vade mecum* carried on the reader's person. The size, preparation, careful structure, use of expensive materials and extensive illustrations suggest that, if completed, the book would have been a commanding addition to Francesco's library. It would not only be a book to read as a kind of structured performance but also, when circulated among other readers, it would be an object that displayed or signified Francesco's taste, cultural heritage and knowledge. Though the *Carrara Herbal* was not a practi-cal tool for Francesco Novello, neither was it simply a 'picture book' for bibliophiles (as Minta Collins alleged of late medieval illustrated herbals in general).[5] Rather, through its text, illustrations and material qualities, the *Carrara Herbal* constructs a reading experience that draws attention to itself as a valuable object – valuable for the knowledge it contains and for how it conveys that knowledge visually and materially.

Textually, the manner in which the scribe, rubricators and penwork artists adorned Serapion's work emphasised the pattern in which Serapion presented his material. Like Dioscorides in *De materia medica*, Serapion presented his material according to a formula, making his text accessible to specialists and nonspecialists alike.[6] The reader quickly becomes familiar with this formula, finding a pattern in Serapion's presenta-tion of content. Serapion begins with the plant's name and any synonyms, describes the plant's characteristic visual features, tastes and smells (often by way of comparison to other plants), and provides its primary, secondary and often tertiary *qualities* and their *power*. Then, he lists the plant's curative *properties* (often citing his sources), gives examples of these effects and offers instructions on how to best prepare medicines. Finally, he notes the different results of these medicines when given to various patients, depending on their sex, age and temperament or dominant humour.[7]

The illustrative and scribal techniques used in the creation of the *Herbal* respond to this textual rhythm, creating a syncopation in colour and line that invites the reader to engage with the very words as well as with their meanings.[8] Writing pri-marily in dark-brown ink, the scribe, Jacobus Philippus,[9] reproduced Serapion's work in easily legible and beautifully formed regular gothic miniscule script. He arranged the text on the full page with wide margins to better display the text block against the pale vellum, emphasising the fine quality of the parchment and making it easy to read. Likewise, the book's rubricators added alternating blue and red pilcrow signs (¶) to distinguish certain phrases, especially phrases that name Serapion's sources. Further, they used red ink to delineate the chapter number, the initial mention of the plant's name and its primary *vertù* (virtue) and, sometimes, highlighted larger capital letters buried deep in the text block with pale yellow.[10]

So, for example, when reading the entry for *melissa* (*Melissa officinalis* L., lemon balm, f. 18r) in the *Carrara Herbal*, readers encounter Serapion's formula for presenting information and these methods used by the scribe and rubricators to further structure the experience of the text. I have preserved these marks in the entry, which reads:[11]

¶ Melissa. ¶ Chapter XXIII

Melissa is called citraria according to others. ¶ Dioscorides says that melissa is an herb over which the bees delight. ¶ The stem of melissa and its leaves resemble the stem and the leaves of marubio savègo [*Marrubium vulgare* L., common horehound]. And its branches and its stems are quadrangular, so that it has four cantons [quarters/corners]. And the leaves themselves are greater [i.e.: larger], which is not like the leaves of the marubio savègo, nor are they [the leaves] completely hairy like the leaves of the marubio. ¶ Melissa has a characteristic scent of lemons, and for this [reason] it is called citraria. The ***primary virtue*** of this herb is hot and dry in the first degree. ¶ Galen says that the virtue of this [plant] is like the virtue of marubio. But it is of more minor virtue. ¶ Dioscorides says that when one drinks the leaves [steeped] in wine, or when they are made into a poultice, the sting of the scorpion and the bite of a spider called rotella are lessened. And so when the decoction of this herb is poured over the painful bite, it does the same thing. And when women consume [it] in this decoction it will provoke menstruation. And apply a wash to the mouth, and it lessens pain in the teeth. And when the leaves are mixed with nitro [sodium carbonate], it lessens the ulceration of the intestines. And made into an electuary [lozenge], [it helps] those who can neither pull the air into themselves nor send it away [i.e.: who have difficulty breathing]. ¶ And when it is made into a poultice with salt, it resolves scrofula and ulceration. And when a poultice is made of this herb, it lessens the pain of contusion. ¶ Another author says that it has the property to alleviate anaemia and comfort a weak heart. And when it is made into a decoction it soothes the cold and humid stomach and helps it digest fatty food. And [it] helps the obstruction of the brain. And [it] lessens fear and the maladies caused by the melancholic humour and burning phlegm.

In addition to the rubricators' work, a penwork artist or artists adorned many of the opening initials of chapters with flourishing lines and floral motifs. In several instances, although not in the case of *melissa*, these initials begin the name of one of Serapion's sources. Serapion was careful to cite his sources throughout

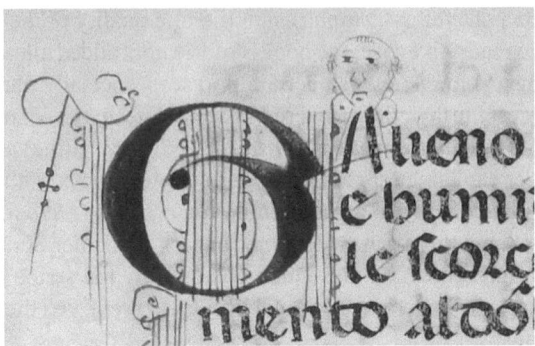

Figure 2.1 Detail of penwork face from entry on *çucha* (*Cucurbita lagenaria* L., bottle gourd)

Carrara Herbal
London, British Library, Egerton 2020, f. 165r
Gouache on vellum, Padua, ca. 1390–1400

his work, noting 'Dioscorides says', 'Galen says', and, more rarely, 'Rhazes says'.[12] These citations bolster Serapion's authority and show him as a member of the lineage of ancient medical writers spanning the Greek and Arabic traditions. The most delightful element of the penwork is the adornment of many of these names: the artist accompanied the name with a tiny face, usually peeking out from the second letter of the source's name, as though Dioscorides, Galen or Rhazes personally appeared to share his ideas with the reader (Figure 2.1). These small faces not only charm the readers, but, like the highlighted information and the colourful pilcrow signs, they also give the readers a convenient place to stop or start reading, look at an accompanying image or seek out a specific piece of textual information, and then pick up where they left off. These visual cues mark out especially relevant information within the text block while simultaneously providing a memorable stopping or starting point for experiencing the book in other ways.[13]

The manuscript's illustrations further attest to the book's quality and value, but it is the artist's varied use of style and composition in the illustrations – not the simple fact of the illustrations' existence – that most distinguishes the experience of reading the book: it deliberately cues readers to their simultaneous role as viewers. As I discussed in Chapter 1, throughout the *Herbal*, the artist used combinations of techniques in his representations of the plants that refer to the many illustrative types used across the history of the genre.[14] In conjunction with this technical elasticity, however, the artist also used compositional variants in which he extended the plant images off the page, grew them up out of the text, encircled a text block or made them appear pressed into the pages of the book.[15] These diverse compositions engage the readers at every turn of the page, halting or prompting their progress through the textual content.

The illustration of *formento* (*Hordeum hexastichum* L., six-row barley, f. 21r, Plate 4) demonstrates how the relationship between image and text functions in the *Herbal*. Together, these elements orchestrate a specific reading experience that draws attention to the materiality of the manuscript and so to the act of mentally and physically engaging with it. In this illustration, the artist depicted four detailed barley heads growing up from behind the text of the following entry on barley flour (*de la farina* [*del formento*], unillustrated). He portrayed the barley heads' ladder-like pattern of growth and the feathery awns that spread outward like rays to surround them. He also carefully observed and recorded the thin, hollow cylinder-shape of the barley's leaves that grow around the stalk and extend outward upon maturity. The curving width of an extended leaf causes it to fold over itself and droop downwards.

The artist's composition emphasises this distinctive feature of the barley's pattern of growth to unify the image with its surrounding text. He represented the flag leaf of the far left barley spike folding gracefully across the width of the page, which creates a visual break between the text entries, stopping the reader's progress through the text. Further, he extended the barley stalk and leaf off the page, producing a frame for the subsequent text block. This compositional frame visually divides the textual information even as it reminds the viewer of the conceptual connection between the barley heads and the barley flour they can become. It provides both a visual break and a sense of continuity between the entries.[16] By deliberately emphasising the textual content through its connection with the visual imagery, the composition reminds the reader of the part the illustration plays in the creation of meaning and of an experience of the book as an object. It makes readers more consciously aware of the object they hold by pulling them out of complacent reading and viewing.

Whether one is reading the text or looking at the images, each aspect continuously interrupts the other. By pausing to admire an image, the reader's progress through the text is broken. As the reader stops reading to wonder at the naturalistic image of the pressed *meliloto* (*Lotus corniculatus* L., bird's foot trefoil, f. 15r, Plate 2) or clump of *viola* (*Viola odorata* L., violet, f. 94r), or to marvel at the exacting pictorial demarcation of genera of *malbavisco* (*Althaea officinalis* L. and *Lavatera thuringiaca* L., marshmallow, f. 52v, Figure 1.1), the plant fictions compel the reader to dwell on the page. Readers know these plants are not truly contained within the book's pages, but they surrender to the illusion despite this logic. In between the states of knowing and disbelieving lies a moment of pleasant deception, a moment of pleasure that – like the penwork faces – captures readers away from the text and delights.

The result is similar when the appearance of a schematic plant picture or a picture that combines representational techniques interrupts the readers' progress through the text. The insertion of plant representations drawn from earlier or contemporary sources suggests to readers the book's place within a lineage of illustrated herbals. These illustrations may even pull at the readers' memory of specific illustrated books of *materia medica* they had read. Conversely, and perhaps more simply, the very differences between the pictorial types give readers pause and, in their variety, enrich readers' experience of the book with inflections of pleasure. In different ways, the interruptions in the text caused by the illustrations and the unexpected diversity of the imagery please the readers and keep them engaged – not just with Serapion's teachings, but with the book itself. They guide the readers' consciousness back to the book as a material object to be experienced and so to its place in Francesco's book collection. In this way, the illustrative apparatus in the *Herbal* becomes a vehicle for the dissemination of pleasure's attendant sets of social, medical and aesthetic mores at the Carrara court.

On beauty, nature and the illustrated book (of *materia medica*)

In Chapter 1, when considering the roles illustrations could play in books of *materia medica*, we encountered Pliny's cautionary remarks about the potential pedagogical dangers of such imagery.[17] The traditional medical authorities Theophrastus and Dioscorides seem to accord implicitly with Pliny's assessment when they advocate the importance for students of medicine to recognise plants as they appear across their lifecycles – something a single image of a plant cannot adequately record. Despite his reservations, however, Pliny acknowledged the attractiveness of the plant imagery. In noticing the illustrations' beauty, Pliny opened up a different avenue of interpretation for the role images could play in books of *materia medica*, perhaps a role less central to the effective study of medicinal plants but one important to the history of the genre nonetheless.

In his *Naturalis historia* (*Natural History*), Pliny also introduced two influential ideals about nature that complement his view of plant imagery's 'attractions', ideals that would colour the interpretation of nature and its role in daily life from Roman antiquity through the seventeenth century. First Pliny praised *otium*, the privileged, solitary life of retreat from the city to the countryside, as valuable for the development of a good leader's mind and body, and, second, he urged his readers to value the pleasure found in a garden for its healthful benefits. For Pliny, the garden was a natural arena shaped and enjoyed by noble hands, an idea that associated the moulding of nature by human invention – by art – with social privilege. In Book 19, on the pleasures of the garden, Pliny established the antique pedigree of the pleasure garden (in Epicurus' thought) and its long association with nobility and privileged leadership (with the legendary kings of Rome, no less). To emphasise the connection between *otium* and the pleasures of a garden, Pliny also pointed out that, historically, the very term for 'garden' (*hortus*) was conflated with the term for 'villa' or 'family estate', the site of rural retreat for the aristocracy.[18]

In his discussions of *otium* and gardens, Pliny embraced cultivated nature as a pleasurable means to promote a healthy and balanced lifestyle. He considered the pleasures of a garden an important aspect of the life of an aristocratic man, especially a leader, and in this context emphasised the fanciful delight, rather than the medicinal practicalities, of plants. For instance, in Book 16, in his discussion of the cypress tree (*Cupressus sempervirens* L.), Pliny gives an example of the role of human invention in shaping nature solely for the delight of the viewer. He remarked that, in Roman gardens, cypress trees were clipped 'and made into thick walls or even rounded off with trim slenderness, and even made to provide the representations of the landscape gardener's work, arraying hunting scenes or fleets of ships and imitations of real objects with [their] narrow, short, evergreen leaf'.[19] The cypress topiary has no practical role in the garden; yet, in a space designed to promote pleasure and engage fantasy, Pliny celebrates topiary as a vehicle for artful invention meant solely to evoke pleasure.

Illustrated herbals connect to Pliny's observations on pleasure and plants and to two facets of Roman *otium* and their history in particular. On the one hand, the enjoyment of plant imagery parallels the enjoyment of a pleasure garden as a garden dedicated to sensory pleasure alone. The garden provided a transitional space in which the retreat from the work-a-day world of *negotium* into the oasis of villa *otium* occurred for the Romans and for their cultural and political successors across the Mediterranean world.[20] On the other hand, as a book, the illustrated herbal itself provides a point of access to another important facet of *otium*: the ideal of studious leisure (*otium litteratum*). For Pliny and for many of his contemporaries, *otium* included the pleasure of cultivating the mind while in retreat from the duties of the city.[21] The *Carrara Herbal* and other illustrated books of plant *materia medica* engage both these elements of *otium*: their illustrations provide an avenue for the pleasure of viewing nature as shaped by the artful hands of human invention, and, as physical objects, they provide the material necessary for studious leisure – the book, the very emblem of study.

For Pliny, and for many physicians and scholars after him, the cultivation of pleasure through nature and through reading had philosophical and corporeal value.[22] By offering both the delights of nature and the benefits of reading, illustrated books of medicinal plants engaged different sets of reader expectations than those tied more closely to the books' textual content did. These sets instead were tied to status, to notions of studious leisure and leadership, and to the pleasures of *otium* and of beauty and nature more generally. Moreover, and as we will see, the theory and practice of medicine and the ideas connected to these other sets of expectations were not mutually exclusive. Considered in this way, the textual content of illustrated herbals complements reader expectations but does not govern them. Illustrated herbals had their own distinctive purpose and attending expectations.

Nature in gardens and in books

The continuous history of collection of illustrated books of *materia medica* – across varied geographic locales around the Mediterranean and among different communities of collectors – points to enduring ideals about social privilege, the pleasures of nature, and traditions of rural *otium* and contemplative study. For instance, the history of gardens and of Mediterranean garden culture shows the celebration of these ideals.[23] Well into the seventeenth century, the illustrations and texts in botanical books and treatises on rural life and gardens commissioned by aristocratic patrons, in particular, reflected the idealisation of country living. In his popular early fourteenth-century treatise on agriculture, the *Liber ruralium commodorum* (*On Rural Life*), Piero de' Crescenzi (1233–1321) brought this idealisation into conversation with established social hierarchies about reading, nature and health in a new way.[24] De' Crescenzi's ideas circulated widely, as the numerous extant manuscripts and printed editions of the *Liber ruralium commodorum* attest.[25] By the close of the fifteenth century, many royal and noble households in Italy, France and England owned copies of his work, which suggests the currency of his views into the Early Modern period.[26]

Over the course of 12 books, de' Crescenzi discussed the practicalities of plant cultivation and animal husbandry and the curative properties of plants.[27] The majority of the work appropriated ancient Roman ideas about agriculture, viticulture, plant medicine and animal husbandry gleaned from such sources as Cato (234–149 BCE), Varro (116–27 BCE), Columella (4–70 CE), Pliny (23–79 CE) and Palladius (late fourth century – early fifth century CE) and mediated through the works of Avicenna (ca. 980–1037) and Albertus Magnus (ca. 1200–1280).[28] In Book VIII, however, de' Crescenzi abandoned these sources and made explicit the connection between divisions of labour and lifestyle at court and types of gardens.[29] In this book, de' Crescenzi surpassed earlier associations between gardens and class. He hypothesised that certain types of gardens were appropriate to different social groups specifically because of the groups' particular status and health and hygiene requirements.

De' Crescenzi outlined the physical characteristics and corresponding social distinctions of three classes of garden that correspond to three social classes of people. The description of the small garden, with fragrant herbs and flowers and a small spring and healthy breezes, is not associated immediately with a particular class.[30] However, the succeeding chapter on moderately sized gardens explicitly states that the garden's size should be calculated in relation to its owner's social status. De' Crescenzi wrote: 'Let the space of the earth set aside for the garden be measured according to the means and rank of persons of moderate means, namely, two or three or four or more *iugera* or *bubulcae*'.[31] He then proceeded to describe the distinguishing features of the moderate garden. It should be 'surrounded with ditches and hedge of thorns and roses . . . [or] of pomegranates'.[32] Finally, de' Crescenzi considered the pleasure garden, with its expansive lands, open meadows, ponds, pergolas or summer lodges, and displays of the wonders of nature and of sensual artifice, as appropriate for persons of great means.[33] For de' Crescenzi, wonders of nature and of art ought to adorn the most prestigious gardens, and he considered grafting as the epitome of both. He advocated the need to experiment, engineer and transform plants into new flora. Further, he described experiments and natural wonders wrought from creatively engineering ordinary plants, like watercress (*Nasturtium officinale* W.T. Aiton), lettuce (*Lactuca sativa* L.), leek (*Allium ampeloprasum* L.), radish (*Raphanus sativus* L.) and cucumber (*Cucumis sativus* L.). The sole function of these 'unusual things' – literally things of no use (*inusitatas*) – was to evoke delight from the garden's owner and his guests.[34]

Perhaps the most remarkable aspect of Book VIII is that de' Crescenzi assumed his prior discussion of the traditional medicinal virtues of plants into a discussion of the garden itself as a natural *space* that possessed healing properties. His approach to the role of plants in a garden is very different from the way that earlier authorities on medicine approached plants. De' Crescenzi prefaced Book VIII by noting that he intended to show how plants in a garden space can heal the mind and, in doing so, can preserve the health of the body (a view of the mind/body relationship humanists would later echo). He wrote:[35]

> In the previous books, trees and herbaceous plants were discussed according to how they can be useful to the human body; but now the same ones must be discussed according to *how they give pleasure to a rational soul and consequently preserve the health of the body*, since the humoric state of the body is always closely related to the disposition of the soul.

In this passage, de' Crescenzi transitioned from a discussion of plants' medical utility to their pleasures but recognised that their pleasures are also medically useful. De' Crescenzi then 'grafted' his ideas about pleasure and plants onto his view of gardens and social status.

De' Crescenzi's theory on the pleasure and utility of plants – like his complementary views on *otium* and villa gardens – provides a useful foil for how illustrated books of *materia medica*, in general, and the *Carrara Herbal*, in particular, could have generated meaning for the reader. De' Crescenzi considered aristocratic gardens a balm for the souls of their owners, a balm that in turn preserved the health of their bodies. He understood the enjoyment of plants, and especially of plants shaped by human invention, as crucial to the overall health of the patrician patient. Considered in this way, the illustrations in the *Carrara Herbal* are a translation of de' Crescenzi's ideas into book form: the illustrations function like the garden, in which the plants are likewise shaped by human artistry. Experiencing the illustrations, the reader reaps the benefits an aristocratic visitor would in a pleasure garden – benefits felt in body and soul.

While de' Crescenzi posited that artful nature was the province of aristocrats' enjoyment, which contributed to their health, individual health regimens for such patrons (*regimina sanitatis*) also advocated leisurely reading as a complementary recreational avenue that promoted health through the cultivation of pleasurable experience.[36] Reading the *Carrara Herbal* brought these tenets of pleasure and health together for the benefit of Francesco Novello and his court intimates. As a beautiful book, the *Herbal* met the requirement for leisurely reading needed to maintain a prince's health and focus. Furthermore, its very subject addressed additional (and quite literal) means for the maintenance of health: reading the *Herbal* itself was an act promoting Francesco's health, while its content augmented his knowledge on how to maintain health and cure disease.

On pleasure and health in Carrara Padua

As an illustrated book, the *Carrara Herbal* was designed, in part, to cultivate pleasurable experiences for its elite audience. But as agents of reading pleasure and purveyors of knowledge, the *Carrara Herbal* and other illustrated books of *materia medica* also functioned within commonplace tenets about health that circulated at court and in medical and humanistic texts compiled for aristocratic readers. Pleasant activities like reading, conversations and storytelling, visiting a garden, and listening to music and viewing beautiful objects warded against melancholy, an emotional state that left one susceptible to poor health.

At university, students of medicine encountered this valuation of pleasure as a purveyor of health in the *al-Qānūn fi'l-ṭibb* (*Liber Canonis*; *The Canon of Medicine*), written by the Persian physician and natural philosopher Avicenna (Ibn Sīnā, ca. 980–1037)[37] and available in a Latin translation perhaps by Gerard of Cremona (ca. 1114–1187) by the late-twelfth century.[38] The *Canon* was a central text on medical theory studied at universities from the thirteenth through seventeenth centuries, and Francesco Novello owned copies of the first, second, third and fifth books as well as two books of excerpts drawn from Avicenna's treatise (one of which was written in the vernacular).[39] The *Canon* was one of three texts by Avicenna available in Latin during the late Middle Ages. The other two texts were: *al-Adwīa al-qalbīya* (*De viribus cordis*; *On the Faculties of the Heart*), translated into Latin in the late-thirteenth or early fourteenth century by Arnaud de Villanova (d. 1311), professor at Montpellier, either from an earlier Hebrew translation or from the Arabic original, and *al-Orjūza fi'l-ṭibb* (*Cantica Avicennae*; *Avicenna's Poem* [*of Medicine*]), translated by Arnaud's nephew, Armengaud Blasius (d. 1312), at Montpellier in the late thirteenth century.[40]

In Book I of the *Canon*, Avicenna discussed his theory of medicine and his view of the physical and emotional causes of health and sickness.[41] Avicenna's concept of health acknowledged a central relationship between emotions and a substance called *rouh*. In the Latin tradition, *rouh* was translated as *spiritus* and associated with breath,[42] but 'breath' in the sense of vital spirit or life energy (what the Chinese call *Qi*)[43] rather than simply just the physical act of breathing.[44] For Avicenna, each organ of the body possessed its own *spiritus*,[45] and the quality and strength of the *spiritus* related to an individual's constitution. In the *Canon*, Avicenna identified the foundation of the 'single breath' – the starting place for the breath in all the other organs – as the heart.[46] Moreover, in *De viribus cordis*, in which Avicenna both incorporated and expanded upon information in the *Canon* about the heart and emotional health,[47] the physician noted that the heart's *spiritus* is influenced by emotional or psychological states, in particular.

Avicenna argued, then, that emotional states can encourage or endanger individuals' health specifically because emotions can alter or imbalance the *spiritus* of the heart, which is central to overall health. He wrote:[48]

> Sages, and those physicians who agree with them, are satisfied that joy and
> sadness, fear and anger, are passions [emotions] peculiarly related to the breath

of the heart. Each of these emotions is maintained or discontinued (1) by the [human] agent; (2) by the persistence or cessation of the disposition exhibited by the substance of the patient [over which humans do not have control].

For Avicenna, strong (and so potentially dangerous) emotions could be continued or stopped either by an individual's agency (things that we do and for which we are responsible) or by an individual's predisposition to feel certain emotions, which is independent of individual choice and premised on one's constitution or circumstance.[49]

Avicenna pointed out, however, that regardless of individuals' tendencies toward certain passions, they could encourage joy and delight through external sources and so promote or maintain physical health through more controllable factors.[50] Avicenna described some sources of joy that influence the body's health and encourage a healthy *spiritus* of the heart. He specifically mentioned reading books on rhetoric and morals as 'gladdening influences'; other sources of joy include conversing with interesting people, doing something peaceful, engaging with unusual or remarkable new things, uplifting the mind and meeting friends.[51] For Avicenna, joy had the potential to balance the heart's *spiritus*, and pleasurable activities – of which reading was a vital component – cultivated joy.

In the late Middle Ages, regimens of health, often originally written for patrons of considerable social standing,[52] and compilations of *consilia* (physicians' case studies) circulated among the educated elite at courts across Europe.[53] These documents offered advice similar to Avicenna's for attaining moderate joyfulness as a guard against the poor health associated with extreme emotions. For instance, the physician Benedetto Reguardati (1398–1469) described the best emotional attitude for preserving health in a regimen written around 1435. He wrote:[54]

> For the preservation of health we should strive most resolutely for moderate pleasures and for gladdening solaces. So that as much as possible we may live happily in temperate gaiety. That condition expands the *spiritus* and natural heat to the outer parts of the body and makes the blood purer; it sharpens one's wit and makes the understanding more capable; it promotes a healthy complexion and a pleasing appearance; it stimulates the energies throughout the whole body and makes them more vigorous in their activity.

While Reguardati did not specify particular 'gladdening solaces', other physicians offered more concrete examples. In a *consilium* regarding a patient suffering from digestive disorders, for instance, the Padua-trained physician Gentile da Foligno (d. 1348) noted:[55]

> Among other things [the patient] should especially take care not to remain alone nor to plunge himself into sadness or heavy thoughts. To this end conversation with good friends works very well, as do a change in scenery, tackling things that seem challenging to complete, and hawking and hunting.

Likewise, the Sienese physician and philosopher Ugo Benzi (ca. 1376–1439) recommended engaging in specific activities to promote health. In a *consilium* written for an unnamed young nobleman, Benzi specifically noted the salubrious values of conversation with friends, looking at beautiful things, listening to music, visiting gardens and reading enjoyable books. He wrote:[56]

> There should be the most diligent effort made to instill liveliness and good hope in him [the patient] and to shift his thoughts on one day to some delightful and fitting thing, on another to something else. Such things include looking at various beautiful and entertaining decorations; hearing music and songs; reading something not too difficult, like a narrative or some other work he likes; perfuming or selecting clothes for himself; preparing houses, pleasure gardens, and estates; and other similar activities.

For these European physicians, as for Avicenna, joyfulness could be encouraged and health preserved or promoted by engaging in pleasant activities. Reading was one of these activities that helped to regulate the emotions, especially the emotions of aristocratic or noble patients.

The ideas expressed in regimens of health and *consilia* were echoed in other late medieval literary contexts as well. After the Black Death pandemic in 1348, in particular, the regulation of emotions became an important tactic used to ward against the plague, an idea recorded in the widely read and disseminated plague manuals but also in other medical and humanistic literature.[57] For instance, the handbook on health known as the *Tacuinum Sanitatis* (*Tables of Health*),[58] which includes dietetic, hygiene and lifestyle advice along with information on select *materia medica*, records (in text and in image) ways of managing difficult emotions in order to achieve the temperate joyfulness associated with health and the avoidance of plague. Storytelling, walking, horseback riding, hunting or hawking, and sitting or talking in the garden were some of the activities prescribed (and, in several cases, illustrated) in the *Tacuinum* that were considered useful to noble patients in promoting joyfulness.[59] These healthy prescriptions became accepted knowledge among the educated class and were echoed in humanistic contexts.

In the *Decameron*, for example, the poet and early humanist Giovanni Boccaccio (1313–1375) incorporated these medical commonplaces into his fictional setting. A group of patricians flees Florence for the Tuscan countryside in hopes of escaping the plague. There, in the beautiful garden of their rural retreat, the Florentines tell stories to lift their spirits and so help to protect themselves from the plague. In the prologue to his French translation of Boccaccio's *Decameron* for Jean, the Duke of Berry (1340–1416), the humanist and poet Laurent de Premierfait (ca. 1380–1418) directly articulated the relationship between health and morality, recreation and status, and reading and storytelling.[60] Perhaps reflecting knowledge of *otium* and *negotium* or a familiarity with *consilia* or other health regimens written for aristocrats, de Premierfait explained to the duke that labour leads to weakness of body and of mind. According to de Premierfait, to restore the body, one must eat nourishing foods and take medicines. To restore the mind, in particular, one must partake of delightful things because they 'gladden and cheer people's spirits' and so prolong healthy life.[61]

In his prologue, de Premierfait noted that peaceful rest and relaxation were especially important to the health of princes, ideas seen in numerous *consilia* and central to the function of *otium* (and listed among Avicenna's 'gladdening influences').[62] Yet, in his assertion, de Premierfait also echoed Aristotle's argument about the value of leisure in the *Ethica ad Nicomachum* (*Nicomachean Ethics*), which explicitly draws together moral and physical health – a synthesis implied in Boccaccio's work, in many health regimens and in Avicenna's *De viribus cordis*.[63] In the *Ethica* and in the medieval commentary on it by the Scholastic theologian and philosopher Thomas Aquinas (ca. 1225–1274), *Ethicorum Aristotelis ad Nichomachum expositio* (*Commentary on Aristotle's Nichomachean Ethics*), recreation and pleasure were seen as vehicles that led to virtuous behaviour as well as to physical health.[64] Aristotle wrote:[65]

> Anacharsis' motto, Play in order that you may work, is felt to be the right rule. For amusement is a form of rest; but we need rest because we are not able to go on working without a break, and therefore it is not an end, since we take it as a means to further [virtuous] activity.

Aquinas glossed this passage in his *expositio*. He wrote:[66]

> according to the opinion of Anacharsis it seems proper for a person to amuse himself for a time so that later he may work harder. The reason is that relaxation and rest are found in amusement. But, since men cannot work continuously, they need rest. Hence it is clear that amusement or rest is not an end because this rest is for the sake of activity in order that afterwards men may work more earnestly.

For Aristotle and for Aquinas, as for Avicenna and the physicians he influenced in the Latin West, joy (pleasure or amusement) was not an end in and of itself. For the philosophers, this affirmation of joy's ethical usefulness in the promotion of further virtuous activity removed potential negative associations of pleasure with idleness; while, for the physicians, joy's usefulness was understood in terms of the promotion of physical and emotional health. Of course, these views of joy are complements: individuals cannot pursue any activity 'more earnestly' if they are suffering from emotional or physical illness. Joy and pleasure, then, both philosophically and medically, were understood as means to promote further virtue and to preserve health.

*

In connection with humanistic and medical ideals about the value of pleasure to a prince's moral and physical health, the *Carrara Herbal* becomes a vehicle for the promotion of Francesco's identity as a 'good' and 'healthy' ruler of Padua.

Through its text, illustrations and material qualities, the *Herbal* embodies the pursuits of studious leisure, restfulness and healthful pleasure – pursuits appropriate to its princely patron and to members of his court. As a book in Francesco's library, the *Herbal* becomes a go-between, a courtly Galehaut exchanged among privileged readers.[67] Understood in this way, the pleasures of reading the *Herbal* – experiences that initially seem chiefly aesthetic – become experiences that affirm its owner as a wise and healthy Carrara prince, a capable heir to his father's successful rule of Padua.

Notes

1 Illustrated herbals – especially those of very fine quality – were not used primarily to identify plants in the field, contrary to Pächt's once influential thesis (1950: 29). Often, they were too large and too valuable for such a – potentially messy – task. Generally, knowledge about the identification of medicinal plants circulated orally among herb-gatherers or in monastic communities. Physicians, whose training focussed principally on the theory and practice of medicine, received the plant material for medicines already harvested and prepared for their use. See Reeds (1991: 74–94); Collins and Raphael (2003: 5); and Givens (2005: 129 and 2006: 117).

2 On how physicians may have used illustrations in herbals as signposts for retrieving therapeutic information or as a means of communication free from the vicissitudes of language, see Givens (2006), and Touwaide (2013b), respectively.

3 On the relationship between the *Carrara Herbal* and the courtly codex book form, see Chapter 3.

4 The *Herbal* contains 289 folios gathered into 32 quires, the majority of which are quiniones (10 folios). There are three paper folia at the beginning of the codex; ff. 1–2 are likely nineteenth-century additions. The Bolognese naturalist Ulisse Aldrovandi (1522–1605) pasted a piece of paper bearing the *ex libris* 'Ulissis Aldrovandi et Amicorum' ('Ulisse Aldrovandi and friends') onto f. 3v, suggesting this folio dates to the sixteenth century. The remaining 286 folios are parchment. For a detailed codicological description of the manuscript and an account of its possible cropping, see Baumann (1974: 25–6).

5 Collins (2000: 310).

6 Nutton (1995b: 193–4) discusses the accessibility of Dioscorides' book to nonspecialists in his analysis of the Renaissance Dioscorides and suggests this accessibility was central to the book's continued popularity.

7 See Serapion (ed. Ineichen 1962–1966), and Dilg (1999).

8 In a similar way, Givens (2006) describes what she calls a 'textual hierarchy' in reading the Egerton 747 *Tractatus de herbis*, noting especially the use of lighter and darker script. For Givens (2006: 123), such textual design decisions made it easier for readers to find information and assess its importance. Use of such markers is visible in other books of *materia medica*, including the *Carrara Herbal*, where the use of red ink or majuscule lettering structures the text.

9 Dilg (1999: 230) discusses the possibility that Philippus served as translator as well as scribe. Philippus identifies himself in the manuscript's closing folio (289v). See Introduction, p. 14n6.

10 The rubricators added pale yellow to some of the larger capital letters within a text block, in names, in the 'Es' (ands) of lists, and in the 'Qs' of the terms 'Questa' (this) and 'Qualle' (that).

11 '¶ **De la mellissa**. ¶ **Capitolo XXIII**. Melissa, citraria, segondo altri, ven chiamà. ¶ Dixe Dioscorides che Melissa è erba sovra la quale se deleta le ave. ¶ Le verçele de la

melissa e le foie someia a le verçele e a le foie del marubio salvègo. E li soi branchi e le soe verçelle sì è quadrangole, çoè ha quatro canton. E le foie suò è maore che no è le foie del marubio salvègo, né no è chosì pellose como è le foie de questo marubio. ¶ La melissa ha propriamentre odore de citron, e per quest oven chiamà citraria. **Le vertù** de questa herba è calda e secha in lo primo grado. ¶ Dixe Galieno che la vertù de questa è como la vertù del marubio. Ma l'è de più menor vertù. ¶ Dixe Dioscoride che quando el se beve le suò foie cum el vino overe quando se ne fa empiastro, çoa a la puntura del scorpion e al morso de uno ragno che ve(n) chiamà rotella. E così la decocion de questa herba, quando la se buta sovra el lugo morsegò, fa questa miesima cosa. E quando le femene sedesse in la decocion de questa, sì ge provocherà li menstrui. E fassene lavanda a la bocha, e çoa al dolore de li denti. E quando el se cuxe le foie cum el nitro çoa a le ulceracion de li intestine. E fassene loch a quili che no pò tirare lo aere a si e a quili [*ch(e)*] no pò tirare né mandarlo fura. ¶ E quando el se fa empiastro cum sale, resolve le scrovole e mundifica ulceracion. E quando el se fa empiastro cum questa herba, mitiga el dolore de le çonture. ¶ Dixe uno autore che la ha proprietà de alegrare l'anema e *de* confortare el core debele. E quando la se magna da deçuno, çoa al stomego fredo e humido e fa pàire el cibo grosso. E avre le opillacion del cerbelo. E çoa a le paure e hà le malicie che ven per humore melanco[*lico*] e de flema adhusto' (Serapion, ed. Ineichen 1962–1966: 1.28. My translation).

12 For instance, in the entry for *de la anguria* (*Citrullus lanatus* [Thunb.] Matsum. & Nakai, watermelon, f. 163r).

13 The colourful lettering, three-line high opening initials, and red or blue pilcrow signs occasionally overlap areas of the illustration, which suggests that they were added after the completion of the plant images (Baumann 1974: 26).

14 See Chapter 1, pp. 24–8.

15 There are variations even within these types of composition. For example, *camomilla* (*Matricaria Chamomilla* L., chamomile, f. 17v) appears to grow up from behind the text describing its virtues, rather than from in between two entries. Instead of portraying the plant below its corresponding text, the scribe broke the text entry in two and the artist inserted this delicate illustration in the middle of it. Baumann accounts for these variations by suggesting that the scribe and artist worked closely together to find the best placement for the text and image blocks. For Baumann, this 'trial by error' method is especially prevalent in the second book and stabilises into the predominant page layout – in which the text block is on top of the page and the image block lies below – midway through the second tract. After the entry for *polvaro* (*Populus nigra* L., Lombardy poplar, f. 23v), all remaining pages are plotted according to this layout.

16 This is also the mode of representation the artist uses when portraying climbing plants, like *volubelle* (*Calystegia sepium* L., wild morning glory, f. 33r) and *cussus* (*Hedera helix* L., ivy, f. 33v). They crawl across the page, sinuously surrounding the text, and often begin and end outside the confines of the page.

17 See *Naturalis historia*, 25.4 (ed. and tr. Jones 1956: 7.140–1). For the complete passage, see Chapter 1, p. 55n17.

18 The passage reads: 'in XII tabulis legum nostrarum nusquam nominatur villa, semper in significatione ea hortus, in horti vero heredium' and later 'primus hoc instituit Athenis Epicurus otii magister; usque ad eum moris non fuerat in oppidis habitari rura' (Pliny, *Naturalis historia*, 19.19, §50–1 [ed. and tr. Rackham 1950: 5.450–3]). On pleasure gardens in the Roman Empire and their relationship to other leisurely pursuits, such as celebrating public and private festivals, dining in community and visiting the baths, see Robert (2011). Robert's lexica of sites, activities and authors associated with the ideals and practices of Roman leisure are especially useful (Robert 2011: 233–88).

19 'nunc vero tonsilis facta In densitatem parietum cocrcitaque gracilitate perpetuo teres trahitur etiam in picturas operis topiarii, venatus classesve et imagines rerum tenui folio brevique et virente semper vestiens' (Pliny, *Naturalis historia*, 16.60, §140 [ed. and

tr. Rackham 1945: 4.478–81]). For another interpretation of this passage, see Pavord (2005: 66).

20 On gardens in Byzantium, see Littlewood et al. (eds) (2002), and Bodin and Hedlund (eds) (2013). On gardens in the Arabic Empire, especially in al-Andalus, see Ruggles (2000).

21 A wide variety of contemporaneous poets and philosophers shared Pliny's view of *otium*: from Cicero (106–43 BCE) and Seneca (4–65 CE) to Horace (65–8 BCE) and Martial (40–102 CE). The idea dates back further to the philosophy of Epicurus (341–270 BCE) and even to the poetry of Homer. Pliny alludes to the value of study for learned men (and names the works of several such men) in his preface to *Naturalis historia*, but his extraordinary encyclopaedia itself best attests to the importance the historian gave to study. Further, the celebration of studious leisure is expressed in the letters of the elder Pliny's nephew, Pliny the Younger (61–113), who not only lionised his uncle's scholarly pursuits but also described his own participation in *otium litteratum*. See, for instance, his letters to Fuscus (*Epistulae* 9.36 and 9.40), which describe his daily activities at his villa during the summer and winter, respectively (eds Melmoth and Hutchinson 1915: 2.258–63 and 2.268–71; tr. Walsh 2006: 238–9 and 241). For a detailed analysis of Pliny the Younger's view of literary *otium*, especially through examples drawn from his letters, see Johnson (2010), and Gibson and Morello (2012: 169–99).

22 The cultivation of health through pleasure and reading were not ideals restricted to Pliny's *Naturalis historia* or to ancient Greek and Roman culture. Humanists, philosophers and medical authorities from across broad geographical and temporal arenas shared these views and valued pleasure and beauty as means to both edify and heal. This diverse group of thinkers included, for instance, Greek and Arabic medical writers (from the Hippocratics to Ibn Buṭlān [d. ca. 1063]) and ancient philosophers and poets, Scholastics and humanists (from Aristotle [384–322 BCE], Horace [65–8 BCE] and Ovid [43 BC–ca. 17 CE], to Hugh of Saint Victor [1096–1141], Thomas Aquinas [1225–1274], Dante [1265–1321] and Petrarch [1304–1374]). These authors all stressed the importance of pleasure to the health and well-being of individuals. The pleasures found in nature and those found in reading often are cited for their healing properties. I will return to the parallels between these literary and medical views in subsequent chapters. For a more-detailed analysis of how reading, especially, was related to health, recreation and pleasure in the late Middle Ages, see Olson (1982). My interpretation of the healthy benefits of reading the *Carrara Herbal* is indebted to Olson's study of the wider social, cultural and philosophical attitudes about the value of literature during this period.

23 On the transmission of ideals about garden-making in the literature of agricultural writers from before Pliny, through Late Antiquity and the Middle Ages, see Rodgers (2002). On agricultural manuals and gardens in the Islamic world, in particular, see Ruggles (2000).

24 Piero de' Crescenzi (Petrus de Cresentiis), *Ruralium commodorum* (eds Richter and Richter-Bergmeier 1995–1998). The association of nature with the ability to govern prudently (i.e. Roman *otium*) was common knowledge by this time, and the possession of land and a country household was part of the everyday life of de' Crescenzi's educated readers during his time and during the Renaissance. See Calkins (1986), and Bauman (2002; Bauman also provides a transcription and translation of Book VIII of de' Crescenzi's treatise). For a brief introduction to de' Crescenzi's life and work, see Toubert (1984).

25 There are at least 141 extant manuscripts in Latin and in Italian, German and French translations, and many more printed editions in different languages (Calkins 1986: 159n9, and Ambrosoli 1992: 43n4).

26 Calkins (1986: 159–62).

27 Book I addresses the best site on which to build a country house; Book II the cultivation of fields; Book III labours of the fields and the harvest; Book IV wine and tending the vines; Book V trees and their fruits; Book VI vegetable and herb gardens; Book VII meadows and copses; Book VIII different types of gardens; Book IX animals; Book X hunting; Book XI summarises the entire work; and Book XII is a calendar of tasks for tending the land. On the treatise's contents and its fortunes from the later Renaissance, see Ambrosoli (1992) (tr. 1997: especially 41–95).

28 For analyses of de' Crescenzi's sources, see Calkins (1986: 158–9), and Bauman (2002: 113).

29 de' Crescenzi, *Ruralium commodorum*, 8.1–8 (eds Richter and Richter-Bergmeier 1998: 3.11–26; tr. Bauman 2002: 100–11).

30 de' Crescenzi, *Ruralium commodorum*, 8.1 (eds Richter and Richter-Bergmeier 1998: 3.11–13; tr. Bauman 2002: 101).

31 'Secundum facultates et dignitatem mediocrium personarum mensuretur spatium terrae viridario deputandae, videlicet duo vel tria vel quattuor aut plura iugera sive bubulcae' (de' Crescenzi, *Ruralium commodorum*, 8.2, §1 [eds Richter and Richter-Bergmeier 1998: 3.13; tr. Bauman 2002: 101]). For scale, 20 *iugera* was approximately twelve and a half acres (noted by Bauman 2002: 102).

32 'Cingatur fossatis et sepibus spinorum vel rosarum et desuper fiat sepis de malis Punicis in locis calidis, et in frigidis de nuzolis seu prunes vel malis citoniis' (de' Crescenzi, *Ruralium commodorum*, 8.2, §1 [eds Richter and Richter-Bergmeier 1998: 3.13; tr. Bauman 2002: 101]). Plants considered more exotic distinguish the moderate space: roses, pomegranate and quince trees, and fig and almond trees planted in long rows accentuated the relative wealth of the owner.

33 de' Crescenzi, *Ruralium commodorum*, 8.3 (eds Richter and Richter-Bergmeier 1998: 3.14–16; tr. Bauman 2002: 102–3).

34 de' Crescenzi, *Ruralium commodorum*, 8.8, §2 (eds Richter and Richter-Bergmeier 1998: 3.24; tr. Bauman 2002: 108–10).

35 'In superioribus libris tractatum est de arboribus et herbis, secundum quod utilia corpori humano existunt; nunc vero de eisdem dicendum est, secundum *quod animae rationali delectationem afferunt et consequenter corporis salutem conservant*, quia complexio corporis animi semper adhaeret affectui' (de' Crescenzi, *Ruralium commodorum*, 8.Praefatio, §1 [eds Richter and Richter-Bergmeier 1998: 3.11; tr. Bauman 2002: 100. My emphasis]).

36 For example, the fifteenth-century revision of a *regimen sanitatis* (*régime du corps*) written by Aldobrandino of Siena (d. 1296; on his life and work see Marti 1960), originally for Beatrice of Savoy (1205–1267), Countess of Provence, and especially popular among the French elite, contains the prescription to read unusual and pleasant things (Olson 1982: 57, and Bertiz 2003: 208). For a brief introduction to *regimina sanitatis*, see Weiss-Adamson (2005).

37 For an introduction to Avicenna's life and works, see Goichon (1999); Aminrazavi (1997); and El-Bizri (2006). For translations of and commentary on the first book of the *Canon*, see, most recently, Abu-Asab, Amri and Micozzi (2013), and the earlier translation by Gruner (1930). The translation by Abu-Asab, Amri and Micozzi draws on Arabic versions of the text. Gruner's translation is from the Latin versions of the *Canon* published in Venice in 1595 and 1608 in consultation with a printed Arabic edition of 1593 (which Abu-Asab, Amri and Micozzi also consult) (Gruner 1930: 18–21). For a discussion of these and other English translation efforts, see Abu-Asab, Amri and Micozzi (2013: 6–9). For a summary of the contents of Books II–V, see Shah (1966: 427–9). These books have not been translated into English and are available in Latin translation only in fifteenth- and sixteenth-century copies and facsimiles thereof.

38 Touwaide (2013a: x) suggests that Gerard of Sabloneta (fl. mid-thirteenth century) may have completed the Latin translation, rather than Gerard of Cremona, as scholars have

long believed. Osler (2007: 211) also discusses the 'second' Gerard's translation of Avicenna. For an introduction to Gerard of Cremona, see Burnett (2005).

39 The books by Avicenna are listed on Zago's 1405 inventory of Francesco's collection (numbers 25, 32, 49, 54, 58 and 59; see Appendix). On the prevalence of Avicenna's medicine at European universities during the late Middle Ages and Early Modern period, see Siraisi (1987a, 1987b: 111 [repr. 2001b: 162–3] and 1994 [tr. 2001]).

40 On the dissemination of Avicenna's text into Western Europe, see Siraisi (1987a). There are several early printed editions of the Latin translations of these three works bound together, including editions printed in Basel (Per Joannes Hervagios, 1556) and Venice (apud Iuntas, 1582). Peterson (1993) includes a partial English translation of *De viribus cordis* along with her analysis of the text, as does Gruner (1930), along with his translation of Book I of the *Canon*. Armengaud Blasius's Latin translation of the *Cantica Avicennae* is available, with a French translation, in Jahier and Noureddine (1956).

41 Avicenna describes 'active causes' of health and sickness, writing: 'Active causes are the ones that change or preserve the conditions of the human body, such as air, food, water, drinks, retentions and evacuation, habitat, residency, movement and rest – both physical and psychological, sleep and wakefulness, age changes, sex differences, occupations, habits, and objects that come in touch with the human body that are natural or unnatural' (Book I, Part I ['First Art'], Thesis [Lesson] I, §2 [eds and tr. Abu-Asab, Amri and Micozzi 2013: 38]).

42 *Canon*, Book I, Part I ('First Art'), Thesis (Lesson) VI, §168–73 (ed. and tr. Gruner 1930: 123–5). Gruner attempts to describe Avicenna's concept of breath, which has no equivalent in Western thought. He writes (1930: 125–6): '[breath is] that which binds the vegetative and sensitive life into one connected whole. It is common to, and like in, *all* living things. . . . Breath is *not* "respiration," "breathing," drawing in breath. . . . By picturing the breath as a sort of aura pervading the body, with a polarity correspondent with the cosmic ether (its source, whence it individualized into the human being), the conception of orientation (in time and space) becomes feasible'. Avicenna describes the breath in *De viribus cordis* as 'that which emerges from a mixture of first-principles, and approaches towards the likeness of celestial beings. It is a luminous substance. It is a ray of light' (§1091 [ed. and tr. Gruner 1930: 353]).

43 Abu-Asab, Amri and Miccozzi (2013: 27).

44 Notably, in their recent translation of the *Canon*, Abu-Asab, Amri and Micozzi seek to translate Avicenna's vocabulary into that of modern medicine. They translate *rouh* as oxygen – one component of the breath, but not its entirety, which, in Arabic, is called *nāfās* (2013: 27) These translators also point out that in Classical Arabic *nāfs* ('soul') and *rouh* ('spirit'), while distinct concepts, often are used interchangeably (2013: 27). Such flexible use of the term allows for both the more literal (corporeal) understanding of *rouh* expressed by Abu-Asab, Amri and Micozzi, and the more philosophical (incorporeal) one connoted in the Latin translation of *rouh* as *spiritus*.

45 Since we are most concerned with the Latin interpretation of this idea, I will use the terms *spiritus* and 'breath' in the following discussion.

46 In the *Canon* Book I, Part I ('First Art'), Thesis (Lesson) VI, §171 (which is also included in *De viribus cordis*), Avicenna wrote: 'There is one single breath which accounts for the origin of the others; and this breath, according to the most important philosophers, arises [its starting place is] in the heart, passes thence into the principal centres of the body, lingering in them long enough to enable them to impart to it their respective temperamental properties' (ed. and tr. Gruner 1930: 124). For analysis of this lesson, see Abu-Asab, Amri and Micozzi (2013: 88–9).

47 Peterson (1993: 3). Gruner (1930) identified sections from Book I, Part I ('First Art'), Thesis (Lesson) VI of the *Canon* that were incorporated in *De viribus cordis* (§168–73 in his translation). Avicenna later excerpted the strictly psychological sections of *De*

viribus cordis (chapters 2–8) and added them to his *Kitāb al-nafs* (*Book of the Soul*), part of his longer treatise *Kitāb al-Shifā'* (*Book of Healing*) (d'Alverny 1952: 348, and Peterson 1993: 4). For a brief introduction to *De viribus cordis* as a vector for medical knowledge about the effects of emotions on bodily health in the medieval Latin West, see Olson (1982: 44–5).

48 *De viribus cordis*, §1093 (ed. and tr. Gruner 1930: 535).

49 Avicenna continued: 'By way of summary, it may be said that when the breath residing in the heart is plentiful (as it is when there is plenty of that material from which it is rapidly and constantly being generated); when it is balanced in temperament; when it is a luminous, beautiful and bright substance – then there is a strong tendency to joy. When the breath is scanty (as occurs in convalescents, in long-standing illnesses, and in old persons); when it is not balanced in character (as in morbid states); and when it is (*a*) very dense and coarse in substance (as in melancholy and old people) – it cannot arouse joy; (*b*) very delicate in substance (as in convalescents and in women), it will not allow of expansion; (*c*) confused (as in melancholy people) – in all these cases there is a very strong tendency to depression, sadness and grief' (*De viribus cordis*, §1103 [ed. and tr. Gruner 1930: 538]).

50 Avicenna allowed that certain sources of joy would appeal to certain people more than others. He wrote: 'All of these [sources of joy] vary in different races according to their affection, habits and ages. None of them is invariably absent. If two agents usually having a gladdening effect occur together, the effect is not so much the greater. All that happens is that the disposition is more drawn to one than the other' (*De viribus cordis*, §1109 [ed. and tr. Gruner 1930: 541]).

51 *De viribus cordis*, §1108 (ed. and tr. Gruner 1930: 541).

52 For instance, Aldobrandino of Siena's popular *Régime du corps* originally written for the Countess of Provence (see p. 83n36 in this volume).

53 Olson (1982: 57). *Consilia* follow a general formula (the degree to which the formula was followed varies by physician, however). They include a description of symptoms followed by a prescription for a regimen of diet and activities and, finally, a description of any accompanying medical intervention. On this general formula, see Lockwood (1951). On *consilia* as a genre of medical writing and on their growing vogue among educated readers in the late Middle Ages, see Siraisi (1981, 1987b [repr. 2001b], 1994 [tr. 2001; especially in relation to the growing interest in Avicenna's medicine] and 2007: 65–79); Agrimi and Crisciani (1994); and Crisciani (2005). For several thirteenth-century examples of *consilia*, see Alderotti (eds Girogi and Pasini 1997).

54 'Pro sanitatis igitur conseruatione summopere ad temperata gaudia et solatia alacriora conari debemus, ut quam possibile sit lete uiuamus moderata cum letitia. Spiritus, naturalem calorem ad exteriora expandit membra; clariorum sanguinem facit; ingenium acuit; intellectum solertiorem efficit; et uiuidum colorem placidumque aspectum inducit, atque totius nostre corporis uirtutes excitat et in eorum operibus agiliores prestat' (*Pulcherrimum et utilissimum opus ad sanitatis conseruationem* [Bologna], 1477, ff. 124v–125r; ed. and tr. Olson 1982: 50).

55 'Inter alia singulariter procuret non remanere solitarius nec profundare se ad tristitiam et cogitamina. Ad hoc multum valet conuersatio cum dilectis et mutatio de terra in terram et tentare aliqua videantur difficilia in consecutione et aucupari et venari' (*Consilia Cermisoni. Consilia Gentilis* [edition of Venice 1495?], f. 63v; ed. and tr. Olson 1982: 59n33). On Gentile's *consilia*, see Thorndike (1959). On Gentile's life and works, and for a summary of earlier historiography on the physician, see French (2001).

56 'Sed sit diligentissimum studium in dando sibi alacritatem et bonam spem et permutando cogitationes suas quadam die ad vnam rem delectabilem et honestam, alia die ad aliam. Et hoc aut videndo diuersa ornamenta pulchra vel ioculatoria, aut audiendo sonos et cantilenas, aut in legend aliquid non difficile sed vel hystoriam vel aliam rem sibi caram, vel odorando vel ordinando sibi vestes, vel aptando domos et viridaria et

possessions, et aliis modis similibus' (*Consilia Ugonis Senensis* [edition of Venice, 1495?], f. 13r; ed. and tr. Olson 1982: 60n36).

57 Bertiz (2003: 100).

58 The illustrated version of the *Tacuinum* was especially popular among the elite of Lombardy. For a brief description of the *Tacuinum* and its historical relationship to the *Carrara Herbal*, see Introduction, p. 8. The scholarly literature on the *Tacuinum* is extensive. The following bibliography is not comprehensive; but, as a starting point, see the classic discussions of the *Tacuinum* in Sarton and Thorndike (1928); Pächt (1950); Unterkircher (1967 and 1986); Witthoft (1973 and 1978); and Cogliati Arano (1976 and 1988); as well as the more recent analyses in Dixon (1990); Elkhadem (1990; especially on the text of the *Tacuinum*); Opsomer-Halleux (1991 and 2003); Sigler (1992); Moly Mariotti (1993); Segre Rutz (2000 and 2002: 123–70); Bertiz (2003); Hoeniger (2006); and Touwaide (2009c–f). Regarding the illustrated copies of the *Tacuinum*, in particular, Bertiz (2003: 14–18) provides concise descriptions of the extant copies and their provenances along with their relevant historiographies.

59 Bertiz (2003: 205–12).

60 Olson (1982: 76–8).

61 De Premierfait's 'spirits' ('esperitz') can be understood both in the sense of improving one's mood (spirit) and in the way Avicenna conceived of *spiritus* (*rouh*), as a literal substance central to preservation of bodily health but fundamentally connected to emotions (to the psychology of an individual). The passage from de Premierfait's prologue reads: 'after difficult and burdensome work, whether physical or mental, it is natural that everyone restore his energy either through the help of food or through some proper pleasure in which the soul takes delight. . . . Since you and other earthly rulers represent divine power and majesty, I say that just as joyful and happy praise from the heart should be sung or spoken before the heavenly and omnipotent Lord, so it is proper before earthly lords that stories be told in an agreeable way and with proper language in order to gladden and cheer people's spirits. For in order to be more fully worthy in the eyes of God, rulers and all men may prolong their lives in any rational way consonant with God and nature' ('selon ordre de Nature, aprez griefves et pesantes besongnes traictees par labour corporel ou par subtillité d'engin, il affiert que chascun home refreschisse ses forces ou par confort de viands ou par aucune honneste leesse, en quoy l'ame prengne delectacion. . . . puisque vous et autres princes terriens portez la representacion et figure de puissance et magesté divine, je di que, ainsi comme devant Dieu celeste et tout puissant doivent ester chantees ou dictes loanges de cueur joieux et esbaudi, aussi devant les princes licitement peuent ester racomptees nouvelles soubz gracieuses manieres et honnestes paroles pour leesser et esbaudir les esperitz des homes, car pour plusamplement meriter envers Dieu il est permis aux princes et aussi a tous homes alongner leurs vies par toutes voies consones a Dieu et a Nature acompaignee de Raison') (de Premierfait, *Prologue* [ed. di Stefano 1998: 3–4; tr. Olson 1982: 76]). Di Stefano's edition of de Premierfait's translation derives from the oldest extant manuscript copy, now Rome, Biblioteca Apostolica Vaticana, Pal. lat. 1989, which dates to 1414–1418, and which may have been created under de Premierfait's direction. See di Stefano (1998: xii–xiii). For an alternative analysis of this passage, see Olson (1982: 75–7).

62 On Avicenna's sources of joy, see p. 77.

63 This idea also features in the Pseudo-Aristotelian *Secretum secretorum*, a treatise to which I will return in the next chapter.

64 Olson (1982: 94–8).

65 Aristotle, *Ethica ad Nicomachum*, X.VI.6 (ii) (1176b34–1177a1) (ed. and tr. Rackham 1934: 611).

66 Aquinas, *Ethicorum Aristotelis ad Nichomachum expositio*, X, lectio IX (tr. Litzinger 1964: 2.900–1). For an edition of the original Latin, see Spiazzi (1964: 538). For another interpretation of Aquinas's gloss, see Olson (1982: 95). Notably, and as Olson (1982: 97) also points out, in Article II of Question 168 of Aquinas's great opus on Christian

theology, *Summa theologica* (written 1265–1274), the philosopher discusses the potential virtue in play (*in ludis*). He suggests that, when strained, the soul tires just like the body. For Aquinas, contemplation is the most tiring because it requires a person to transcend his natural *sensibilia*, which causes greater tiredness. The remedy, for Aquinas as for Aristotle (who also associates virtuous activity with contemplation in the *Ethics*, X.VII.2 [1177a19–25]), is to rest the soul. Pleasure is this rest. Olson (1982: 95–7) likens Aquinas's comment on the relationship between pleasure and the soul to sleep and the body.

67   Written on the back of the 1404 inventory of Francesco's library is a list of books loaned prior to the seizure of Carrara effects and property by Venice's 'Council of Ten' in 1406 (see Lazzarini 1901–1902: 26). For example, on 4 August, Milone, natural son of Francesco Novello, borrowed the *Tesaurus pauperum* (likely the *Thesaurus pauperum* [*Treasure of the Poor*] by Peter of Spain [fl. thirteenth century], a work traditionally bound with the *Secretum secretorum*. See Chapter 3, p. 100). Milone returned the volume on 15 August. This loan history is evidence that Francesco Novello's collection, like that of his father, circulated at court and helped disseminate his self-image.

3   The 'physician prince' and his book

While the *Carrara Herbal* is the only identified illustrated medical treatise from Francesco Zago's partial inventory of Francesco Novello's book collection, it was one among many treatises on medicine.[1] Over two-thirds of the books listed and described by Zago concern the theory and practice of medicine or remedial therapy. In addition to Serapion's work, Francesco's library included Latin and vernacular translations of medical treatises by the canonical physicians Avicenna (Ibn Sīnā, ca. 908–1037) and Rhazes (al-Rāzī, ca. 854–925 or 935).[2] But the library also included treatises penned by contemporary local physicians like Marsilio da Santa Sofia (d. 1405) and Piero da Pernumia (d. after 1393), who was court physician to Francesco's father.[3] These contents point to Francesco's interest in medicine, in general, and to his support of local physicians and the medical schools at the University of Padua, in particular.

The subjects in Francesco's medical books mirror those encountered by the medical students during their training. Students at the university were required to read the works of Galen, Rhazes and Avicenna, along with *consilia* and compendia of medical recipes akin to those in Francesco's collection.[4] The works of Aristotle and those attributed to Hippocrates were also central to the medical school curriculum.[5] In terms of medical botany, the primary sources – in addition to Galen – were Dioscorides and Pliny.[6] By the early fourteenth century, Pietro d'Abano (1257–ca. 1315) lectured on Dioscorides' *De materia medica* – including the original Greek rather than only earlier Latin versions.[7] Furthermore, the Paduan physician noted his consultation of Serapion's work and the use of this material in his teaching.[8] Yet the versions of these books in Francesco's library were far from the humble and generally unillustrated versions acquired and studied by the medical students.[9] Rather, as we saw in Chapter 2, Francesco's books conveyed medical knowledge in a manner befitting a prince.

Part of Francesco Novello's purpose in developing his library was the celebration of medical knowledge and local physicians in light of their specific connections to the Carrara family and to Padua. To do so, Francesco's collection, and the *Carrara Herbal* in particular, defied the strict categorisation associated with book collection in the late Middle Ages. Its hybrid form suggests that it drew from the many aspects of book culture in northern Italy, from the university to the court, from learned study to prestigious and pleasurable entertainment. In its makeup and presentation, the *Carrara Herbal* crossed the boundaries between university textbooks and courtly codices and effectively brought university medicine under the purview of the court. In bridging the conceptual space between the university and the court, Francesco Novello's personal library demonstrated his interest in the university while remaining an indisputable sign of his princely status.

The *Carrara Herbal* enabled its patron and principal viewer, Francesco Novello, to portray himself as the orchestrator of different value systems circulating in Padua. Both in his book collection and in his role as patron, Francesco connected the courtly, social mores established by his father and encouraged by Petrarch with the hierarchy of medical learning epitomised by the university. The development of a new social role at court – that of the court physician – mirrored this fusion. Moreover, by adopting the figure of the court physician as a foil for his identity as prince, Francesco structured his persona in a manner different from and yet akin to that of his father. The making and circulation of the *Carrara Herbal* gave definition to Francesco Novello's self-image not only as a Carrara prince but as a metaphorical physician for the people of Padua as well. Both the form and content of the manuscript provided tools that enabled Francesco to construct an image of himself as a 'physician prince'.

From the university library to the prince's *studiolo*

In its form, the *Carrara Herbal* shares many of the distinctive characteristics of the *libri di banco* (desk books) produced and used in university centres from the twelfth century onward. Like other books of this kind, the *Herbal* is a large volume,[10] subdivided into sections that are demarcated by colourful indicators of various sorts: rubrics and red and blue enlarged initials, for instance. These colourful guides, accompanied by the scribe's clear gothic miniscule script, contributed to ease of reading and memorisation. Abbreviation of common terms and enlargement of margins to allow space for notation were also characteristic of such books.

Although the *Herbal* shares the content of the books studied at the medical school and the initial appearance of a *libro del banco*, it differs from them in a number of significant ways. Firstly, the *Herbal* was written in the Paduan vernacular, the language of court and city, rather than in Latin, the language of the university and scholarship. Secondly, the text block occupies the full width of the page rather than two columns, as in a typical desk book. Thirdly, the book currently bears no evidence of having been chained to a desk, as were many *libri di banco*, for consultation by students and faculty.[11] Likely, readers would encounter the *Carrara Herbal* as part of Francesco's book collection in a secluded *studiolo*, or personal study or library, entrance to which was granted to privileged court intimates and guests. Perhaps most strikingly different of all, the *Carrara Herbal* is heavily illustrated, a characteristic it shares with the so-called 'courtly' codex, a form that developed in the Padovano and the Veneto during the thirteenth century.[12]

The courtly codex was a luxury book reserved for a privileged audience, an identity confirmed by the ubiquitous owner insignias found on these manuscripts. Written in the vernacular, the contents of courtly codices tend toward epic or romance poetry and prose, themes popular among the aristocracy.[13] Generally, they have a smaller format than a desk book, are penned in gothic textura on parchment and contain illustrations in fine pigments. In the *Carrara Herbal*, the artist applied many layers of paint to achieve the levels of opacity, density of colour and tonal variety that characterise the remarkable plant imagery. The opulent illustrations, along with the vernacular rendition of Serapion's treatise and the marked presence of family heraldry, most overtly indicate a shift away from the format of books associated with the universities toward the format of courtly production. Yet, while the *Carrara Herbal* shares the lucid presentation, beautiful illustration and vernacular language of the courtly codex, it does not quite fit into this category of book, either, due to its scholarly subject matter and large size.

The frontispiece to the *erbario* section of the *Carrara Herbal* illustrates this tension between book forms most concretely. It integrates Serapion's text with illustrations of a citron tree and the Carrara family's heraldry, as discussed in the Introduction (see Plate 1). Representations of the family's heraldic arms (*stemma*), centred in the upper and flanking margins, along with the shields of arms (*cimieri*) of the elder and younger Francesco and the personal devices (or 'badges') of Francesco Novello, punctuate a decorative border of stylised acanthus leaves.[14] In turn, this border, crowned with Francesco's initials in the uppermost corners, surrounds both the image of the citron tree and Serapion's textual content about the citron's medicinal significance.[15] In the visual language of the court, the heraldry and initials tell the viewer that although this large version of Serapion's pharmacopeia bears some resemblance to a university textbook, it belongs to the prince and to his ancestral family.

The Carrara *signori* used heraldic signs as markers of possession not only for their manuscripts but also for their architectural and fresco commissions, currency and personal seals. The family symbols provided concise, recognisable signs that represented the individual members of the Carrara family and their histories. In the *Carrara Herbal*, the family heraldry claims the book and its contents as Carrara possessions, but it also prompts the viewer to see Serapion's text and the plant imagery in direct relationship to the heraldry, stretching the boundaries between book types. Further, the artist portrayed the citron tree in a way that parallels the conceptual relationship between the heraldic signs and their owners (in which a symbolic, unreal image signifies a specific, real individual). Doing so, he integrated the types of imagery on the frontispiece and brought the visual rhetoric of the court to bear on the subject matter of the text.

The artist's portrayal of the citron tree is a hybrid of non-naturalistic and verisimilar representational types. The tree's body is disproportionate to the foliage and to the citrons, which the artist rendered naturalistically, emphasising the characteristic lanceolate leaves and the fruits' leathery rind and ovoid shape. This mode of representation, as neither extremely schematic nor highly naturalistic, lends the image an emblematic quality. In addition, the placement of the tree – situated in between two of Francesco Novello's personal devices and two Carrara *cimieri* in the lower margin – accentuates this association and presents the tree as a type of heraldry itself. Like the other forms of heraldry on the frontispiece, which are set against a solid-coloured ground and framed in gold, the citron tree is set against the pale vellum of the page and is framed by a colourful border adorned with gold. The composition of the frontispiece itself imitates that of the heraldry.[16]

Personal heraldic devices are comprised of symbolic designs (usually animals or plants) and accompanying mottos that explain the designs' meaning. If we consider the citron tree as a visual icon of one of Francesco Novello's personal badges (set as it is between two of his other badges), then the textual content above the tree becomes a type of personal motto. The text records Serapion's entry for the citron tree in the formula used for each plant throughout the codex, giving his advice about the tree's medicinal properties and about who will benefit from these properties. As a type of 'motto', such medical knowledge contributed to the prince's persona as an educated benefactor learned in the arts of the medical school he supported. As a new personal heraldic device, however, the illustration of the citron tree colours the perception of the remaining plant imagery in the codex. The illustrations, especially those combining the stylistic cues of both the verisimilar and the schematic modes, function as a different type of heraldry through which readers could mentally connect the image to a real object – not just to the plant portrayed, but to the Carrara lord and to his book.

The frontispiece, then, shows the reader that the *Carrara Herbal* is a courtly codex, while its scholarly content and size mark it as a university textbook. Just as its imagery and text are combinations of different illustrative and knowledge traditions, so the *Herbal* itself is a combination of book forms. This merging of book forms recalls the bond between the university and the court, a bond formed at the beginning of the Carrara seigniory. In order to better understand the significance of the relationship between the Carrara lords and the university, and so the motivation behind the commission of the *Herbal* as a courtly university book, it is necessary first to understand the significance of the university to the city of Padua.

The University of Padua and its scholars: 'Tamquam filios' of the Carrara princes

Considered a crowning ornament of Padua since its inception in the first quarter of the thirteenth century, the university played a large role in the city's economy and its politics during both the communal and seigniorial periods.[17] The statute of election for the first Carrara *signore*, Giacomo I 'il Grande' da Carrara (1264–1324, r. 1318–1320) reflects the importance of this role.[18] When the Major Council (*Maggior Consiglio*) of the Commune of Padua elected Giacomo I as *Defensor, Protector et Gubernator populi paduani* (Defender, Protector and Governor of the Paduan people) on 25 July 1318, he was granted wide-ranging military and legal powers and responsibilities that included the support of the university and protection of its scholars.[19] The statute tells us that Giacomo's role as protector of the university was second in importance only to his role as defender of the city.[20] As Captain General, Giacomo's foremost duty was the defence of Padua against Cangrande della Scala (1291–1329), lord of Verona, and the provision of supplies and food for the city – the principal reasons for his election in the first place.

However, the edicts of the election statute specifically stipulate the relationship between the Carrara prince and the University of Padua: the university's students and faculty were to be like sons ('tamquam filios') to Giacomo.[21]

As Giacomo's 'sons', the members of the university were related to the Carrara ruler. Metaphorically speaking, the university, its students and professors became part of a Carrara genealogy. Giacomo's promise to nurture his generative bond with the university inaugurated the Carrara family's tradition of university patronage, a tradition that continued for the duration of the dynasty. The Carrara prince became a symbolic father whose paternal function was fulfilled by the continued success of his 'sons' – the university students and faculty. As sons of the Carrara, these men were not only products of Padua's great university but also products of Carrara patronage. Their successes reflected positively on their makers.

To legitimate and celebrate their seigniory, subsequent Carrara lords followed Giacomo il Grande's precedent and accounted for the university in their patronage and rule. They pledged to assure its continued vitality, and that vitality brought praise to the family as benevolent and generous rulers. Beginning with Giacomo's election, the family continued and expanded the original privileges granted by the Commune of Padua to students and professors at the university, privileges that included fiscal and tax incentives to settle in the city. The Carrara rulers also actively courted students and professors from other universities, especially from Bologna.[22]

Francesco il Vecchio (r. 1350–1388), for his part, provided funding for a college of disadvantaged international students and, doing so, set a philanthropic precedent of endowment that was followed by other prominent citizens.[23] Earlier in the Carrara rule, Ubertino da Carrara (r. 1338–1345) established an important exchange between Paduan and Parisian medical students to bring fresh knowledge into the medical school.[24] In his biography of the Carrara *signori*, the *Liber de principibus Carrariensibus et gestis eorum* (*The Book of the Carrara Princes and Their Deeds*, ca. 1402), written during Francesco Novello's rule, humanist Pier Paolo Vergerio (ca. 1369–1444) specifically praised Ubertino for his visible support of the city and the university. He praised the lord for commissioning large public buildings and the first clock tower, repairing roads and completing the city walls, securing provisions during famine and spurring the economy through support of the guilds. In the same passage, however, Vergerio also praised Ubertino for increasing financial support to the University of Padua, sponsoring the Paduan students at the University of Paris and persuading the locally renowned professor of law Raniero Arsendi (1292–1358) to settle in Padua and lecture at the university.[25]

For Francesco Novello's part, he continued to entice famous teachers to Padua with property grants. Notably, for 29 parcels of land, Francesco brought the physician and professor Niccolò da Fano (fl. late fourteenth/early fifteenth century) to Padua, where he served as professor of medicine at the university from 1393–1405.[26] In addition, after years of bickering between the judicial and medical schools in the university, the younger Francesco finally made the medical schools' administrative autonomy a reality in 1399. As with all major Italian universities, the University of Padua comprised four schools: the university and doctoral college of jurists and their counterparts in the arts and medicine. The jurists' schools long claimed administrative primacy over their counterparts in the arts and medicine.[27] The official separation of the medical and judicial universities and doctoral colleges was one of the major accomplishments of Francesco Novello's seigniory, and it attested to his championship of medical study.[28] It also attested to the rapid rise of Padua's medical schools in prestige and influence. During the Carrara rule, and especially after 1350, the medical schools expanded rapidly and so demanded greater autonomy from the jurists' regulations. The University of Padua became known widely as a pre-eminent centre of medical study, arguably surpassing Bologna.[29] Respected scientists and physicians, nearly half of whom came from Padua and the Padovano, filled the ranks of the professoriate.[30]

As the various schools grew in prestige and population, students and faculty gained greater prominence in the civic and court life of Padua.[31] Professors of both jurists' and medical schools and members of the medical guilds served as consultants and diplomats in the Carrara government. For instance, the son of Raniero Arsendi, the jurist Arsendino Arsendi (d. ca. 1389), and the scientist and physician Giovanni Dondi dall' Orologio (1330–1388) were part of a war council convened in July 1372 in the early days of the disastrous Border War with Venice.[32] Arsendi also served as an ambassador to Florence, Ferrara and the papacy and as envoy to Venice during the turbulent 1370s.[33] At Francesco il Vecchio's behest, Giovanni Dondi constructed a planetary clock for public display that charted the movements of the celestial bodies according to the Ptolemaic system. The clock brought even more praise to the learned men of the university and to the city of Padua. Such visible participation of the university's jurists and physicians in the governance and civic life of Padua reveals the living relationship between the Carrara and the city's institution of learning.

The increasingly visible role of the university faculty in public processions and family rituals points to the need for continued renewal of the symbolic bond between court and university during times of celebration and transition. Doctors of medicine and law played key roles in the funeral of Petrarch in July 1374, Francesco Novello's wedding to Taddea d'Este (1365–1404) in May 1377, and the funeral procession of Francesco il Vecchio in November 1393. Paduan chroniclers recorded all these events in exceptional detail, testifying to the importance of the university and its members in the official life of the city.

For instance, in the *Cronaca carrarese* (*The Chronicle of the Carrara*), the Paduan chroniclers Galeazzo Gatari (1344–1405) and his sons Andrea (ca. 1370–d. after 1454) and Bartolomeo (1380–1439)[34] described the events surrounding Petrarch's death on 19 July 1374. Gatari recounted that upon learning of the poet's death,[35]

> Signore Francesco da Carrara, Prince of Padua, with many archbishops, bishops, abbots, priors, monks and universally all the clergy of Padua and of the Padovano, and the knights and doctors and scholars of Padua, went together [to the village of Arquà on the mountain in Paduan territory] to honour [Petrarch's] remains.

Likewise, Andrea Gatari noted that Taddea d'Este, 'in a purple gown with the *carri* embroidered in coral' ('vestita di detta porpora con carri ricamati di coralli'), was escorted on the final leg of her wedding procession into Padua beneath a baldacchino carried by noblemen ('con un baldachino simile foderato di varij et portato da gentilhomini'), and surrounded by 'six knights, who guided her horse, and by all the doctors [of the University] on foot in their white gowns with hoods drawn, such that never did a bride to-be appear with such honour, honour enough for an empress' ('sei cavalieri havea atorno, che reggevano il cavallo, et tutti li dottori inanti vestiti di bianco con li suoi bavari et venivano a piedi, che mai fu vista donna andare a marito con simile honore bastevole certamente ad una imperatrice').[36]

Finally, commenting on the ritual procession for the elder Francesco's funeral, Galeazzo Gatari remarked that Francesco's casket was escorted to the church by 'the most famous doctors, in their hooded cloaks, who led the way and carried a baldacchino of gold cloth lined with ermine [above his casket]' ('perfino ala chiesia, sora la qual cassa era per famosisimi doctori, con loro capuzi di varo in testa, portado uno baldacchino di pano d'oro fodrado d'armelini').[37] The presence of these esteemed doctors in the funeral procession orchestrated by Francesco Novello – like their presence at the arrival of Taddea d'Este – visually connected the physical bodies of the Carrara with the physical bodies of the doctors, the tangible, living embodiments of the knowledge pursued in practice and perfected at the university. The doctors of medicine and law served as physical emblems of the university and its schools, and their participation in these significant rituals publicly acknowledged the university's importance to Padua and to its governing lords.

The *Carrara Herbal* provided a tangible point of access to the metaphorically generative union between the *signore* and the university. It was both a product and an emblem of the particular economy of knowledge and pleasure that defined Paduan culture under the Carrara. Where Francesco's library represented the collected knowledge of court and university, the *Herbal* represented the bringing together of this knowledge in a tangible way that befit the *signore* of Padua. If the *Carrara Herbal* was one product of the union between the Carrara seigniory and the university medical schools under Francesco Novello, another – although not one unique to Padua – was the growing social position of court physician.

The court physician was a practicing medical doctor and often a university scholar who served as a confidant to the *signore* and was part of his extended court family.[38] The position he came to occupy at court bridged the role of the physician and the role of the educated, humanist advisor. Along with promoting health regimens and prescribing medicines to treat any illnesses, the court physician was responsible for fostering the prince's moral character, and – like Petrarch and the humanist teachers of earlier generations – he promoted the study of history and the use of its great men as *exempla* for the prince.[39]

In his person and practice, the court physician merged the two defining patronage trajectories and social identities of the last two Carrara lords: he connected Francesco Novello's support of the university medical schools with his father's promotion of humanist ideals, especially of Petrarch's *viri illustres* as the exemplary predecessors of the Carrara rulers. As an ideal, the court physician embodied both the continuity between the Carrara rulers and the new direction of patronage particular to Francesco Novello's identity as ruler: it was the perfect complement to the *Carrara Herbal* and foil for the book's owner.

The court physician in Padua

The career and writings of University of Padua-trained professor and physician Michele Savonarola (1385–1466) reflect the fusion of university and court values in the last days of the Carrara rule of Padua.[40] Savonarola, who left his post as a professor of medicine at the University of Padua in 1440 to pursue a position as court physician to the d'Este rulers of Ferrara, wrote two treatises, in particular, that reveal his background very clearly. The *Libellus de magnificis ornamentis regie civitatis Padue* (*Book of the Magnificent Ornaments of the Regal State of Padua*, ca. 1446)[41] is a guide to the city's monuments and a biography of Padua's prominent citizens – living and dead – written in the tradition of Petrarch's *De viris illustribus* (*On Famous Men*).[42] This work illustrates the social hierarchy at the Carrara court and the place of medical doctors within it. Savonarola's treatise, *Del felice progresso di Borso d'Este* (*The Felicitous Progress of Borso d'Este*, ca. 1455),[43] written for the lord of Ferrara – Borso d'Este (1413–1471; r. 1450–1471) – and his court intimates, provides further evidence of how physicians worked at court.[44] Although Savonarola wrote his treatises in Ferrara, he drew upon his experiences in Padua for their content, which makes his work important evidence of the Paduan cultural milieu in the early fifteenth century.[45]

Savonarola's earlier work, the collection of biographies, provides concrete evidence of the high status accorded to physicians during the Carrara rule and afterwards, when Padua became part of the Venetian republic. In the *Libellus*, Savonarola ranked contemporary Paduans and Paduans of recent history according to the perceived social value of their professions and occupations – including arts and letters, medicine and law.[46] At first glance, it appears that Savonarola ranked the study of law above that of medicine, which was customary; however, his placement of Padua's most renowned medical son, Pietro d'Abano, as the leader in his category of (natural) philosophers complicates the initial picture of the social hierarchy.[47] Philosophers, both moral and natural, had a higher position on the social scale than military and political leaders, jurists, and physicians.[48] Savonarola placed Pietro d'Abano in a social position second only to that of theologians. That is, he placed Pietro at the height of the secular social ladder.[49] In doing so, Savonarola demonstrated for his reader that he considered medicine a truly worthy pursuit, one that was highly valued by the court.

Following Pietro, Savonarola ranked Petrarch and the local humanists, Albertino Mussato (d. 1329) and Lovato Lovati (ca. 1237–1309), among the (moral) philosophers. This placement prefigures (perhaps even predetermines) Savonarola's own association between medicine and moral history in his work at Borso's court. Savonarola placed Pietro, as the most esteemed practitioner and theorist of medicine, alongside Petrarch, Mussato and Lovati, poet-chroniclers whose works

Savonarola lauded for their moral authority and as historical record.[50] All three poets employed history as a moral guide for their readers. Alternatively, Pietro d'Abano's medical theories discuss the relationship between medical treatment and a patient's history, astrological chart, behavioural and moral tendencies, and elemental complexion. The proximity of these figures at the height of the secular social hierarchy presented in Savonarola's work points to the evolution of the new role of the court physician. Their elevation also marks the value invested in the court physician as a figure who combined the characteristics of these great men to the benefit of the prince and his court.[51]

In the sense that he occupied a social role that combined the knowledge and values of Pietro d'Abano with those of Petrarch and the local humanists, the court physician himself occupied the pinnacle of the secular social hierarchy. In *Del felice progresso*, Savonarola provided a glimpse into this role, revealing his place as a privileged member of the court's most intimate circle. While it was not a *consilium* of medical prescriptions, *Del felice progresso* complemented Savonarola's traditional health regimen for Borso by combining observations and advice on the prince's good health with a moralistic history that narrates his life and government.[52] In effect, *Del felice progresso* is a moralised chronicle of the prince's life that, by virtue of its author's profession, also contains prescriptions for the maintenance of his moral and physical health.[53] In its form and in its content, *Del felice progresso* is representative of the marriage between the role of the physician and that of the moralising poet-historian.[54]

As Borso d'Este's physician, Savonarola composed a *regimen sanitatis* in the vernacular, entitled *Libreto de tutte le cose* (*The Little Book of All Things*), which prescribed exercise and dietary methods to help keep the prince's body healthy.[55] But, as Savonarola's *Del felice progresso* demonstrates, the court physician's role did not stop with such corporeal prescriptions. In his narrative of Borso's life, Savonarola prescribed methods to keep the prince's morality healthy, describing 18 virtues necessary for a good ruler and focussing especially on prudence.[56] He urged the prince to study history's exemplars, including the recent history of successful rule of Ferrara, under Leonello d'Este (1407–1450; r. 1441–1450), and of Padua, under Francesco il Vecchio. Savonarola's programme for the maintenance of the prince's well-being combined ethics, devotion and physical health. It included dietetic, educational and spiritual advice written specifically for the prince.[57] Yet Savonarola modelled his advice on that compiled in other popular guidebooks for rulers, especially the Pseudo-Aristotelian treatise known as the *Secretum secretorum* (*The Secret of Secrets*) and in its more literary and philosophical cousin, *De regimine principum* (*On the Government of Princes*).[58]

The tools of the court physician's trade: Secretum secretorum *and* De regimine principum

The *Secretum secretorum* is a Latin translation of an Arabic treatise, the *Kitāb sirr al-asrār*, which has both long and short versions. The Arabic versions developed between the eighth and eleventh centuries and were in circulation in Latin translation in fragmentary form from the early twelfth century, and in a longer version from the thirteenth.[59] In the late thirteenth century, Giles of Rome (Egidio Romano, ca. 1243–1316) wrote *De regimine principum*.[60] Giles' treatise is a contribution to the *Speculum principis* (*Mirror of Princes*) literary genre; its content draws upon Thomas Aquinas's commentary on Aristotle's politics and ethics.[61] Savonarola references the *Secretum* directly, both in his earlier work on physiognomy, the *Speculum phisionomie* (*The Physiognomic Mirror*, 1442),[62] written for Borso's brother, Leonello d'Este, the former *signore* of Ferrara, and in *Del felice progresso*.[63] While he does not refer to Giles' treatise openly, Savonarola copied the work almost word for word in many instances, especially in Book III of *Del felice progresso*, which deals with how to choose wise counsellors.[64]

Both the *Secretum* and *De regimine* were advice manuals addressed to privileged readers, often to a prince, and were popular with scholarly and lay audiences during the late Middle Ages. They both participate, to different degrees, in the *Speculum principis* tradition: both discuss political matters, provide detailed advice on statecraft, emphasise a relationship between princely conduct and the health of the state, and give examples of proper ethical behaviour. The *Secretum*, however, distinguishes itself from other works in the *Speculum principis* tradition because it also includes detailed (if sometimes contradictory) medical information and a wealth of other arcana.[65] Considered in a different way, the *Secretum* adds the flesh of a medical textbook and encyclopaedia of lore to the skeleton of a *Speculum principis*. The combination of these genres was central to Savonarola's *Del felice progresso*[66] and would become the hallmark of the court physician's approach to medicine and his role in court society.

The *Secretum* is meant to be a letter from the aging Aristotle to his former student, Alexander the Great (356–323 BCE), sent during Alexander's campaign to conquer the Persian Empire (ca. 334–328 BCE). The history of the *Secretum*'s transmission is complex: its structure is heterogeneous, and it appears in various forms in its many translations and revisions. The work may have begun as a behavioural treatise (a *Speculum principis*) comprised of Aristotelian pseudepigrapha of either Hellenistic or Roman origin.[67] Yet, over its lengthy history, the *Secretum* accrued its encyclopaedic content, likely from a variety of Greek and Syriac sources, making it what Regula Forster aptly terms 'an encyclopaedic mirror for princes'.[68] However, while no original text can be identified and its recensions are highly diverse in their thematic foci, the *Secretum* – in all its manifestations – gives some advice on how to preserve the prince's health as well as advice on statecraft, learning and the importance of virtuous behaviour.[69]

In its Latin short version, dating to ca. 1120, Johannes Hispaniensis (perhaps better known as John of Seville, fl. 1120–1153) translated parts of the Arabic version and married it to a set of dietetic and hygienic advice.[70] John addressed the treatise to a recipient identified only as 'Lady T., by the grace of God Queen of the Spains',[71] who may be Teresa (1080–1130), the Countess of Portugal and illegitimate daughter of Alfonso VI (1040–1109), King of Léon and Castile.[72] In his prefatory remarks, John described the work as his response to Lady T.'s request for a dietary regimen to preserve her health. He tells the lady that after she made her request, he (felicitously) remembered an example of just such a regimen found in Aristotle's letter to Alexander, 'that is', he writes, in 'the *Secret of Secrets*'.[73] Here, John plays to the epistle's legendary authority to convey his rather mundane dietetic advice.[74]

As Forster argues, the form of the text – what she calls the *mise en scène* of the epistle from Aristotle as 'the first teacher' – cloaks what amounts to basic information about health (and, in its longer forms, other commonplace knowledge) with the allure of exclusivity and secrecy.[75] Whether applied to issues of health maintenance or to any of the other categories of advice included in the *Secretum*, this exclusivity appealed to elite readers and ensured the genre's longevity. The large number of extant manuscripts produced in the Latin West attest to the work's popularity: in its 'short form', about 150 Latin manuscripts and many others in European vernaculars are extant.[76] In its 'long form', the more complete translation from the Arabic into Latin made by Philip of Tripoli (fl. 1227–1259) in the early 1230s, over 350 Latin manuscripts are extant.[77] Indeed, it was a 'medieval bestseller'.[78]

In the long version of the *Secretum*, Book I and part of Book II describe the ideal relationship between ethics and politics – that is, they form a traditional *Speculum principis*, content paralleled in Giles of Rome's later *De regimine principum*.[79] Yet, beyond describing the prince's behaviour, physical bearing and ideal moral qualities, the author of the *Secretum* provided additional medical knowledge specific to a prince's constitution. Midway through Book II, the author deviates from his discussion of the prince's moral character and turns to a detailed account of his health, diet and hygiene (a *regimen sanitatis*). He then closes the book with an account of the importance of physiognomy – the art of divining people's characters based on features of their bodies and behaviours – to the prince's body of knowledge. The treatise's later books contain information about plant medicine (an herbal) and medicines derived from stones (a lapidary), as well as information on the 'secret arts' of alchemy, astrology and oneiromancy allegedly preserved from long-lost Greek sources.[80]

After its introduction (in its long form) in the 1230s, the *Secretum* joined a growing corpus of translations of Aristotelian works studied and circulated at the universities.[81] Initially, the *Secretum* was read and annotated mostly by university doctors and scholars of medicine and ethics: by the mid-thirteenth century, it was a prized addition to scientific and moral teaching at universities, especially at Paris and Oxford. Roger Bacon (ca. 1214–1294), Albertus Magnus (ca. 1208–1280), Pietro d'Abano and Jean Buridan (ca. 1300–1361), among many great Schoolmen, all commented on or extensively cited the treatise.[82] With such a legacy, Savonarola's familiarity with the book is unsurprising.

As William Eamon has discussed, although the popularity of the *Secretum* waned at the university throughout the fourteenth and fifteenth centuries, it continued to grow at court, especially among the educated lay readers of the aristocracy.[83] Thus, it is likely that Savonarola would have known the *Secretum* through a more courtly context, as well. Young university graduates – perhaps even Savonarola himself – often used the work as an introduction into court life after leaving the academy.[84] With its allure of mystery and promise of shared secrets, the *Secretum* became a type of heraldic badge that represented the new graduates' privileged knowledge while advancing their identity as trustworthy intellectuals and allies to the prince.[85] A scholarly ally, as the *Secretum* also notes, is important to the prince's well-being and to the success of his rule. Using metaphors of the healthy body, the author of the *Secretum* noted that 'understanding' (*intellectus*) or knowledge[86]

> is the head of government. It is the health of the soul, the preserver of virtue, and the mirror of vice. By it are hateful things cast off and worthy things chosen. It is the fountainhead of virtue and the root of all good, praiseworthy, and honourable things.

The court physician was the point of access to this knowledge for his prince.

Michele Savonarola – as just such a court physician – also turned to the often-complementary work by Giles of Rome, *De regimine principum*, when composing his advice for Borso d'Este. Savonarola considered *De regimine principum* required reading for any prince, and for Borso in particular. Borso's father, Niccolò III d'Este (1383–1441), owned a copy of the treatise, so it was in circulation at the court of Ferrara during the rules of both his sons, Leonello and Borso.[87] While undoubtedly influenced by Giles' treatise, Savonarola ameliorated parts of it to suit his needs.[88] For instance, in Book III, which incorporated Giles' brief foray into dietetics, Savonarola added advice premised on his own observations. He also tailored Giles' discussion of princely virtues to show Borso as an exemplary prince (or, more likely, to encourage such exemplarity).[89] Furthermore, like Petrarch in his letters to Francesco il Vecchio and in his *De remediis utriusque fortunae* (*On the Remedies for Different Fortunes*), Savonarola discussed politics in medical terms; but, unlike the humanist's metaphors, Savonarola's comparisons were grounded in experience.[90]

In *Del felice progresso*, Savonarola argued that the moral and physical health of the prince was essential to the health of the city. He even compared the role of the physician to that of the prince, explaining that the arts of healing and healthy living directly related to the art of governing well.[91] The true prince must be like a (court) physician to his people. Savonarola, following the humanistic example, emphasised the need for Borso to study the lives of great men and to emulate them in order to prepare for the future, nurture his soul, and secure the moral health of his community. He advised Borso to study Roman history in the humanistic sense, the sense of 'historia magistra vitae est', as a guide to life; specifically, as a guide to a Christian life.[92] But Savonarola's advice did not stop with ethical recommendations based on historical accounts, as Petrarch's and other humanists' had done. Savonarola coupled his moral and intellectual prescriptions with physical ones. Not only could he promote the 'health of the soul' and the prince's virtues with his humanistic knowledge; as a court physician, Savonarola promoted the 'health of the body' with his medical skills as well. Providing the keys to the health of the prince's body and soul, Savonarola helped to secure the health of his government.

While the *Secretum* and Giles' *De regimine principum* (and other treatises written in the *Speculum principis* tradition) share and convey ethical, medical and political advice, the detail and emphasis placed on this advice differentiates them.[93] Part of Savonarola's genius in writing *Del felice progresso* was his ability to blend these genres – among others – to create a new form of advice manual tailored to Borso's strengths (and weaknesses) and to court life in Ferrara. These genres, however, have a history of such hermeneutical flexibility. The treatises bound to the *Secretum* in the construction of individual codices clarify some of the similarities and differences between the *Secretum* and other works written in the tradition of the *Speculum principis*. Moreover, they show how these genres often intertwined.

In manuscripts produced during the thirteenth century, the first century of the treatise's circulation in long form, the *Secretum* was bound to medical compendia (such as Peter of Spain's *Thesaurus pauperum* [*Treasure of the Poor*]) or to Aristotelian or Pseudo-Aristotelian moral treatises (such as the *Ethica ad Nicomachum* [*Nicomachean Ethics*], *Physiognomonica* [*Physiognomonics*], *Politica* [*Politics*], *Ars rhetorica* [*Rhetoric*], *Œconomica* [*Economics*], *Magna moralia* [*Great Ethics*], and *Liber de Pomo* [*Kitāb al-Tuffāḥa*, *The Book of the Apple*]) or to commentaries on these moral treatises (like Giles of Rome's *De regimine principum*).[94] The treatises to which the *Secretum* was bound often reflect the principal interests of their owners – either in medicine and the 'secrets of nature' or in ethics and politics – and suggest the many roles the *Secretum* played both in university and court settings.[95] These flexible roles are central to understanding the development of the figure of the court physician, more generally, and to Savonarola's blending of genres in *Del felice progresso* in particular.

The idea of the healthy body of the prince and the use of his body as a metaphor for the state connects the *Secretum* and *De regimine principum* – regardless of their titles. The health of the prince's body is the literal subject of the medical contents in the *Secretum*, but it is also the metaphorical subject of the moral contents. Similarly, the *Speculum* tradition is concerned with the relationship between the prince's ethics and the overall health of his kingdom: the 'body' of his territories. In the sections dedicated to the prince's morality in both literary traditions, the authors use corporeal metaphors and references to sickness and health in order to describe the invisible moral system that supports good governance. This rhetorical strategy provides a point of continuity between the moral treatises of the humanists and philosophers and the medical ones of the physicians, a point to which I will return.[96] It also prefigures the court physician's role as a combination of the two.

The *Carrara Herbal* as the court physician's book

Considered through the lens of the developing role of court physician, the context within which to judge the form, style and content of the *Carrara Herbal* is far richer. Like all other medical treatises indebted to Galen's theory of medicine, Serapion's *Liber aggregatus de medicinis simplicibus* contains information on plants to complement the management of the external factors that influence an individual's health – the so-called six non-naturals.[97] For physicians like

Savonarola, as for Pietro d'Abano before him, the material contained in the *Carrara Herbal* would have been a source for the prescriptive medicines used to help patients regain their constitutional balance – their health – in response to an imbalance caused by one of the non-naturals.⁹⁸

More than simply accounting for the contents of the *Herbal*, however, there are aspects of Savonarola's writing that shed light on the remarkable pictorial language used in the *Herbal*. Along with his specific moral and medical prescriptions, Savonarola peppered the historical narrative in *Del felice progresso* with vivid details characteristic of contemporary chronicles. For instance, when he described court festivals, Savonarola specifically noted the colourful tapestries that hung on the walls, the beautiful clothing worn by the other courtiers and the identities of the important people attending the festivities.⁹⁹ He also inserted into his text local anecdotes taken from daily life in Ferrara and proverbs in current circulation at court. As Chiara Crisciani argues, in rhetorical practice, the use of such details legitimised Savonarola's narrative and aided in its persuasive efficacy.¹⁰⁰ It also allied his work with the chronicle tradition in Padua.

Savonarola employed an ornamented rhetoric, one filled with lengthy descriptions of contemporary experiences and culture, not simply to better persuade his audience but also to make his message more immediately relevant and memorable. His insertion of specific details of local concern into his writing served as an indicator of authorial objectivity, a technique broadly characteristic of the Paduan chronicles and the humanist milieu under Francesco Novello.¹⁰¹ Whereas Petrarch advocated and practiced an unornamented rhetoric to convey his moral messages, as his prose works demonstrate, Savonarola followed a different path. Rather, his use of verisimilitude stemmed from a tradition of moral storytelling particular to Padua: the chroniclers used inflated rhetoric to convey the moralistic histories with which they aimed to guide the moral life of the community.¹⁰² Likewise, Savonarola embellished his rhetoric to better convey his concern for the health of the prince, and so for the health of the prince's kingdom.

In all the Paduan chronicles from the thirteenth and fourteenth centuries with which I am familiar (and those from across northern Italy more broadly), the authors used verisimilar details to energise the past, to make it memorable and accessible to their audiences, and to suggest their authorial reliability. For instance, in his detailed description of Francesco il Vecchio's funeral procession mentioned earlier, Gatari emphasised the familial and communal heraldry used in the funeral procession. He used descriptive rhetoric to stress the apparent unity of the people under the Carrara lords – old and new. To get a sense of how his rhetoric accomplishes this goal, it is worth citing the passage at length. The *Cronaca* reads:¹⁰³

> On the 20th of the month [of November], being the fated hour and the grand congregation of clergy being therein, [the clergy] commenced to issue forth from the court and to process around the *piazze*, that is to [the *piazza*] of the Fruit and to [the *piazza*] of the Herbs [which flank the Palazzo della Ragione, the town hall] and on to the cathedral; after the clergy, one-hundred horsemen wearing sable [clothes of mourning] followed, each accompanied by a

servant dressed in black, with a shield bearing the arms of the Carrara hanging down from his neck, and a large banner shaking with his great grief. (Beside each horse walked two poor persons all dressed in grey cloth, and each carried a torch in his hand, given to him in charity. Four horsemen wearing the arms of the four quarters of the city followed them with banners, shields, and squires on foot as attendants). . . . After these, followed the multitude [of citizens] with candles burning . . . after these, followed the family of the *signore* all dressed in black crying out with plaintive voices, which shook the sky. There were, by numbers, 800 people; after them followed the bier that bore the body of the deceased. The casket was covered with a pall of cloth of gold lined with ermine, and was carried by noble knights to the church[;] around the casket were the most famous doctors, in their hooded cloaks, who led the way and carried a baldacchino of gold cloth lined with ermine [above the casket]: to the right of the casket, in profound dolour, came the *signore* dressed in sable [clothes] with two ambassadors from the *signoria* of Venice; after him, [followed] misser Francesco Terzo with ambassadors from the Commune of Florence; after him, followed Giacomo da Carrara with the Bolognese ambassadors; after him, [followed] Nicollò da Carrara with the Marchese ambassadors; after them, followed the other children of the House of Carrara . . . after these, the multitude of the people [followed], of which the majority were dressed in sable [clothes], [and] with cries and infinite wails, they all accompanied the casket to the cathedral, where the wife of the *signore* [Taddea d'Este] along with all the women of Padua cried out and wailed such that it was near impossible for me to write; . . . After accompanying the body to the church, the *signore* returned to court, where it was already the twenty-second hour, and he had begun the day at its first hour. After this, from the high portico of the palace, misser Giovanni Aluise de' Lambertazzi pronounced a sermon to laud the deceased *signore* and the house of the Carrara and the *signore* present therein, and to thank the noblewomen and noblemen there on the part of the *signore*. (Thus finished the sacred office, [and] not even for twenty-four hours was the body laid in the sepulchre in the baptistery, in the Chapel of Saint John the Baptist, when it was placed in an *arca* of red marble atop four columns in the middle of the chapel, where every day the office [for the dead] was celebrated with masses and orations for the soul of *signore*.)

Gatari's highly detailed description reveals that the procession maintained a strict order, an order designed to reflect the social and political hierarchy of Carrara Padua. His account also records that key components of the former lord's public character were emphasised visually through the choice of costumes and classes represented in the procession. Most notably, in his description of the procession's participants, Gatari highlighted Francesco il Vecchio's commitment to defending Padua militarily ('one hundred horsemen . . . all displaying the "del Carro" arms') and diplomatically ('[and then came] the Venetian ambassadors . . . with those of Florence and Bologna [and] . . . the ambassadors of Ferrara'), as well as his support and love for the university ('sixteen of the most learned doctors of the city') and the Church ('not fewer than twenty-four mitres [were present]').

Similarly, in the two orations he composed for Francesco il Vecchio's funeral,[104] Vergerio described in detail the rituals Francesco Novello organised in honour of the former *signore*, and he demonstrated the importance of visual details to memorialising and moralising the past in Carrara Padua.[105] A member of the third generation of early humanists (those after Boccaccio [1313–1375] and Lombardo della Seta [d. 1390]), Vergerio was Francesco Novello's court humanist and a tutor of the Carrara children during the last years of the dynasty. Vergerio's approach to language is not Petrarchan and may have influenced Michele Savonarola's rhetorical choices. Vergerio enlivened his orations with detailed descriptions and use of verbs associated with seeing and imagining, qualities central to the Paduan chronicle tradition.[106] As John M. McManamon has argued, Vergerio's principal rhetorical strategy as a teacher and orator was to create mental images that inspire using words, a Ciceronian technique aimed at making oratory more persuasive.[107] Like the chroniclers, Vergerio's writing style demonstrates a belief that vision was the most persuasive and authoritative of the senses.

In his description of the funeral rites in *De dignissimo funebri apparatu*, Vergerio – like Gatari – emphasised the structure and arrangement of the procession as a hierarchy of the proper, healthy body of the *signoria*.[108] Unlike Gatari, however, Vergerio directly connected his description of the funeral rites with an illustrious Roman history of Padua – a connection that Francesco il Vecchio had encouraged through his use of ancient Roman imagery in his artistic and literary commissions.[109] This association between Carrara Padua and Roman Padua articulated in an oration commissioned by Francesco Novello reveals that the younger Francesco was aware of how his father portrayed himself through his patronage choices. The form of Vergerio's detailed descriptions, however, shows Francesco Novello's own patronage strategy – characterised by the collection of chronicles and local histories (rather than legendary Roman ones) and books dedicated to knowledge of a healthy, ideal body. In effect, the description of Francesco il Vecchio's funeral illustrates a meeting of the two Carrara lords' self-images: in its content, Vergerio's oration connects Francesco il Vecchio's funerary rites to his legacy of patronage associated with the Roman world. In its use of the chroniclers' detailed language and in its portrayal of the body of the *signoria*, Vergerio's description highlights the new direction of Francesco Novello's patronage.

A visual rhetoric in the *Carrara Herbal*

In *Del felice progresso*, the *Cronaca carrarese* and *De dignissimo funebri apparatu*, Savonarola, Gatari and Vergerio all used details from daily life and personal experience to help convey their messages and to persuade the reader of their authorial objectivity. Savonarola's use of the chroniclers' rhetorical strategies in *Del felice progresso* most strikingly parallels the connection between chronicle culture and medical culture visualised in Francesco Novello's book collection. Like all good chroniclers and storytellers, Savonarola captivated his readers with his detailed descriptions of Borso's history and the events in which the *signore* participated. He appealed to his readers' sense of vision and borrowed a form associated with contemporaneous moral storytelling that would have been familiar to them. But Savonarola's use of visual details to capture his readers' attention also speaks in relative context to the varied use of representational techniques in the *Carrara Herbal*'s plant imagery.

The *Herbal* presents a distinctive reading and viewing experience in part through its diverse illustrations, which delight the readers, hold their interest and disrupt a passive reception of the book's content.[110] Like the use of highly detailed descriptions in Savonarola's work and in the Paduan chronicles and orations, the illustrative corpus of the *Herbal* certainly makes the book more memorable and impresses its textual and visual contents more firmly onto the readers' minds. The use of visual detail, in rhetoric as in illustration, suggests its currency as an effective and memorable communication device in Paduan court culture.

*

When Francesco Novello first came to power in 1390, after regaining Padua from Giangaleazzo Visconti (1351–1402), he had medals struck in celebration.[111] The medals provide another example of the visual and textual rhetorics in circulation in Paduan culture and their blending by the Carrara *signore*. In a way Vergerio's funerary oration for Francesco il Vecchio would reflect, the obverses of the medals show profile portraits of Francesco Novello and of his father in the tradition of the emperors' portraits on the bronze *sesterces* of early Imperial Rome.[112] The profile portraits mirror one another, drawing attention (on the one hand) to the lords' visual similarities as father and son and as members of the ruling family and (on the other) to the importance of a moralised vision of Roman culture to the Carrara sense of self (Figures 3.1 and 3.2). The portraits emphasise the importance of family genealogy to Francesco Novello and hint at the parallels he would deliberately construct between his rule of Padua and that of his father.

On the reverses of the medals, an inscription encircles a representation of the *carro*, the family's heraldic arms. It reads 'recuperavit Paduam' and gives the date of 19 June 1390. Of course, the inscription commemorates the date on which Francesco Novello 'recovered Padua' from Giangaleazzo Visconti. However, considered within the context of Francesco's book collection and the development of the figure of the court physician, it also celebrates Francesco's 'recovery' of Padua in a therapeutic sense. As a 'physician prince' and exemplar to his people, Francesco cured them from the ailment of Visconti occupation. He ousted the foreign occupier, physically purging the city of its 'illness', while his careful patronage and construction of personal exemplarity would project a moral recovery, too. In his role as benevolent ruler, Francesco recovered the health of his people and healed the city from the infection of bad government. Francesco would continue to cultivate this narrative of self throughout his rule using patronage strategies that associated him, alternatively, with the University of Padua's medical schools (as we have seen) and with the legacy of his father's support of the humanist poet Petrarch, to which we now will turn.

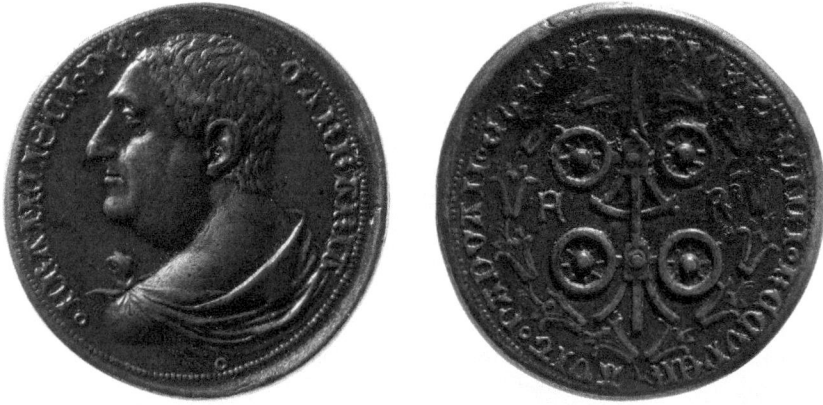

Figure 3.1 Anon., medal with portrait of Francesco il Vecchio

Obverse: FRANCISCI. DE CARRARIA.
Reverse: 1390. DIE. 19 IVNII. RECVPERAVIT. PADVAM. ET C.
Padua, Museo Bottacin, Inv. 89
3.5 cm diameter, bronze, Padua, ca. 1390

Su gentile concessione del Comune di Padova – Assessorato Cultura e Turismo

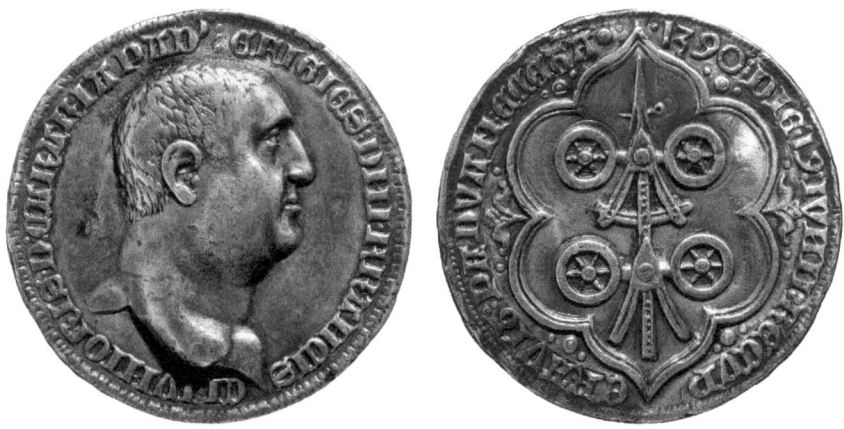

Figure 3.2 Anon., medal with portrait of Francesco Novello

Obverse: EFIGIES. DNI. FRANCISCI. IVNIORIS. D. CARARIA. PAD.
Reverse: 1390 DIE. 19. IVNII. RECVP-ERAVIT: PADVAM: ECETA.
Padua, Museo Bottacin, Inv. 796
3.3 cm diameter, silver, Padua, ca. 1390

Su gentile concessione del Comune di Padova – Assessorato Cultura e Turismo

Notes

1   Venice, Biblioteca Nazionale Marciana, lat. XIV, 93 (coll. 4530), fol. 147r. See Introduction p. 13n3, and Appendix.

2   Rhazes was a practicing physician and medical theorist in Baghdad. His theoretical works and commentaries were required reading at Islamic and European centres of medical learning. For an introduction to his life and work, see Richter-Bernburg (2006). On Avicenna and the Latin transmission of his work, see Chapter 2, pp. 76–7 and notes. Francesco Novello's collection included at least 24 treatises by Rhazes and Books I–III and V of Avicenna's *Liber Canonis* (*The Canon of Medicine*), along with two additional books of excerpts from Avicenna's work (see Chapter 2, p. 84n39, and Appendix).

3   The inventory lists two treatises written by respected local professors of medicine at the University of Padua: the *consiglio*, or book of collected medical advice and counsel, by Marsilio da Santa Sofia (number 36 on inventory) and a book of medical maxims on diet by Piero da Pernumia (number 38) (Lazzarini 1901–1902: 27).

4   For details of the university medical curriculum (as recorded in the earliest extant statutes from the University of Bologna in 1405), see Grendler (2002: 314–24). For a list of subjects specifically taught at Padua, see Grendler (2002: 24). From the thirteenth century on, the *Canon* by Avicenna was the basic medical theory taught at Italian universities during the Early Modern period (Siraisi 1987a, 1987b: 111 [repr. 2001b: 162–3] and 1994 [tr. 2001], and Crisciani 2005: 308). As Pesenti Marangon (1999) and Ongaro (2005: 192–3) have discussed, Avicenna's *Canon* was in circulation at the University of Padua by 1316, when the physician and professor Giovanni Mondino da Cividale (ca. 1275–1340), contemporary and colleague of Pietro d'Abano, wrote a commentary on its first book. Avicenna presented a view of medicine that complemented the prevailing Aristotelian natural philosophy taught at universities and integrated it with Galenic medicine (Grendler 2002: 320).

5   Grendler (2002: 314–18).

6   Grendler (2002: 343).

7   Pietro travelled to Constantinople and may have seen the illustrated Greek copy of Dioscorides' *De materia medica* now known as the *Vienna Dioscorides* (Vienna, Österreichische Nationalbibliothek, *medicus graecus* 1) (Reeds 1991: 16, and Touwaide 2008c: 601–3). On the *Vienna Dioscorides* and the illustrative traditions of the Greek herbals, see Chapter 1, pp. 32–6.

8   Siraisi (1973: 161); Bettini (1974: 57n11); and Grendler (2002: 343). Is it a coincidence that Padua's pre-eminent medical son, Pietro, would single out Serapion, the author of the text housed in the *Carrara Herbal*, as a reference and an illustrated version of Serapion's treatise would assume a vaunted position in Francesco Novello's library?

9   The university students often owned small, portable, inexpensive and unillustrated handbooks with similar medical content for individual study and practice. Records of the gate-toll (*gabella*) paid by book merchants when they came to sell their wares reveal a market for books of many different values, from illuminated manuscripts to everyday, unillustrated books for students, merchants and lay-people. Petrucci (1995: 189) cites the gate-tolls paid by book merchants entering Perugia in 1379. The toll varied according to the value of each book. He notes that the toll for bringing large missals, ecclesiastical books, bibles and breviaries into Perugia was 3 *soldi*; 2 *soldi* for law books, smaller format grammar and poetry books, and 6 *denari* for small books.

10 Petrucci (1995: 171–3) considers any book with a length over 30 cm a large format book.

11 The *Herbal* has been rebound at least twice, making it difficult to know with certainty whether the book originally was chained. The current binding, which did not alter the

size of the leaves, is the British Library's from 1965. However, during an eighteenth-century rebinding, the leaves of the *Herbal* likely were trimmed. The title page illumination and a number of the plant illustrations show slight loss on the interior margin, which attests to the resizing of the manuscript. This resizing could have removed evidence that the manuscript once was chained; however, this practice would have been unusual for a volume associated with a patrician book collection. In addition, the adornment on the title page of the interior margin of the *Carrara Herbal* is cut only fractionally compared to the corresponding marginalia on the exterior margin, which suggests that the current state of the manuscript still conveys a close approximation to the original. See Baumann (1974: 25–6), and Collins (2000: 279n162).

12 Petrucci (1995: 179–80).

13 Petrucci (1995: 181).

14 For heraldry types and associated vocabulary, see Boulton (1990). For detailed descriptions of the Carrara *stemma*, the *cimieri* and the badges on the frontispiece, see Introduction, pp. 6–7.

15 This addition was the final step in the manuscript's illustration, which was likely the work of three painters – one responsible for the plant images and two others dedicated to the additional ornament and heraldry (Baumann 1974: 26).

16 For further analysis of the frontispiece's imagery and a discussion of its rhetorical implications, see Kyle (2014).

17 For the history, economy and politics of Padua, see Hyde (1966b) (for communal Padua), and Kohl (1968 and 1998) (for seigniorial Padua). On the rise of the University of Padua, in particular, see Siraisi (1973).

18 For an introduction to Giacomo 'il Grande', see Ganguzza Billanovich (1977c).

19 His powers included command of the army, jurisdiction in court cases (civil and criminal), and the ability to appoint the commune's magistrates, its *podestà* (chief magistrate) and the *podestà*'s staff, as well as executive power over the treasury, the university, the election of officials and the development of new laws. The commune did enact safeguards to protect its rights: Giacomo swore to maintain his duties in public assembly, and a panel of eight jurists (*sapientes*) was commissioned to set and limit his salary (Kohl 1998: 39–41).

20 A copy of the statute of election, now Padua, Archivio Papafava dei Carraresi 39, parchment 1, reads: 'That the nobleman Lord Giacomo da Carrara, son of the late nobleman Lord Marsilio da Carrara, be and ought to be and is understood to be by the authority of the present law and statute, and with every measure and right by which he best can be the Defender, Protector and Governor of the Paduan people, and of the City and District, and Captain General of their inhabitants' ('Quod nobilis vir Dominus Jacobus de Carraria, natus quondam nobilis viri domini Marsilii de Carraria, sit et esse debeat, et esse intelligatur auctoritate presentis legis et statute, et omni modo et iure quo melius esse poterit, Defensor, Protector et Gubernator populi paduani, et civitatis et districtus, et in eis habitantium Capitaneus generalis') (ed. Colle 1824–1825: 1.30; tr. Kohl 1998: 39). For another view of Giacomo's election as it relates to the end of the communal era, see Hyde (1966b: 276–83 and, on the election statute in particular, 279n4). Lazzarini (1934: 285n1), in his article that includes a transcription and discussion of Francesco il Vecchio's statute of election (Padua, Archivio Papafava dei Carraresi 35, parchment 2), noted that the later statute in many ways parallels the 1318 statute in the rights and responsibilities it conveys to the *signore*.

21 Kohl (1998: 37–8 and 41). This section of the statute reads, 'Doctores, et Scholares, et totum Studium Paduanum tamquam filios recommendatos' (Archivio Papafava dei Carraresi 39, parchment 1 [ed. Colle 1824–1825: 1.32]). In a letter to Francesco il Vecchio (*Rerum senilium* XIV.1), Petrarch used this very metaphor to describe the prince's obligations to his citizens as well. See Chapter 5, pp. 156–7.

22 Kibre (1962: 63–6), and Siraisi (1973: 29).

23 Kohl (1998: 34). In 1362, Francesco il Vecchio endowed a college for 12 poor students of civil law. A medical professor, Bartolomeo Campo, followed suit in his testament of 1369 and endowed a college for students of medicine (Kibre 1962: 66–7).

24 Kibre (1962: 65), and Siraisi (1973: 150).

25 Vergerio wrote: 'duodecim adulescentes Patavinos, qui ad disciplinas apti viderentur, deligi mandavit, eosque praebitis in omne tempus large commeatibus Parisius misit, quae urbs litterarum studiis famosissima tunc erat, uti, cum liberalibus disciplinis imbuti essent, medicinae operam darent'. And later, 'Hec urbem et munivit muris et aedificiis ornavit, et studiis atrium bonarum instruxit. Nam opera quidem murorum, quae Marsilius inchoaverat, pro magna parte perfecta reddidit. . . . Horologium, quo per diem et noctem quattuor ac viginti horarum spatia sponte sua designarentur, in summa turri constituendum locavit. . . . In primis vero studia litterarum fovit magnopere, Raineriumque de Forlivio [Raniero Arsendi of Forlì], ejus temporis jurisconsultum insignem, interpretendarum legum gratia magna mercede conduxit. Agri quoque curam praecipuam gessit. Hoc auctore, via, qua itur ad Campum S. Petri, strata est' (*Liber de principibus*, IV, 'De Ubertino de Carraria, tertio ex ea Familia Principe Paduae', §101 and §105–6 [ed. Gnesotto 1924: 427 and 431–2]). Kohl (1998: 199) examines Ubertino's accomplishments in detail, and McManamon (1996: 112) discusses Vergerio's praise of the Carrara lord in the *Liber de principibus*.

26 Kohl (1998: 291). In return for the land, Francesco charged the professor a nominal rent of one ducat per year.

27 Kibre (1962: 65–6); Siraisi (1973: 23); and Kohl (1998: 33).

28 Kohl (1998: 33). For at least forty years prior to Francesco Novello's intervention, the debate over the schools' autonomy had raged at the University of Padua as the medical school continued to grow in student numbers and in prestige.

29 Ongaro (2005: 192).

30 Kohl (1998: 34).

31 Siraisi (1987b: 107–8 [repr. 2001b: 159]).

32 On the war council, see Kohl (1998: 172 and 199–200). Despite a much-lauded victory in May 1373 at the Battle of the Brenta Canal at Lova, the Border War with Venice (24 June 1372–September 1373) ended with the routing of Padua and its allies (principally the Habsburgs of Austria and King Louis of Hungary) at the Battle of Buonconforto (1 July 1373). The terms of peace with Venice were harsh: *La Serenissima* claimed the Paduan cities of Cittadella, Camposampiero and Solagna (to the north), Mirano, Stiano and Castelcarro (on the eastern frontier), and Anguillara and Borgoforte (on the Adige). Francesco il Vecchio was ordered to raze a number of fortifications along the frontier with Venice and publicly to admit war guilt before the Doge and the Major Council, and Padua was made to pay 250,000 ducats as reparation. On 2 October 1373, Francesco Novello and Petrarch travelled to Venice to fulfill the public admission of guilt. An ailing and frail Petrarch praised the peace between Venice and Padua and called for a renewal of their friendship. See Kohl (1998: 119–31).

33 Kohl (1998: 200).

34 When Galeazzo died in 1405, his sons continued their father's chronicle, adding to and embellishing the history Galeazzo began. The version of the *Cronaca* published by Medin and Tolomei (1931) contains the work of Galeazzo and Bartolomeo drawn from the copy of the *Cronaca* now Paris, Bibliothèque nationale de France, it. 262, which was written in Bartolomeo's hand. This version is compared to one penned by Andrea (now Padua, Biblioteca Civica, MS 1490).

35 'Morí adunque nella villa d'Arquà sula montagna del tereno di Padoa, dove ad onorare fu il ditto corpo a sopelire miser Francesco da Carara, prinzipo di Padoa, con quanti arcivescovi, vescovi, abadi, piori, munixi e universalemente tuta la chieresia di Padoa e dil padoano disstreto, e cavalieri e dotori e scolari, ch'era in Padoa, andarono tuti ad onorare il ditto corpo' (Gatari, *Cronaca*, 'La morte de misser Francesco Petrarca', 19 luglio 1374 [eds Medin and Tolomei 1931: 138; my translation]).

36 Gatari, *Cronaca*, 'Quando Madona Tadia venne a marido', 28 maggio 1377 (eds Medin and Tolomei 1931: 143; my translation).

37 Gatari, *Cronaca*, 'Come il Signore fe' aportare el corpo de suo padre a Padoa e l'onore che li fu fato, che fu a dí XVIII de novenbre 1393', 18–20 novembre 1393 (eds Medin and Tolomei 1931: 442–3; my translation). For further discussion of this passage in the *Cronaca*, see pp. 101–103 in this volume.

38 Francesco Novello's book collection and his use of the 'most learned doctors' of the university in public ritual processions suggest that the ideal of the physician as counsellor to princes and 'doctor of the soul', believed to be a fifteenth-century development, was present in fourteenth-century court culture as well.

39 While Francesco Novello fashioned his identity to echo this growing role, it is unknown whether an actual court physician served in Padua under Francesco Novello. Likewise, although we know the identity of Francesco il Vecchio's physician (Piero da Pernumia), it is unknown whether he practiced medicine in a way similar to later court physicians, like Michele Savonarola.

40 Although Savonarola left Padua to work for the d'Este family in Ferrara in 1440, he continued to hold his birth city and the medical training and political views he learned there in high regard. On Savonarola's life, family, and the development of his thought, see Pesenti Marangon (1976); Crisciani (2003 and 2005); and Crisciani and Zuccolin (2011).

41 Ed. Segarizzi (1902).

42 Savonarola's use of the biographical genre in his *Libellus* stemmed from the humanist tradition of collective biography, a Classical genre revived by Petrarch in *De viris illustribus* and continued by second-generation humanists Boccaccio (1313–1375) and Giovanni Colonna (d. 1348). The prerequisite for inclusion in a collective biography, as a form of exemplary literature, was social status. The individuals included were limited to distinguished men and women of their respective societies or cities. See Siraisi (1987b: 106, 115–16 and 128–9 [repr. 2001b: 158, 167 and 179]).

43 Ed. Mastronardi (1996). Mastronardi's edition was prepared from the manuscript now Ravenna, Biblioteca Classense, Cl. n. 302. When citing Savonarola's text, I have included the book number, chapter (when applicable), and the corresponding folio number from the Ravenna manuscript, as denoted in Mastronardi's edition.

44 Savonarola wrote this treatise in both vernacular (*Del felice progresso*) and Latin (*De felici progressu*) versions, as he also did for many of his medical treatises. It is unknown which version was written first (Zuccolin 2007: 238–9).

45 Crisciani (2005: 301).

46 Savonarola subdivided his category of medical doctors into *medici theorici*, the theoretical branch of medicine, which he considered a higher pursuit than the secondary division, the *medici practici*. These subcategories were necessarily fluid since most doctors were both theorists and practitioners. Savonarola determined the doctors' placement on the social hierarchy according to his perception of their occupational emphasis (Siraisi 1987b: 130 [repr. 2001b: 180–1]).

47 Siraisi (1987b: 129–30 [repr. 2001b: 179–81]), and Crisciani (2005: 304). As Siraisi (1987b: 130n70 [repr. 2001b: 181n66]) notes, the other physicians listed in Savonarola's category of medical doctors can be found in Gloria (1888). Andrea Gloria (1821–1911), director of the Museo Civico in Padua, gathered and published archival documents related to the history and monuments of Padua, especially to its university (both before [Gloria 1884] and during [Gloria 1888] the Carrara seigniory) and to the Carrara palace (see Chapter 4, p. 136n9). Regarding the physicians noted by Savonarola, all of those listed in the first group (*theorici*) received formal training at a university and taught medicine at the University of Padua (Gloria 1888: 1.369–444; and Siraisi 1987b: 129–30 [repr. 2001b: 180]). Of the eight *practici* noted by Savonarola, four are not identified as professors of medicine, while three are identified as such (Gloria 1888: 1.369, 1.399–402, 1.413–14), and one is identified as a professor, but his subject

of specialisation is unspecified (Gloria 1888: 1.375–6; and Siraisi 1987b: 129–30 and 130n70 [repr. 2001b: 180 and 181n66]). The *practici* identified as professors likely taught a branch of the university curriculum known as 'practica', while the other *practici* likely made a living by strict practice (Siraisi 1987b: 130n70 [repr. 2001b: 181n66]). In 1391, the University of Padua began to appoint professors of 'practica' alongside those of 'theoretica' (Gloria 1888: 2.252; and Siraisi 1987b: 130n70 [repr. 2001b: 181n66]).

48 Notably, Pietro d'Abano himself sought to combine medical theory and natural philosophy in his work. This combination is visible perhaps most clearly in his treatise, *Conciliator differentiarum philosophorum et praecipue medicorum* (*Reconciling the differences of Philosophy and Medicine*, ca. 1300–1307). The work is divided into 210 'differences', and, over the course of the treatise, Pietro proposed ways in which Greek and Arabic medical teaching could be reconciled with philosophical teaching about nature. In the first 10 of these differences, Pietro addressed the shared problems of practical and theoretical medicine. In the next 100 he addressed specifically theory, and in the final 100, practice. Within the section dedicated to concerns of theory, Pietro addressed questions about the elements, humours and complexions, the naturals, non-naturals and preternaturals, the concepts of *membrum, virtus,* and *spiritus,* portents and the uses of signs, and the concepts of crisis and critical days. Within the section dedicated to practice, Pietro addressed procedures to conserve and maintain health, restore health, and cure disease. See Wallace (1988: 231–2).

49 Savonarola's praise of Pietro d'Abano is not the whole story. Pietro's medical theory was controversial; like many of the time, it included astrology and an adherence to the Aristotelian belief that the natural world was subject to a hierarchy of causes. The end result of this line of thinking is a philosophy of astral and natural determinism known loosely as Averroism. The Inquisition tried Pietro three times on charges of heresy, once in Paris (where he was acquitted) and twice in Padua (where he died in prison while awaiting trial) (Klemm and De Leemens 2005: 404; on the trials, see Alessio 1976: 180–97). Allegedly, the Inquisition found Pietro posthumously guilty and ordered the exhumation and burning of his remains. His friends or supporters, however, already had removed Pietro's body to thwart the Inquisitors, so an effigy was burned in his stead (on Pietro's relationship with the Inquisition and on the legends regarding the fate of his body, see Thorndike 1923–1958: 2.938–47). Perhaps this legendary act of resistance sheds light on why Pietro's followers tend to downplay the charges of heresy against the physician. Savonarola was not alone in his high praise of Pietro or in his reticence to accept him as a heretic (Jacquart 1990: 153n47). Chroniclers and historians, as well as fellow physicians, praised Pietro in their works for the following two centuries (Thorndike 1923–1958: 2.882–3 and 2.914–16). For an introduction to Pietro's life and works, see Thorndike 1923–1958: 2.874–947; Premuda 1970; Alessio 1976; Siraisi 1985; and Klemm and De Leemens 2005).

50 Lovati's poems address moral problems that related to public life as well as political events. Lovati's student, Mussato, in his prose histories of contemporary regional politics, emulated the Roman historian Livy (59 BCE–17 CE). In his verse tragedy, *Ecerinide,* which attacks the recent tyranny of Ezzelino da Romano (d. 1259), Mussato emulated Seneca. Both Lovati and Mussato pay homage to the over-century old Paduan chronicle tradition in their works as well (Hyde 1966b: 290–7).

51 Savonarola's hierarchy points to a connection between Pietro d'Abano and Petrarch. The connection he makes between the medical doctor and humanist reflects the growing importance of the court physician's role as a combination of the professional qualities these men exemplify. It also maps the connection that Francesco Novello longed to make between his support of the medical schools and his father's patronage of Petrarch.

52 Prescribing individualised regimens of health (*regimina sanitatis*) for elite patrons was not a new practice. As discussed in the previous chapter, many late-medieval

physicians wrote specific medical plans for aristocratic or royal patients. For instance, in the mid-thirteenth century, Aldobrandino of Siena (d. 1287) wrote a regimen at the request of Beatrice of Savoy (1205–1267), Countess of Provence, and, in 1308, Arnaud of Villanova (ca. 1240–1311) penned a well-known and often imitated regimen for James II (1267–1327), king of Aragon, known as the *Regimen sanitatis salernitanum*. University students, physicians' apprentices and practicing physicians themselves studied and shared compilations of these *consilia* as part of their ongoing training. See Siraisi (1987b: 112–13 [repr. 2001b: 163–4]), and Bertiz (2003: 76–8).

53 Zuccolin (2007: 239) memorably describes *Del felice progresso* as a combination of 'the *speculum principis*, the *laudatio Urbis*, the confrontation of the arts, the *regimen sanitatis*, and the historical chronicle'.

54 The structure of the treatise shows its thematic flexibility. In Book I, Savonarola debates the best forms of government. In Book II, he describes the visits of the Holy Roman Emperor, Frederick III (1415–1493; r. 1452–1493), to Ferrara in 1452 and Borso d'Este's investiture as duke in May of that year. In Book III, Savonarola gives advice on how to govern well, which includes, among other things, 'prescriptions' for areas of study that a wise prince ought to pursue, characteristics he ought to look for when choosing his counsellors, and the kinds of foods he ought to eat to preserve and augment his health.

55 Ed. Nystedt (1988).

56 Zuccolin (2007: 249–58).

57 Crisciani (2005: 301).

58 On Savonarola's debt to the *Secretum* tradition, see Crisciani (2003 and 2005). On Savonarola's debt to *De regimine principum*, see Zuccolin (2007).

59 The literature on the *Secretum*, its genesis and its transmission is extensive. As a starting point, see Manzalaoui (1974); Williams (2003 and 2008); and Forster (2006 and 2010). On the transmission and translations of the *Secretum*, in particular, see Forster (2006).

60 On Giles of Rome's treatise and its influence in the Renaissance, see Briggs (1999).

61 Zuccolin (2007: 239–43).

62 Currently, there is no critical edition of Savonarola's *Speculum Phisionomie*; however, Gabrielle Zuccolin is preparing one, and she generously shared her work with me. See Chapter 5, p. 161n1.

63 In *Del felice progresso*, Savonarola specifically praised Alexander the Great for following Aristotle's advice on prudent governance, advice allegedly given in the *Secretum*: 'E vogly, pregotte, signuor mio, a la memoria rivocare quanto splendore e quanta gloria recevuto ha e tutavia receve Alexandri Magno per haver havuto sempre apresso di sé Aristotile e per havere la doctrina di quello con gran diligentia observata. O principi moderni, considerate biene dentro da vuy se 'l vostro principare è somegliante a quello morale e philosophico di Alexandre e se di tale expectati tanta gloriosa fama quanto luy per il suo conseguitato ha!' (*Del felice progresso*, I, f. 6r [ed. Mastronardi 1996: 84]). For a discussion of this passage as evidence of Savonarola's debt to the *Secretum secretorum*, see Crisciani (2005: 301 and 319n32).

64 Zuccolin (2007: 241).

65 For commentary on the contents of the *Secretum*, see Williams (2003: 7–30).

66 Crisciani (2005: 301) describes *Del felice progresso* as a 'renewed' *Secretum secretorum*, a combination of encyclopaedic knowledge and a *Speculum principis*.

67 Williams (2003: 28–30) gives a hypothetical line of descent.

68 Forster (2010: 104). On dating, original language and sources, see Forster 2006: 11–19.

69 Pritchard (1989: 209).

70 For Latin text and English translations, see Burnett (1995: 255–7), and Williams (2003: 353–7).

71 'Domine T. gratie dei Hispaniarum regine' (*Prologue* to 'short form' translation [ed. and tr. Williams 2003: 354 and 357]).

72   Forster (2010: 104).
73   'id est *Secretum secretorum*' (ed. and tr. Williams 2003: 355 and 357).
74   Forster (2010: 104).
75   Forster (2010: 102–3). See also Manzalaoui (1961: 83).
76   Williams (2003: 368–88), and Forster (2010: 104–5).
77   Williams (2003: 388–413), and Forster (2010: 105n29).
78   Forster (2010: 105).
79   Manzalaoui (1977: x), and Williams (2003: 11).
80   The translator of the 'long form', Philip of Tripoli, noted in his prologue that the *Secretum* was a 'most precious philosophical pearl' ('preciosissima philosophie margarita') that 'contained something useful about almost everything' ('in quo fere de omnibus aliquid utile continentur') (ed. and tr. Williams 2003: 364). The 'long form' version contains a proem, two introductions, and ten books: I. *On the Kinds of Kings*, II. *On the Position and Character of a King* (which includes subsections on the use of astrology, and the section on health and the body), III. *On Justice*, IV. *On Ministers* (which contains subsections on cosmology, astrology, the soul, sensation and numerology and advice regarding the characters of ministers and political advisors), V. *On Scribes*, VI. *On Ambassadors*, VII. *On Governors*, VIII. *On Army Officers*, IX. *On the Conduct of War* (which includes subsections on the role of astrology and onomancy [a type of divination using names] in war), and X. *On the Occult Sciences* (which contains subsections on talismans, alchemical theory and the Emerald Tables of Hermes, the lapidary and the herbal) (listed by Williams 2003: 10–11).
81   Williams (2003: 111).
82   For a list and discussion of the other well-known scholars who commented upon and owned the *Secretum* (up to 1400), see Williams (2003: 183–297).
83   Eamon (1994: 43–4). As it gained popularity outside of the universities, the *Secretum*'s credibility became more and more suspect within them, and it was considered definitively spurious by the sixteenth century. Eamon argues that the *Secretum*'s significance was much larger outside of the university than within it. He suggests that the 'learned magus' persona projected through the possession of the book helped new graduates from the universities to secure prestigious jobs as advisors at court or within civil administrations.
84   Eamon (1994: 49–50).
85   Perhaps these young graduates pointed out the passage in the *Secretum* in which the author discusses the ideal character of a prince's advisor, a passage that advocates their suitability for the job (Eamon 1994: 49–50). The author advised his reader, the prince, to choose his company carefully. Per Roger Bacon's translation and commentary on the *Secretum*, the worthy advisor must possess 'a good understanding, and a quick apprehension of what is said to him' ('bonitate apprehensionis et voluntatem ad intelligendum id quod dicitur'), and he should be 'skilled in all sciences' ('penetrabilis in omni sciencia') (Bacon, *Secretum*, III.14 [ed. Steele 1920: 5.141–2; tr. Eamon 1994: 49]). Eamon (1994: 49–50) also cites and further discusses the significance of this passage. The *Secretum* author's description of the ideal advisor for a prince suits the role of the university graduate, and especially that of the court physician. As privileged counsellor and confidant to the prince, the court physician possesses wit and an exclusive 'understanding' of the moral and natural sciences. Similar descriptions of ideal advisors to princes can be found in Petrarch's letter to Francesco il Vecchio (*Rerum senilium* XIV.1) and Paduan court humanist Giovanni Conversini's description of his role as advisor to the elder Francesco (in a letter dated 13 September 1385), which suggests the *Secretum*'s corresponding influence on humanist court culture during the fourteenth century in Padua. See Conversini, *De primo eius introitu ad aulam* (*Of his Earliest Introduction to Court*) (eds and tr. Kohl and Day 1987: 29). On Conversini (1343–1408) and his role as teacher at the *Studium* in Padua and chancellor at the Carrara court, see Kohl (1983: 574–8).

86 'Scias itaque quod intellectus est capud regiminis, salus anime, servitor virtutum, speculator viciorum: in ipso siquidem speculamur fugienda, per ipsum eligimus eligenda: ipse est origo virtutum et radix omnium bonorum laudabilium et honorabilium' (Bacon, *Secretum*, I.7 [ed. Steele 1920: 45; tr. Eamon 1994: 49]). Eamon (1994: 49) further discusses the significance of this passage.

87 Zuccolin (2007: 240–1).

88 Zuccolin (2007: 240–3) charts the many parallels between Savonarola's work and Giles' through multiple examples, some of which show that Savonarola borrowed verbatim from Giles.

89 Zuccolin (2007: 241).

90 Zuccolin (2007: 255). Notably, the moral philosophy in Giles' *De regimine*, as a *Speculum principis*, parallels aspects of Petrarch's own contribution to the genre, *De viris illustribus*, which Francesco il Vecchio used to articulate his sense of self as a Carrara prince.

91 Crisciani (2005: 317 and 324n101). For example: 'che certo né il principio, né il medico, biem che seppano le regole di l'arte, non puoteno conseguire di sua opera degna laude senza exercitio et experientia' and 'che molto vale la experientia nel rezere e governare i stati, come quella vale nel medicare d'i corpi' (Savonarola, *Del felice progresso*, I, f. 7r; and III, 'capitolo quarto', f. 40r [ed. Mastronardi 1996: 87–8 and 213, respectively]). Crisciani (2005: 317) further discusses the significance of these passages.

92 Crisciani (2005: 304). The original source for the idea of history as a guide to life is Cicero (*De oratore*, II.9 [eds and tr. Sutton and Rackham 1942: 1.222–7]). In his work, Savonarola encouraged Borso to study the exemplary lives and deeds of ancient heroes and leaders as well as those from recent history. For instance, Savonarola pointed to Francesco il Vecchio and Borso's father, Niccolò III d'Este, as modern *exempla* for Borso to follow. For examples of the use of history and historic figures – including the Carrara and d'Este princes – to mould Borso's character and ameliorate his government, see Savonarola, *Del felice progresso*, I, ff. 4v and 8v; and III, 'capitolo secondo', f. 37v (ed. Mastronardi 1996: 78, 92–3 and 203–4, respectively). On Savonarola's view of the study of history and its relationship to prudent governance, see Zuccolin (2007: 256–8).

93 Chiefly, the *Speculum* differs from the *Secretum* in its narrower scope and in its focus on the ethics of power. Olson's comments on the long version of the *Secretum* reflect the relationship between the two forms (1982: 54). He calls the long version 'a kind of middle ground' between the ethical advice central to the *Speculum principis* tradition and medical advice central to a physician's regimen of health.

94 Williams (2003: 263–5). Slightly less often, the treatise was bound with generally scientific, philosophical or theological texts during this period (especially Aristotle's *De animalibus* [*On Animals*] or the Aristotelian *Problemata* [*Problems*]).

95 Scholars referred to their copies of the *Secretum* with alternative titles, which often emphasise certain aspects of the text and so reveal the owners' personal interests (Williams 2003: 269–71). For instance, Albertus Magnus, who was concerned primarily with the ethical and political advice in the *Secretum*, referred to it as *De regimine dominorum* (*The Regimen of Lords*) (Williams 2003: 310). Williams (2003: 269–71) argues that by referring to a copy of the *Secretum* as *De regimine principum* (or similar variations), the owner of the copy revealed his primary interest in the text's connection to the aspects of the *Speculum principis* tradition that address ethics and moral guidance. Conversely, to refer to the text as the *Secretum secretorum* reflected the owner's primary interest in its natural philosophy.

96 On this dynamic, see Chapters 5 and 6.

97 According to Galenic medicine, the six non-naturals (which he called 'necessary causes') affecting health are air, exercise, sleep, diet, evacuation and repletion, and the passions of the soul (emotions). See Galen, *Ars medica* (*The Art of Medicine*), 23

(ed. and Latin tr. Kühn 1821–1833: 1.367–9; English tr. Singer 1997: 374–5). All six must be regulated and balanced in accord with the patient's elemental constitution or temperament (hot, cold, moist or dry). For a brief introduction to this vast topic, see Nutton (1995a: 141 and, on the non-naturals in Galenic medicine more generally, 2013: 242 and 246–8).

98   Francesco's *Herbal* contains material that Pietro d'Abano studied and taught. Pietro specifically commented upon his study of Serapion's *Liber aggregatus* (Siraisi 1973: 161, and Bettini 1974: 57n11).

99   See Book II of Savonarola's *Del felice progresso* in which he describes the pomp and circumstance of Holy Roman Emperor Frederick III's visit to Ferrara and Borso's investiture ceremony (ff. 28v–32v [ed. Mastronardi 1996: 169–84]).

100   Crisciani (2005: 317).

101   Crisciani (2005: 301–5).

102   Crisciani (2005: 305–6).

103   'a dí XX del mexe, esendo del dí fato tuto'iaro e la grande turba dela chierexia esendo ivi, cominiò a usire fora dila corte e andò intorno le piaze, cioè a quella dele Frute e a quela dela Biava e andò al Domo; dopo la ierexia seguí cento cavalla coverti de bruno, su cadauno uno famiglio vestido a nero, con uno scudo al collo apicado al'arme da Carara, e una gran bandiera stravolta con grandinisimi pianti (a cadauno cavallo andavano a lato due poveri tutti vestiti di panno bigio, e cadauno un torcio in mano acceso, dato loro tutto per limosina. Dopo questi andavano IV cavalli coperti all'arma de i IV quartieri della città, con le bandiere, scudi e famigli a piedi, come gli ante-detti). . . . Dopo questi, seguí la moltitudine de la cerra che ardea . . . dopo questi, seguí la famiglia dil signor tuta vestida a nero con voxe de pianti, che tonava il ciello, ch'era per numero cercha VIIIc persone; dopo questi seguí la chassa dove'era el corpo del perfato. Era la cassa coverta de uno rechisimo 'panno d'oro fodrado d'armeliny, e fu la detta cassa portada da nobilli cavalieri perfino ala chiesa, sora la qual cassa era famo-sisimi doctori, con loro capuzi di varo in testa, portado uno baldachino di pano d'oro fodrado d'armelini: driedo la cassa venia pieno di grave dolglia il signore vestido di bruno tra mezo due anbasadori dela signoria di Vinexia; dopo luy, misser Francesco Terzo tra mezo anbasadori del comun de Fiorenza; dopo lui, seguia Iacomo da Carara tra mezo li anbasadori Bolognexi; dopo lui, Nicollò da Carara tramezo anbasadori del Marchexe; dopo questi, seguí la prole da Carara . . . dopo quisti, la moltitudine del povolo, ch'era la magior parte tuta vestida di bruno, con stridi e pianti infiniti, e aconpagnarono perfino al Duomo la detta cassa, dove li era la donna dil signor con tute le donne di Padoa, e i pianti e stridi che fu per le donne fatti saria inposibelle a me a scrivere; . . . Aconpagnado adunque el corpo ala chiesia retornò il signore ala corte, che già era ore XXII, e aveasi comenzado a prima ora de dy. Azunto adunche in corte nel brolo [i.e.: portico] suso ad alto per misser Zuane Luixe dî Lanbertazi fu fato uno sermone a laude dil prefato signore e di la caxa da Carara e dil signor ivi presente, e rengraciando le signorie e signori ivi azonte per parte del signor. (Così finito il santo uffizio, non prima delle XXIV hore, fu sepolto il detto corpo nel battistero, nella cap-pella di santo Giovanni Battista, il quale fu messo in un'arca di marmot rosso sopra Quattro colonne nel mezzo di detta cappella, nella quale ogni giorno si celebrava l'uffizio con assai messe et orazioni per l'anima del detto signore)' (Gatari, *Cronaca*, 'Come il Signore fe' aportare el corpo de suo padre a Padoa e l'onore che li fu fato a dí XVIII de novembre 1393', 18–20 novembre 1393 [eds Medin and Tolomei 1931: 441–4; my translation]).

104   *De dignissimo funebri apparatu in exequiis clarissimi omnium principis Francisci Senioris de Carraria* (*On the most worthy funereal preparation for the funeral [rites] of Francesco the Elder of Carraria, most famous prince of all*) (ed. Muratori 1730: cols 189A–194A) and *Oratorio in funere Francisci Senioris de Carraria, Patavii Principis* (*Oratory on the Funeral of Francesco il Vecchio da Carrara, Prince of Padua*) (ed. Muratori 1730: cols 194B–198C).

105 On the role of vision in Vergerio's funeral orations for Francesco il Vecchio, see McManamon (1996: 43–7). Throughout his work, McManamon (1996) comprehensively analyses the important role vision played in Vergerio's theory of education and his practice of oratory. See, especially, McManamon's Chapters 3, 5 and 6.

106 On this literary method, see McManamon (1996: 44n33). Savonarola's use of detailed description mirrors Vergerio's use of it in his orations. For instance, in the second oration composed to honour Francesco il Vecchio at his death (*Oratorio in funere Francisci Senioris de Carraria* [ed. Muratori 1730: cols 194B–198C]), Vergerio used the rhetoric of vision to empower his speech. He began the oration with a panegyric description of Padua and its territories – the geographical body of the *signoria* – and argued that Francesco il Vecchio created its peace and prosperity. Based on this vision, Vergerio urged the mourners to take comfort in Francesco's legacy. By celebrating Francesco il Vecchio's virtues, Vergerio created a 'blueprint' for Francesco Novello's rule in the tradition of the *Speculum principis* (McManamon 1996: 46–7). Vergerio used a similar technique in an earlier oration commemorating the anniversary of Francesco Novello's restoration to power, written ca. 1392 (*Ad Franciscum Juniorem de Carraria* [*To Francesco Novello da Carrara*] [ed. Muratori 1730: cols 204–15]) (McManamon 1996: 43–6).

107 McManamon (1996: 49). Unlike his contemporary humanists, Vergerio preferred to use the epideictic (celebratory) oration rather than the favoured judicial and deliberative forms to make his points. He believed that this form would evoke an emotional response (*pathos*), which would connect his listeners to his subject more intimately (McManamon 1996: 43).

108 Vergerio, *De dignissimo funebri apparatu* (ed. Muratori 1730: 190A–92C). For a more detailed analysis of this aspect of the oration, see McManamon (1996: 42–3).

109 Vergerio told his listeners/readers that the Romans had commemorated their dead with funeral masks and tombs in order to remind themselves continuously of the greatness of their dead ancestors. He argued that the living Romans sought to emulate their ancestors' great deeds, especially by serving the noble state, in order to better commemorate them (Vergerio, *De dignissimo funebri apparatu* [ed. Muratori 1730: 189A–B]). McManamon (1996: 42) cites and further discusses this strategy in the oration.

110 See Chapter 2 for a discussion of this experience and its significance.

111 On the medals, see Marvin (1880); Rizzoli (1932); Cessi (1974); Gorini (2005); and Richards (2007: 134–5). Gorini (2005: 260) posits that the medal of Francesco il Vecchio may have been struck in 1393, at the time of the elder Francesco's death, rather than in 1390, at the time of the younger Francesco's recovery of Padua.

112 Kohl (1998: 268).

4 Portraits of the Carrara

By the time Francesco Novello came to power, the Carrara already had done a great deal of thinking about how to construct and circulate a positive image of the family through artistic and civic patronage. So, when the younger Francesco regained Padua from Giangaleazzo Visconti in 1390, he concentrated his patronage on recognisable avenues associated with his family's earlier strategies, and especially on supporting the university and collecting books. Both avenues were, in part, tributes to his father and to Paduan culture under his father's rule. As heir to the Carrara house, Francesco Novello had grown to adulthood within a *mythos* deliberately constructed and successfully circulated by his father's patronage.

Over the course of his father's nearly forty years as *signore*, Francesco Novello witnessed the use of civic and artistic patronage to advance an image of the lord and the Carrara family as magnanimous, learned and just rulers of Padua with a long-standing, noble pedigree and a history of supporting the city. In particular, the elder Francesco used monumental fresco imagery, his public friendship with Petrarch, and his book collection to encourage this impression. His efforts, however, built upon those of previous Carrara lords who used their patronage, in part, to revise older, more critical and even deprecatory accounts of the Carrara family. Chronicles written during Padua's last communal era, which dates from the fall of the Ezzelino III da Romano (1194–1259) in 1259 to the election of Giacomo il Grande (1264–1324, r. 1318–1320) in 1318, present a less than ideal view of the dynasty and its history.[1] Certainly, they do not corroborate the vision of self and family put forth in the patronage of Francesco il Vecchio or his son.[2]

For instance, in his account of the commune's citizenry, *De generatione aliquorum civium urbis Padue, tam nobilium quam ignobilium* (*On the Generation of Some Citizens of the City of Padua, both Noble and Common*, ca. 1311), the local judge and historian, Giovanni da Nono (1276–1347), organised the great Paduan families into categories of nobility.[3] In his work, da Nono described the Carrara family as neither the most prominent nor the most wealthy citizens of Padua. Rather, he placed the Carrara in the second tier of nobility. They were not ranked among the oldest, powerful magnate families, the tier to which they clearly belonged by the time Francesco Novello claimed power.[4]

Da Nono noted that the Carrara owned property in Padua and around the towns of Carrara and Pernumia and that the family had formed advantageous marriage

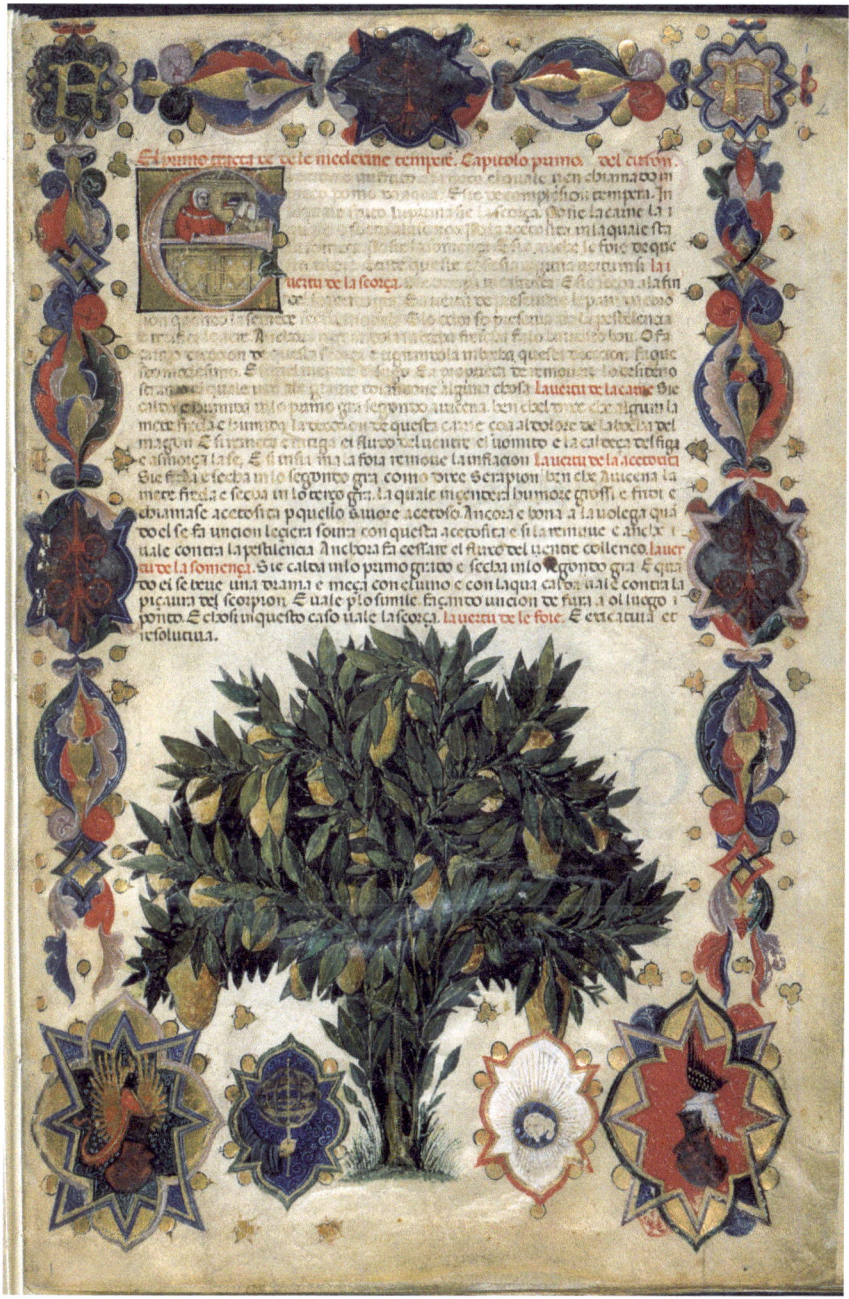

Plate 1 Frontispiece with Carrara heraldry and *citron* (*Citrus medica*, L., citron tree)

Carrara Herbal
London, British Library, Egerton 2020, f. 4r
35 × 24 cm, gouache on vellum, Padua, ca. 1390–1400

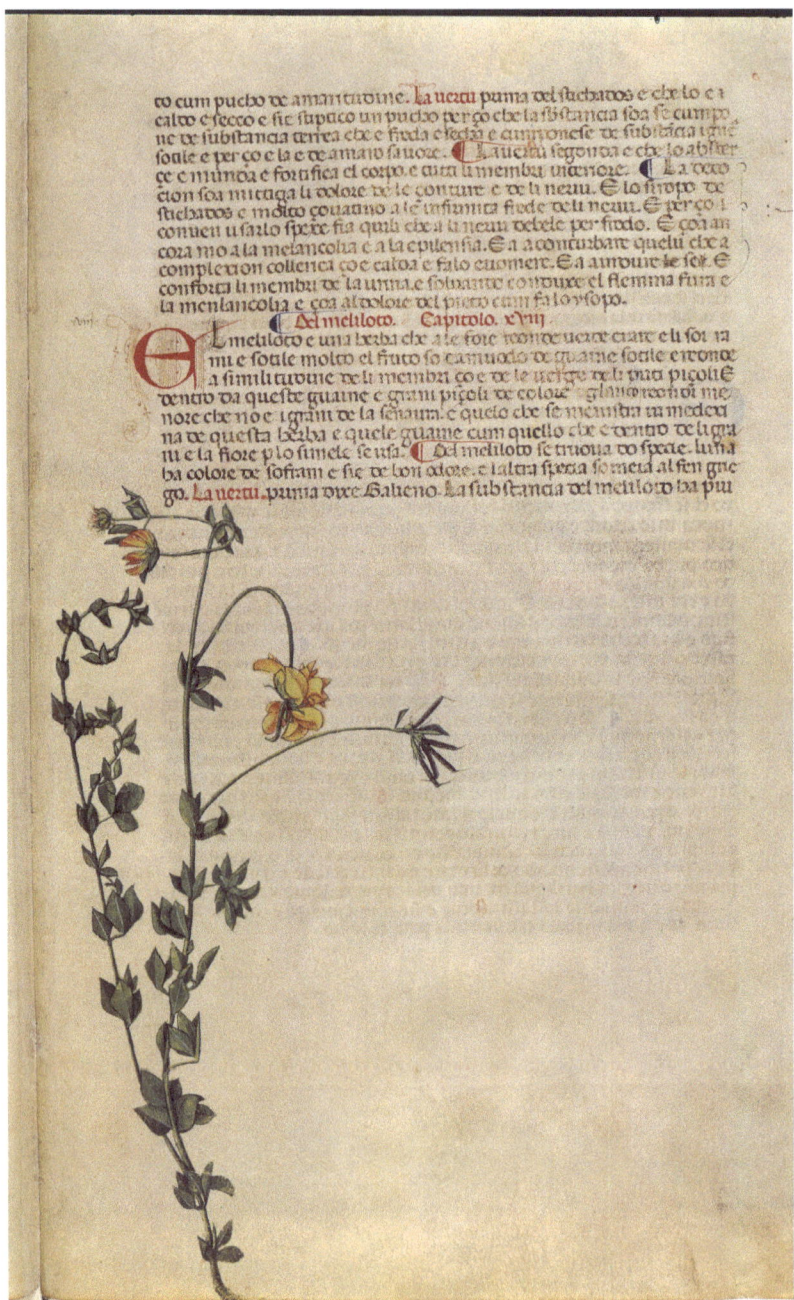

Plate 2 Meliloto (Lotus corniculatus L., bird's foot trefoil)

Carrara Herbal
London, British Library, Egerton 2020, f. 15r
35 × 24 cm, gouache on vellum, Padua, ca. 1390–1400

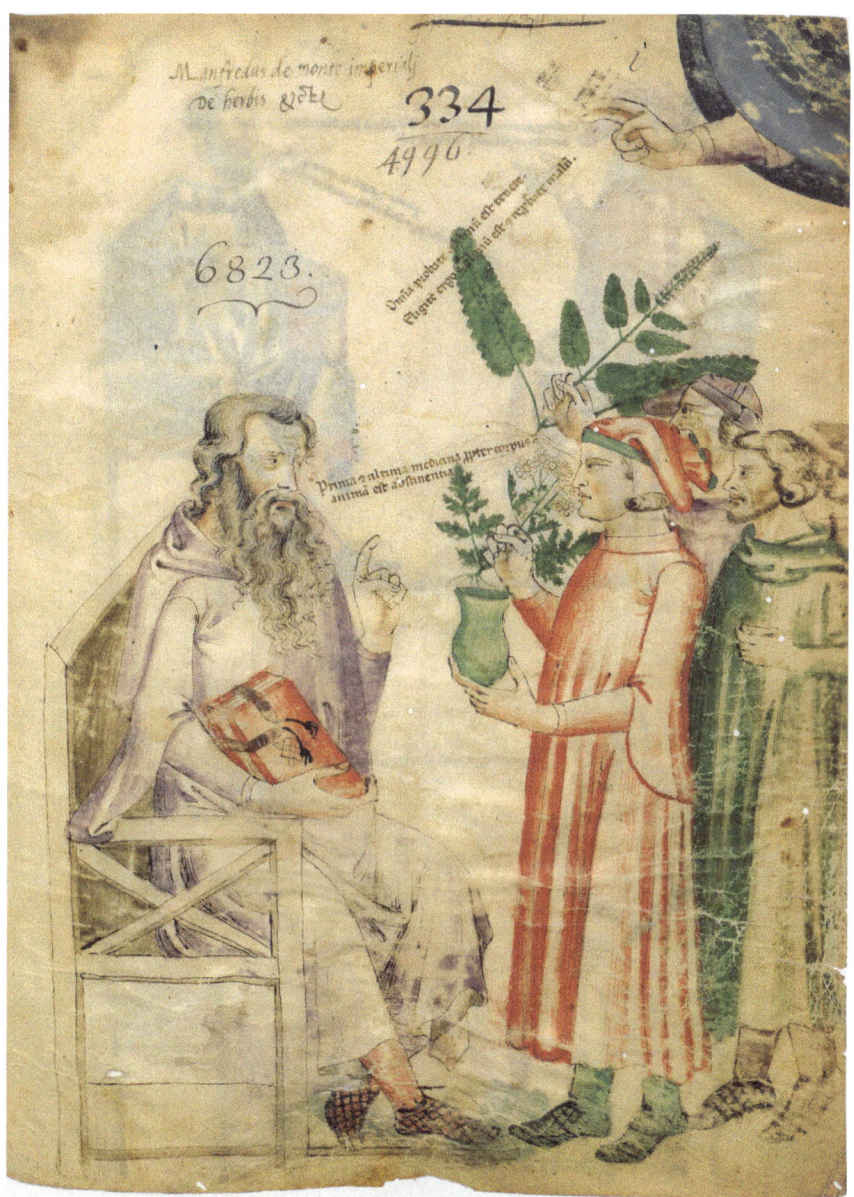

Plate 3 Author portrait of Manfred de Monte Imperiale

Lippo Vanni or Roberto d'Oderisio, *Tractatus de herbis*
Paris, Bibliothèque nationale de France, lat. 6823, f. 1r
34.5 × 24.7 cm, Southern Italy, ca. 1330–1340

Source: Bibliothèque nationale de France, Département des manuscrits, Latin 6823

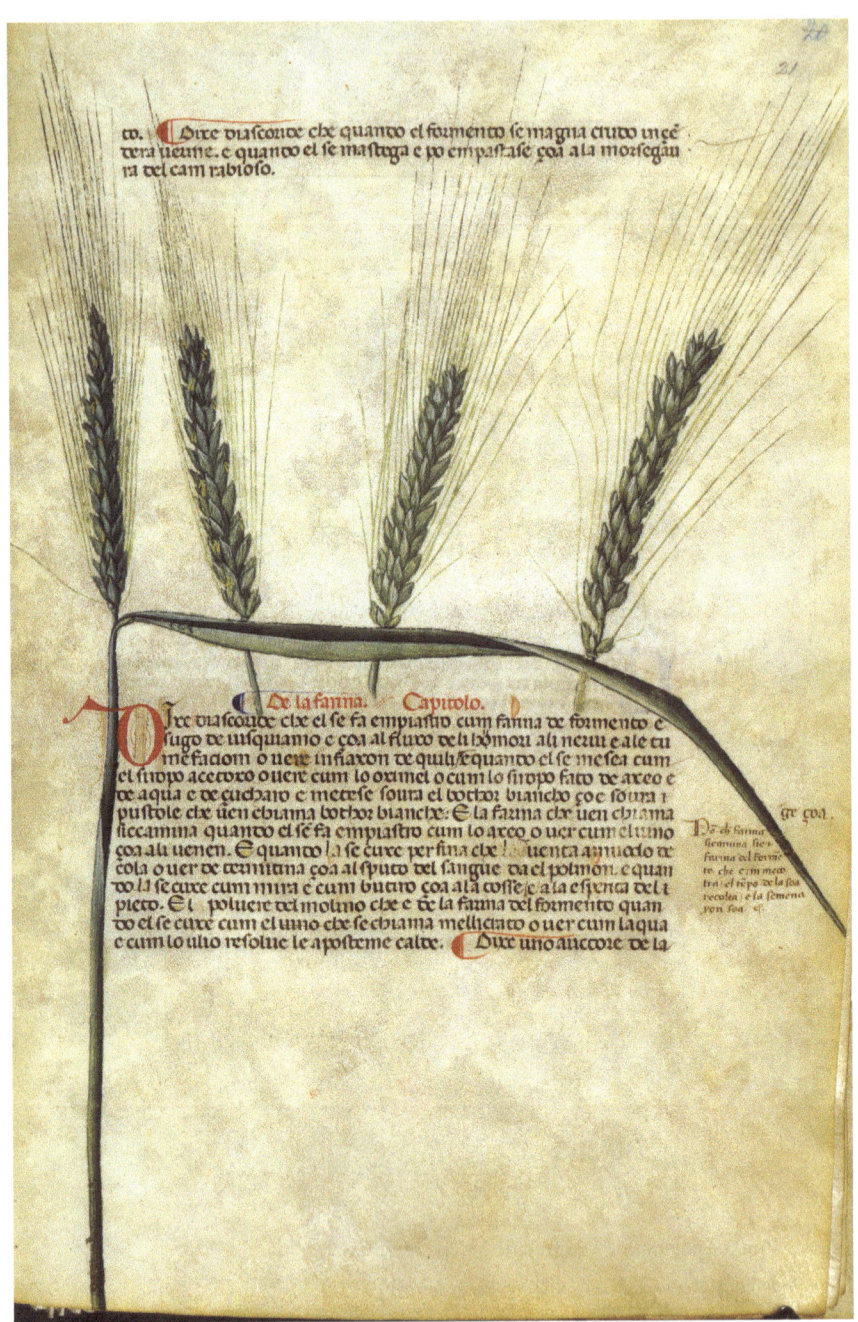

Plate 4 Formento (*Hordeum hexastichum* L., six-row barley)

Carrara Herbal
London, British Library, Egerton 2020, f. 21r
35 × 24 cm, gouache on vellum, Padua, ca. 1390–1400

© British Library Board, Egerton 2020

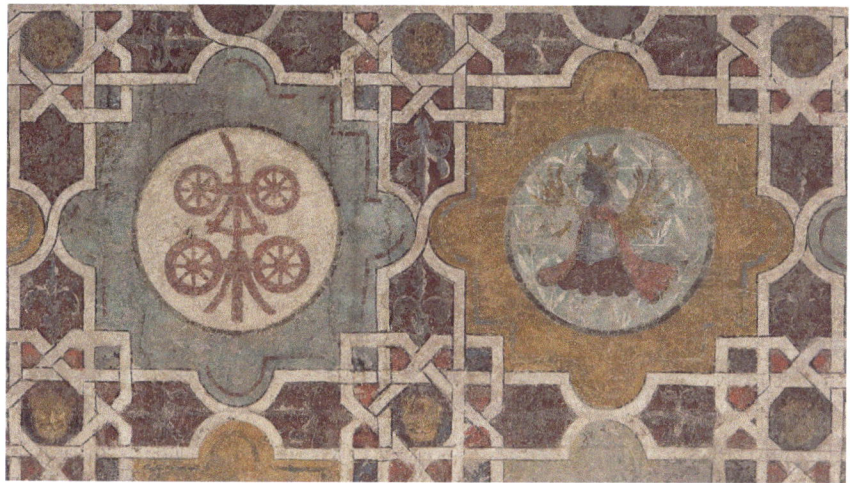

Plate 5 Carrara emblems

Stanza Terrena B (formerly *Anticamera dei Cimieri*)
Padua, Accademia Galileiana di Scienze, Lettere ed Arti
Fresco, Padua, ca. 1340–1343

Reproduced with permission of the Accademia Galileiana di Scienze, Lettere ed Arti in Padova

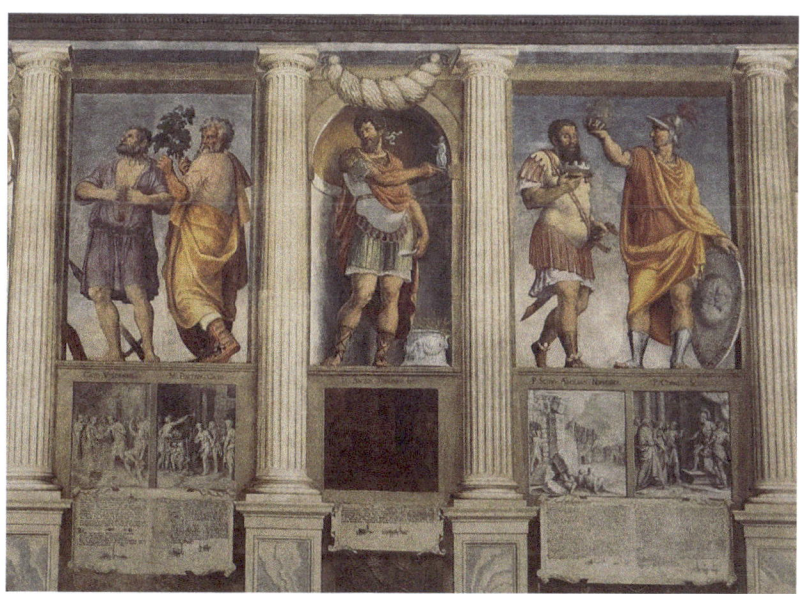

Plate 6 Domenico Campagnola and Stefano dall' Arzere, *Sala dei Giganti* (formerly *Sala virorum illustrium*)

Padua, University of Padua, Palazzo Liviano
Fresco, Padua, ca. 1540

Photo: Federico Meneghetti © Federico Meneghetti / Reda&Co

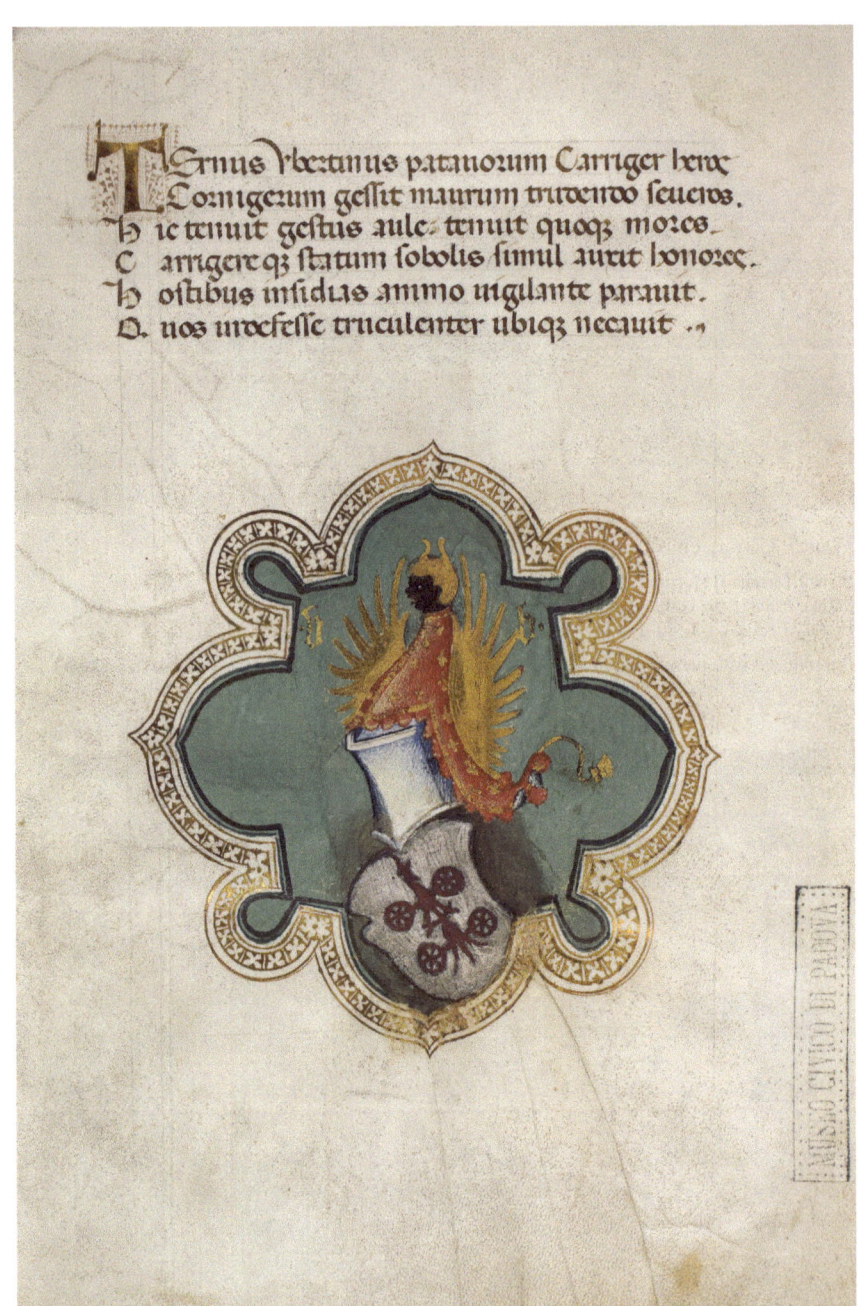

Ternus Vbertinus patauorum Carriger herox
Cornigerum gessit maurum tridendo seueros.
Hic tenuit gestus aule: tenuit quoqz mores.
Carrigere qz statum sobolis simul aurit honoree.
Hostibus insidias animo uigilante parauit.
Quos indefesse truculenter ubiqz necauit .,

Plate 7 Personal arms of Ubertino da Carrara

Liber cimeriorum dominorum de Carraria
Padua, Biblioteca Civica, B.P. 124, XXII, f. 16r
27 × 20 cm, Padua, ca. 1390

Su gentile concessione del Comune di Padova – Assessorato Cultura e Turismo

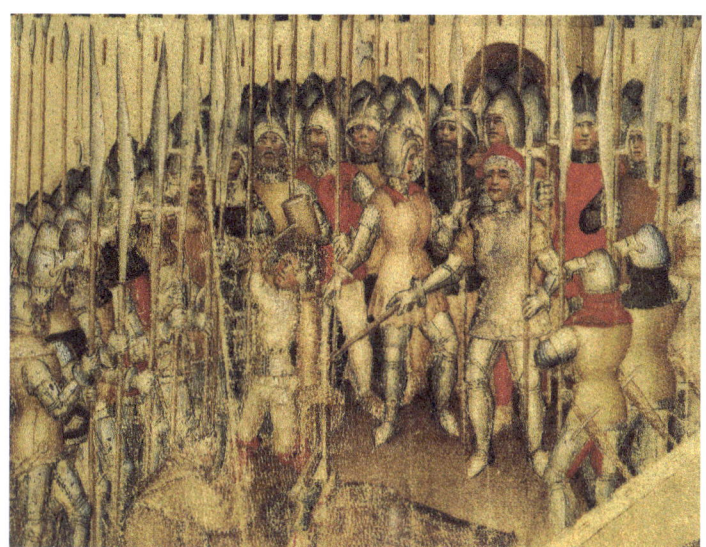

Plate 8 Scene of the execution of Giacomo da Carrara in 1240

Gesta magnifica domus Carrariensibus
Venice, Biblioteca Nazionale Marciana, lat. X, 381 (coll. 2802), f. 2r
Folio 58 × 43 cm, Padua, ca. 1390

Photo credit: Gianni Dagli Orti / The Art Archive at Art Resource, NY

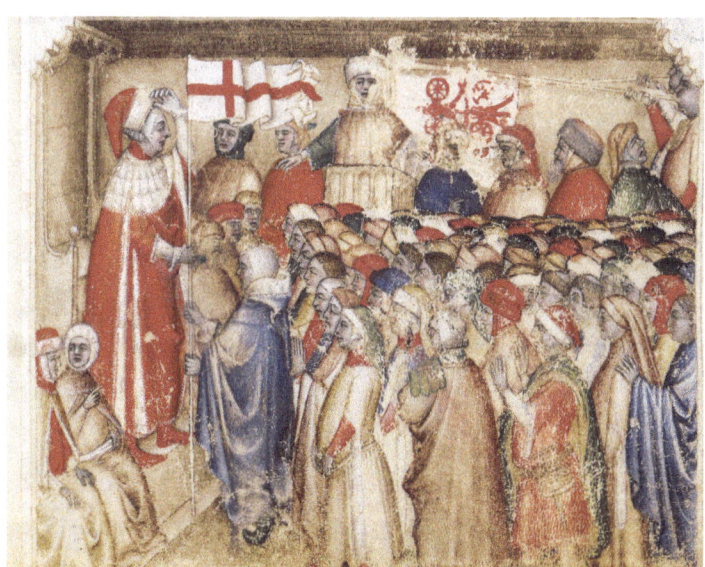

Plate 9 Scene of the election of Giacomo 'il Grande' da Carrara in 1318

Gesta magnifica domus Carrariensibus
Venice, Biblioteca Nazionale Marciana, lat. X, 381 (coll. 2802), f. 2r
Folio 58 × 43 cm, Padua, ca. 1390

Photo credit: © DeA Picture Library / Art Resource, NY

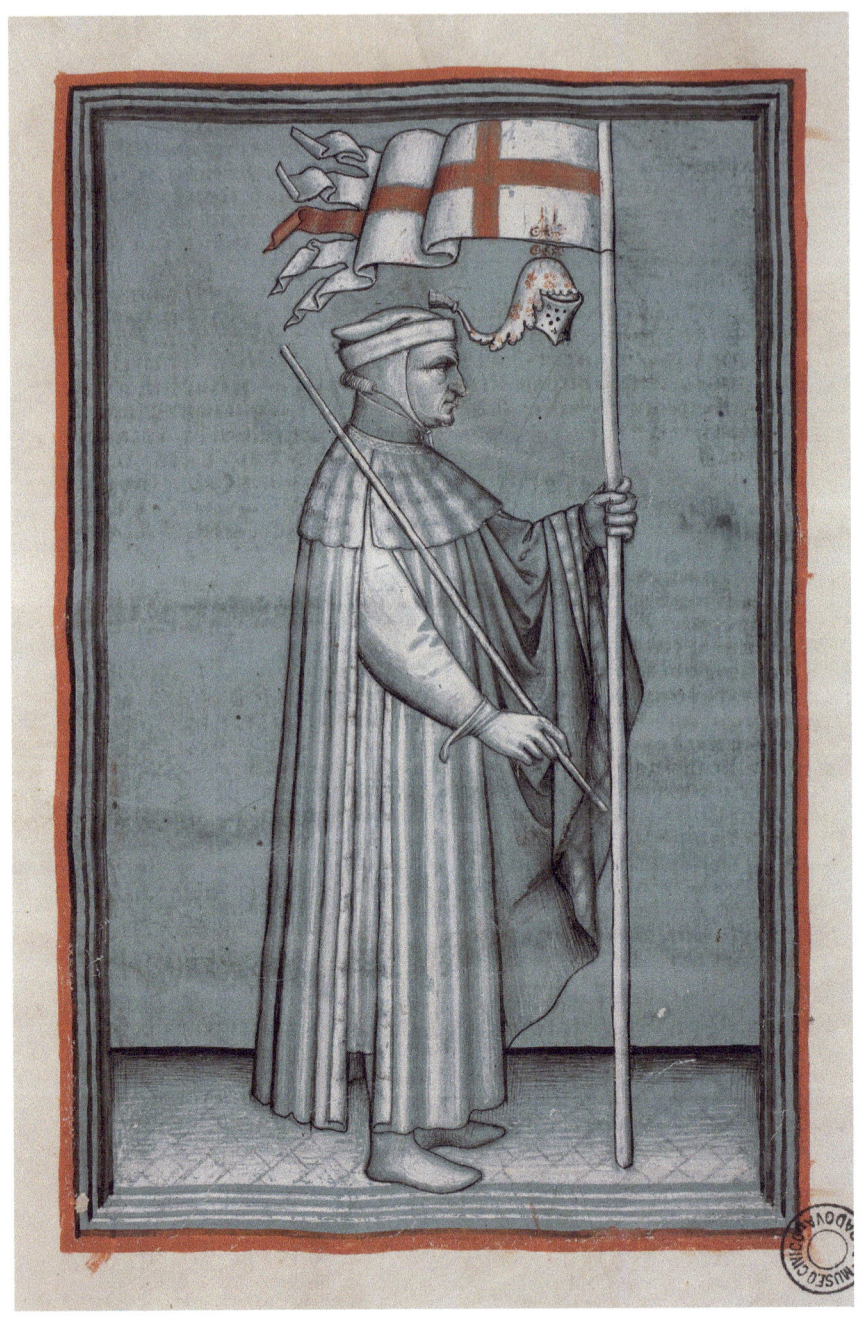

Plate 10 After Altichiero (?), portrait of Giacomo 'il Grande' da Carrara

Liber de principibus Carrariensibus
Padua, Biblioteca Civica, B.P. 158, f. 4v
Folio 34.2 × 24.8 cm, Padua, ca. 1402

Su gentile concessione del Comune di Padova – Assessorato Cultura e Turismo

alliances with many prominent families in northern Italy. These facts accorded the Carrara the designation of nobility by da Nono's criteria. However, the chronicler also noted that the common people did not believe the current members of the Carrara family were descendants of an ancient noble house.[5] Paduans considered the Carrara as citizens of the *popolo* (people), likely because of the fragmentation of the family's estates and the growing divisions within the family itself at that time.[6] The chronicle *De traditione Patavii ad Canem Grandem* (*On Paduan Tradition until Cangrande [della Scala's Usurpation in 1328]*), written by the poet, historian and political opponent of the Carrara, Albertino Mussato (1261–1329), confirmed the family's factional divides and described its lawlessness. Mussato especially complained of the fear mongering, assaults and murders committed by Ubertino da Carrara before Ubertino became *signore* (in 1338).[7] Both Mussato's and da Nono's accounts of the early Carrara are strikingly different from the presentation of the family and their history found in the art and literature commissioned by the Carrara after they assumed leadership of Padua.

The patronage strategies used by the Carrara *signori* sought to redefine the family's history according to a different vision, one that aggrandised them and supported their aspirations for power. In addition to the family's important civic patronage, which – as we saw in the previous chapter – included the support of the university, several different campaigns of their artistic patronage over the course of the seigniory developed a positive image of the family.[8] These campaigns illustrate the familial and artistic contexts that shaped Francesco Novello's collection of books and his commission of the *Carrara Herbal*. In particular, Francesco il Vecchio's extensive artistic and literary patronage and the earlier architectural and decorative commissions for the family palace, the Reggia Carrarese, most influenced the trajectory of Francesco Novello's patronage and his portrayal of self as the new ruler of Padua after 1390.

The Reggia Carrarese as site of identity-building and exchange

The Reggia Carrarese was a complex of buildings that served as both the centre of court politics and the family residence.[9] Three Carrara lords commissioned monumental fresco cycles for the Reggia prior to the seigniory of Francesco Novello, and each of these lords used the palace as the site for important court business and festivities. Over the course of the dynasty, artists decorated the large complex using various types of imagery, by turns, with heraldry, figural portraits and narrative cycles.[10] Francesco il Vecchio commissioned frescoes that depicted ancient heroes from Petrarch's *De viris illustribus* (*On Famous Men*) in the 1370s.[11] The elder Francesco's father, Giacomo II da Carrara, the fifth lord of Padua (r. 1345–1350), commissioned frescoes that drew their imagery from ancient Roman literature. Francesco's more distant kinsman, Ubertino da Carrara, the third lord of Padua (r. 1338–1345) and Giacomo II's cousin, commissioned not only the building of the Reggia but also its first decorative fresco cycles, which depicted Carrara family heraldry within tapestry-like and illusionistic architectural settings.[12] Each lord commissioned frescoes in a different style of representation that complemented his public persona as *signore*. Each style reflected the lord's individual circumstances and ambitions while building upon the political achievements of his predecessors.

Commissioned by Ubertino in the 1340s, the Reggia increased the visible presence and prestige of the family at a critical time in the development of the Carrara *signoria*. The status of the Carrara family in Padua during Ubertino's lifetime was quite different from its status during Francesco Novello's. Although the family's seigniorial power in Padua was established, it by no means was secured. The road to Carrara seigniorial rule had begun two decades before Ubertino came to power, when Giacomo 'il Grande' was elected as *Defensor, Protector et Gubernator populi paduani* (*Defender, Protector and Governor of the Paduan people*) by the commune's Major Council (*Maggior Consiglio*), a council made up of the city's elders (*Anziani*).[13] Between that date and the time of Ubertino's election, however, the family had ruled Padua independently only for about three years.

The history of the Carrara family before 1337 – when the seigniory became established more firmly – is complex and involves a host of shifting alliances and betrayals. Historian Benjamin Kohl explores the nuances of this time in the family's history.[14] As noted in Chapter 3, Giacomo il Grande, the first Carrara *signore*, was elected in part to defend the city against Cangrande della Scala (1291–1329), *signore* of Verona. The Major Council granted Giacomo wide-ranging power over the city, its government and its military in the hope that he would be able to preserve the Commune's independence and unite its people. However, Giacomo was unable to stop the della Scala advance. By the summer of 1319, Cangrande had gained control of the southern Padovano (the larger Paduan territories surrounding the city) and its strongholds (Monselice, Montagnana and Este) and was moving in on Padua. So, with the blessing of Padua's Major Council, the *signore* appealed to the Duke of Austria and King of the Romans, Frederick the Fair of Habsburg (ca. 1289–1330), and asked him to place Padua under the protection of the Holy Roman Empire, effectively thwarting Cangrande's ambitions. By the end of the year, Frederick had accepted Padua into the empire, appointed Ulrich von Walsee (fl. mid-fourteenth century) as Padua's imperial vicar, and sent him to negotiate peace with the della Scala.

From 1320–1328, Padua remained under the protection – and governance – of Frederick's vicars, while Cangrande continued his attacks on the city. Further, Padua was plagued with factional violence that the German overseers could not or would not curb. At this time, the Carrara family also fought among themselves, especially after the death in 1324 of the family's leader, Giacomo il Grande, without an heir. Marsilio 'il Grande' (1294–1338),[15] Giacomo's nephew, assumed nominal leadership of the family but was increasingly opposed by Niccolò da Carrara (d. 1344),[16] who aspired to power within both the family and the city. Primarily on account of this rivalry, the Carrara house divided into the branches of Marsilio I (d. ca. 1292),[17] from which Giacomo il Grande and Marsilio il Grande descended, and that of Niccolò and Ubertino (r. 1338–1345), from which Giacomo II and Francesco il Vecchio descended.

In 1328, allegedly in response to the brutality of German governance, Marsilio il Grande secretly allied the Carrara house with their former rivals, the della Scala, through the marriage of Taddea Carrara (d. 1328), Giacomo il Grande's daughter, to Mastino II della Scala (1308–1351), Cangrande's nephew. At the same time, Marsilio agitated for leadership within Padua. He argued that peace could be achieved only by electing him as *signore* and by placing the city under Cangrande's protection. The Major Council agreed, and, on 3 September 1328, elected Marsilio as Captain General of Padua. On 8 September, Marsilio met Cangrande in Vicenza, and two days later the men triumphantly entered Padua together. Cangrande accepted lordship of Padua on 11 September and appointed Marsilio as his vicar the same day. Marsilio's compromise brought a period of peace and prosperity to Padua.

After Cangrande's death in the summer of 1329, however, the lord's nephews and heirs, Mastino II and Alberto II (1306–1352), 'demoted' Marsilio and became more involved in Padua's governance. For several years, Marsilio continued to serve an administrative role in the della Scala government, but he grew increasingly restless. Seeing an opportunity to secure leadership of Padua for himself, Marsilio secretly allied with Venice and Florence (enemies of the della Scala) and betrayed Mastino and Alberto, ousting them from Padua on 3 August 1337. On 6 August, the Major Council elected Marsilio as *signore*, and the Carrara rule of Padua began again. By the spring of the following year, however, Marsilio was dying. Without a legitimate heir, the *signore* pronounced his cousin Ubertino as his successor, and Ubertino assumed leadership of Padua after Marsilio's death on 21 March 1338.

It is against this background of the family's more tenuous hold on power that Ubertino's extensive civic patronage and his use of architectural and decorative commissions can best be understood. Ubertino was the first *signore* to use architectural and civic patronage campaigns – and monumental fresco cycles in particular – to help consolidate the family's rule and to elevate its standing in Padua and the surrounding territories. Ubertino's patronage efforts are important, among other reasons, because they enabled the later *signori* to portray themselves, the family and its history more positively in subsequent chronicles and artistic commissions.

The Reggia Carrarese was built in stages over the course of Ubertino's seven-year rule. It encompassed several buildings spread over the site originally planned as the residence for Giacomo il Grande (which was never built), and the site selected by Alberto II della Scala for his family's palazzo during their rule of Padua (1328–1337). Positioning the Carrara palace on these sites was a strategic choice for two reasons. First, by building on the site chosen for the residence of the first elected Carrara lord of Padua, Ubertino signalled his connection to Giacomo il Grande and the continuity of the dynasty. Second, building on the site chosen by the della Scala rulers suggested that Ubertino was an opponent of their occupation and a proponent of a Padua free from foreign domination.

Construction began with the so-called *Palazzo di Ponente* (West Palace), the initial, secure family residence. Its main living area comprised a large rectangular block, the long sides of which faced north and south. Its northern, more public face consisted of a two-storey trabeated (post and lintel) loggia, which remains extant, giving access to the apartments on the upper and lower levels. The *Palazzo di Levante* (East Palace), built on the site originally planned for the della Scala residence, was the palace closest to the urban environment and primarily served administrative functions.[18] While little remains of this palace, Vergerio described its architectural design in his *Liber de principibus Carrariensibus*. He wrote that, after Ubertino had finished the city walls,[19]

> [he] built a square portico with tall columns all round, in the place where Can-grande had at first begun his palace. He wanted the loggias to be two storeys high, so that it was possible to walk around, upstairs or downstairs, while sheltered from the rain. Furthermore he made another [portico] in the interior of the building, of the same height and with the same distance between the columns, but composed of only two such sides, facing north and west, so that he could freely view those regions of the heavens.

Ubertino's choices for his decoration of these buildings complemented his legacy of civic patronage (which Vergerio also described in his *Liber de principibus Carrariensibus*)[20] by promoting a message of family strength and stability. The decoration of Ubertino's halls began almost immediately after construction of the Reggia in the early 1340s, which suggests the important role ornamentation played in establishing the complex as the seat of Carrara governance. Fragments of the monumental fresco cycles located in the two rooms on the lower level of the *Palazzo di Ponente* are all that remain of Ubertino's fresco commissions. Known as the *Camera dei Carri* (*Room of the Carri*) and the *Anticamera dei Cimieri* (*Anteroom of the Cimieri*), these rooms were located directly behind Ubertino's personal loggia and facing his gardens.

The decoration of both rooms likely dates to between 1340 and 1343. Frescoes of an illusionistic tapestry inlaid with the family's heraldic arms encircled the *Camera dei Carri*. The red *carro* set against a white ground is featured alongside Ubertino's personal shield of arms, a *cimiero* also adopted by both the elder and younger Francesco, which depicts a golden-horned Saracen atop a helmet. Frescoes of illusionistic, architectural quatrefoil frames that enclose similar alternating depictions of Carrara shields of arms and *carri* adorned the *Anti-camera dei Cimieri* (Plate 5). Pairing his personal shield of arms with the family arms used by the previously elected *signori*, Giacomo il Grande (r. 1318–1320) and Marsilio II il Grande (r. 1328–1337, independently 1337–1338),[21] Ubertino emphasised both his individual lordship and his membership within the govern-ing family.

The frescoes in Ubertino's rooms may have been the sole example of this type of heraldic decoration in Padua at the time. However, the damaged state of the frescoes and the limited survival of contemporaneous fresco cycles preclude any certainty of the designs' uniqueness. On the one hand, we know that the della Scala – *signori* of Verona – and other patrician families in the region used similar motifs, which points to a currency in this type of imagery.[22] The presence of illusionistic fresco imagery adorned with heraldry likely denoted dynastic prestige at the courts of the northern Italian princes.[23] On the other hand, Ubertino's decorative choices may consciously have drawn attention to Marsilio il Grande's victory over Padua's most recent foreign occupiers, the della Scala, only a year before Ubertino was elected.

In September 1337, the month following the expulsion of the della Scala, the notaries guild of Padua had the gates of the communal palace's church painted with the arms of the allied forces responsible for Padua's liberation: the white lily of Florence, the winged lion of Venice, the red cross of Padua and the *carro* of the Carrara, recognising the Carrara family and their regime.[24] To my knowledge, this is the first recorded use of the *carro* to adorn a public building as a sign for the family and in support of the family as rulers of Padua. By echoing the public use of the *carro* as an emblem of victory in the family's apartments, Ubertino reminded visitors of the family's role in 'liberating' Padua from foreign occupation.[25]

Giacomo II: Petrarch and the Theban room

The decorative commissions of Ubertino's cousin and successor, Giacomo II da Carrara (r. 1345–1350), continued to cultivate an image of the family as liberators of Padua. Giacomo commissioned four frescoed halls for the Reggia. The decorative schemes for two of them – the *Sala Thebarum* (*Theban Room*) and the *Camera Neronis* (*Nero's Room*) – differed greatly from those commissioned by his predecessor, Ubertino. For these halls, Giacomo seems to have preferred narrative frescoes that drew their subjects from Classical sources. The decoration of the other two halls commissioned by Giacomo, the *Sala delle Bestie* (*Room of Beasts*) and the family's private chapel, was more traditional and indebted to Ubertino's decorative schemes.[26]

When he came into power in 1345, Giacomo II commissioned the decoration of a new hall of state for the Reggia, the *Sala Thebarum*. Likely, the fresco cycle for the hall was executed during the period immediately following Giacomo's election and the completion of the upper storey of the peristyle courtyard in the first half of 1345.[27] The *Sala Thebarum* remained the central hall for court business at the Reggia until Francesco il Vecchio commissioned the fresco cycle for the *Sala virorum illustrium* (*The Hall of Famous Men*) in the early 1370s. A document dated 17 July 1347 first mentioned Giacomo's hall.[28] The document, a record of state business, described the location in which it was written: 'in eius sala nova superiori, ubi depicta est ystoria Thebana' ('in his [Giacomo's] new great hall where the history of Thebes is depicted').[29] Documentary sources on Giacomo's great hall are scant, and no physical evidence of the frescoes remains. However, as the hall's name and the document from 1347 imply, the frescoes likely depicted episodes from the *Thebaid*, a tragedy about the downfall of the city Thebes, as written by the Roman poet Statius (ca. 45–96 CE).[30]

As a possible record of the fresco cycle's imagery, modern scholars have turned to a copy of the *Thebaid* produced in Padua and illustrated by Jacopo

Avanzo (1350–1416) in the late fourteenth century.[31] In this manuscript, each of Statius' 12 books begins with a monochromatic grey-scale (*grisaille*) scene of the book's principal event, highlighted with blue and red pigments. As art historian John Richards rightly notes, regardless of their relationship to the fresco cycle, the illustrations do not tell us anything about how the frescoes might have been organised.[32] Yet whether they formed a continuous narrative, like Guariento's contemporary treatment of the Old Testament frescoes in the Carrara chapel (1349–1354),[33] or represented the story in distinctive sections is inconsequential here. The important point, corroborated by modern scholars and contemporaneous documentation alike, is that Giacomo II turned to the *Thebaid* as the subject matter for his commission. Perhaps the most important question that remains is why.

Like Ubertino, Giacomo II's seigniory faced challenges to its legitimacy, although for different reasons than his predecessor. When Ubertino died on 9 March 1345 without a legitimate heir, he had not appointed Giacomo II as his successor. Rather, Ubertino recommended to the city council that his distant cousin Marsiglietto (d. 1345),[34] from the Papafava branch of the Carrara family, be elected the next lord of Padua.[35] Ubertino may have done so to thwart the seigniorial ambitions of Giacomo II and Giacomino (d. 1373), the sons of the 'traitorous' Niccolò da Carrara (d. 1344).[36] The Council elected Marsiglietto as lord of Padua on 27 March 1345. The new *signore* quickly moved to secure Venetian protection and support by renewing the alliance of 1337, which originally had helped bring down the della Scala and put the Carrara into power, a renewal witnessed by Giacomo II.[37] At the same time, however, Giacomo II and his brother, Giacomino, assembled a group of powerful local families to support their bid for power.[38] According to Guglielmo Cortusi's *Chronica de novitatibus Padue et Lombardie* (*Chronicle of the Restored State of Padua and Lombardy*, ca. 1360s), on the night of 6 May 1345, after bribing the guards to leave the doors of the Reggia unmanned, Giacomo II entered Marsiglietto's bedroom and murdered him in his sleep.[39] The following day, the Major Council unanimously elected Giacomo II as Lord and Captain General of Padua.[40]

Later apologists downplayed Giacomo II's ignominious entrance into Paduan politics and his uncompromising attitude toward his detractors. In the accounts of Giacomo's life given in chronicles commissioned by Francesco Novello, the anonymous *Gesta magnifica domus Carrariensis* (*The Magnificent Deeds of the Carrara House*)[41] and Vergerio's *Liber de principibus Carrariensibus et gestis eorum* (*The Book of the Carrara Princes and Their Deeds*), the authors commemorate Giacomo II as an active governor with an aptitude for foreign policy, qualities that ensured peace and prosperity for Padua.[42] However, Petrarch's esteem for the Carrara lord, documented in the poet's letters, most helped to cultivate a positive image of Giacomo's character.[43]

Petrarch first came to Padua in March 1349 at the invitation of the Carrara *signore*, a fact the poet acknowledged and commemorated in his last will and testament.[44] Giacomo welcomed him warmly and, among other honours, the Carrara *signore* endowed Petrarch with a canonry that included a home near the cathedral in hopes that the poet would remain in Padua rather than returning to Parma. Petrarch accepted Giacomo's gifts and relocated to Padua, where he lived, intermittently, until Giacomo's death.[45] The *signore* was killed on 19 December 1350 while he was warming his feet after lunch in the *Camera Neronis* – one of the rooms in the Reggia Carrarese that he had had frescoed.[46]

The version of Giacomo's death written by Gatari for the *Cronaca carrarese* gives a dramatic account of the murder. He wrote:[47]

> Gulielmo da Carrara (a bastard) not remembering God, but having the devil in his heart in the morning of the day of S. Antonio, 19 December, while standing beside the Signor Giacomo, drew a knife and stabbed him in the belly. The Signor turned round to the fire, looked hard at Gulielmo, and uttering only these words, 'seize him!' fell dead. Nor did Gulielmo escape. He was cut in pieces where he stood, and his body was flung in fragments into the court. Marsilio, the infant son of the murdered Signor, was placed upon a horse, brought into the public Place, and proclaimed. This was done because Giacomino, the brother, and Francesco the eldest son of the deceased, were absent from the city, having gone to kill wild boars for the Feast of the Nativity.

Shortly after Giacomo's assassination, Petrarch wrote to Giovanni Boccaccio and revealed his sadness at the lord's ignominious death.[48] In the letter, dated 7 January 1351, Petrarch told Boccaccio that he wanted to commemorate Giacomo's benevolence and generosity for posterity, and he lauded the *signore* as 'the great friend of learning, the cultivator and just critic of talents'.[49] He described Giacomo as an enlightened, modern leader and patron, one who supported poets and the study of the liberal arts at his court. Moreover, Petrarch called the Carrara lord his 'dearest and sweetest comfort and support . . . [w]orthy of every praise and distinguished by a uniquely angelic sweetness of manners'.[50] Similarly, in a letter to his friend Giovanni Aretino (d. ca. 1358), dated 4 May 1351 and written after the poet's departure from Padua earlier in the month, Petrarch honoured Giacomo's memory, calling him 'a brave and noble man deserved of praise . . . [who was] the true father of his country'.[51]

In his final will and testament,[52] Petrarch perhaps most clearly showed his admiration for Giacomo and the esteem in which he held the Carrara lord and his family. The poet requested that if he should die in Padua, he be buried alongside Giacomo at the Church of San Agostino. Petrarch wrote:[53]

> If I should die in Padua where I am now, I should wish to be buried in the Church of San Agostino, which the Dominicans now hold. For not only is this place dear to my soul, but it is also there that that man lies who loved me very much and who, through his devoted entreaties, brought me to these parts, Giacomo da Carrara of most illustrious memory, sometime Lord of Padua.

Petrarch's will tells us that the poet believed Giacomo reciprocated his admiration and that the Carrara *signore* viewed him as a friend and ally. Together, Petrarch's will and his letters to Boccaccio and Giovanni Aretino reveal a relationship between the poet and the Carrara lord built upon mutual respect and a shared love of learning, a relationship that sheds light on Giacomo's choice of subjects for his artistic commissions. The character of the visual rhetoric Giacomo employed to adorn his halls also points to his knowledge of Petrarch's moralising view of history. It attests to the poet's influence – if not his direct involvement – in the Reggia's decoration.[54]

Returning to Statius' *Thebaid*, part of Giacomo's reason for choosing the epic poem as the subject for the decoration of his hall was likely because Petrarch and other early humanists had read and admired it.[55] The *Thebaid* is a Latin epic poem written in 12 books.[56] The story Statius recounts, however, belongs to the so-called Theban cycle – a collection of four archaic Greek epic poems known only in fragments which address the mythic history of the city of Thebes. Statius' poem tells a version of the same tale known from the fragments of the Greek *Thebaid*:[57] it is the story of the war between Oedipus' cursed sons, Eteocles and Polynices, for control of the city. The tragedy *Septem contra Thebas* (*Seven Against Thebes*),[58] by the Greek tragedian Aeschylus (ca. 525–455 BCE), also takes this tale as its subject.

Statius' poem begins with the brothers' struggle for power, shows the suffering of the innocent citizens of Thebes as the fraternal war escalates and culminates with the brothers' deaths by each other's hand and the fallout that ensues. However, after Eteocles and Polynices kill one another on the fields of battle outside the city, their mother, Jocasta, commits suicide, and Eteocles' self-proclaimed successor, Creon, cruelly denies the mourning citizens of Thebes the right to build funeral pyres to honour their dead, Theseus, the good and just king, arrives to reinstate order in the final book (XII). He kills Creon, restores the citizens' rights to proper funeral rituals and finally brings a lasting peace to Thebes.

For the Carrara *signore*, Statius' tragedy provided a fitting narrative vehicle through which Giacomo could justify his violent actions and legitimate his rule.[59] Unlike his legally elected predecessors Giacomo il Grande and Marsilio il Grande, Giacomo II came to power through a betrayal. He could not present his rule as unsolicited or legal. As Richards points out, in 1345, when Giacomo plotted against Marsiglietto (whom he considered a usurper who had stolen his rightful position as ruler), Giacomo could well have been likened to Polynices, who was denied his rightful rule by Eteocles (a metaphorical Marsiglietto). Conversely, later in his rule, when Giacomo's court appeared the epitome of order and luxury celebrated by Petrarch and Vergerio, Giacomo could have been associated with the just king, Theseus, who restored order by killing the usurper Creon (a metaphorical Marsiglietto).[60] However, if Giacomo intended to associate himself metaphorically by turns with Theseus and Polynices, and to associate Marsiglietto with Eteocles and Creon, the shifting analogies had the potential to confuse more than to clarify any message about the rightful nature of his rule. The potential for misunderstanding the imagery's metaphorical associations suggests that a more atmospheric reading of Statius' narrative was at play in the *Sala Thebarum*.

In its first 11 books, the story reveals the toll that social and political unrest brings to families and townspeople, scenarios well-known to Paduans and ones that Giacomo II, like his namesake Giacomo il Grande, promised to remedy.[61] Accordingly, the use of Statius' narrative may have provided an avenue for a less specific analogy between Giacomo's circumstances and the themes established in the tale: fraternal conflict, war and tragedy are contrasted with the arrival of a just ruler. Richards argues that by employing narrative imagery from Statius' tragedy in a public hall, Giacomo portrayed himself as another Carrara 'saviour', bringer of peace and prosperity to Padua.[62] Giacomo could present himself as a hero, not in the tradition of Theseus *per se*, but in the tradition of Giacomo il Grande and Marsilio il Grande, who both 'liberated' Padua from the claws of tyranny.[63]

The anonymous *Gesta magnifica domus Carrariensis* also portrayed the Carrara as Padua's liberators. The chronicler described Marsilio il Grande and his libera-tion of Padua in July 1337 in salvific terms. He wrote that 'lux apparuit in tenebris', that light appeared from the shadows, when Marsilio gained control of Padua.[64] The chronicler further recorded that the people of Padua thanked God for the return of the Carrara, and they cried out: 'Benedictus Deus, qui fecit redempcionem plebis sue' ('Blessed God, who brings redemption to his people').[65] In addition, Richards posits that Giacomo II's seizure of power may have been perceived – by Giacomo, if not by the citizens of Padua themselves – as a righting of the unjust treatment of his ancestor and namesake, Giacomo (d. 1240),[66] who was executed by Ezzelino da Romano.[67] In its narrative of Giacomo II's life, the *Gesta magnifica* cements this parallel between Giacomo II and his unfortunate ancestor. The text portrays Marsiglietto as an usurper (like Ezzelino) who deprived Giacomo II of his rightful inheritance of power, which paved the way for Giacomo's violent, but justified, reclamation of it.[68]

By incorporating imagery from the *Thebaid* into his hall of state, Giacomo could associate himself with a hero from Greek mythic history – by way of an ancient Roman author – and simultaneously emphasise his descent from his own 'heroic' ancestors. In a fashion that Petrarch would have approved, Statius' narrative served as a cautionary tale. It provided an ancient example – Theseus – for Giacomo II, the modern ruler, to emulate and yet, by association with Carrara history, posi-tioned Giacomo's ancestors as exemplary men as well.

Notably, Giacomo commissioned another fresco cycle that may also have served to associate the lord with an exemplary leader. The *Camera Neronis*, the room in which the lord was assassinated in 1350, was first mentioned in a document dated 12 December 1347.[69] Because of the room's name, scholars have struggled with the potential subject or protagonist of the frescoes. Roman history has two prominent Neros: the infamous Emperor Nero (15–68 CE) and the lesser-known Republican Consul Gaius Claudius Nero (fl. 207 BCE), who defeated Hannibal's brother, Hasdrubal, at the Battle of Metaurus (207 BCE). Richards argues that while the virtuous actions of Consul Nero in his reconciliation with co-Consul Marcus Livius Salinator (254–ca. 204 BCE) would have been an appropriate foil for the themes of upheaval and betrayal in the *Sala Thebarum*, it seems more likely that the room was named after the despised Emperor Nero. He suggests that the emperor may have served as a negative *exemplum* – illustrating correct moral behaviour through examples of what *not* to do.[70]

The less familiar alternative is more likely, however: the room represented the episode of reconciliation between the Roman consuls and the victory over Hasdrubal. Consul Nero's life as a gifted military strategist, saviour of Rome from Hannibal's armies and conciliatory co-consul likely would have appealed to Giacomo. Further, the Roman historian Livy (59 BCE–17 CE), Padua's 'son', recorded the story of Consul Nero's defeat of Hasdrubal and praised him as a sav- iour of the Republic.[71] Similarly, and perhaps most importantly, Petrarch praised the consul and included him among the virtuous men of Roman antiquity in his *De viris illustribus*.[72]

Patronage and exemplarity under Francesco il Vecchio

The decorative schemes of Giacomo II's halls provided the thematic model that truly began the Carrara use of a Petrarchan view of (primarily) ancient Roman history and its characters as foils for the dynasty's vision of its own history and values. Petrarch's continued involvement in Carrara Padua would lead to the most overt celebration of *Romanitas* – the culture of ancient Rome – and its connection to the Carrara concept of self and government in the patronage of Giacomo's son, Francesco il Vecchio (r. 1350–1388). When he came to power after the murder of his father in 1350,[73] Francesco il Vecchio built upon the strategies of patronage established by Giacomo II and Ubertino. He continued to adorn the halls of the Reggia, and, like his father, Francesco shifted the style of representation both to reflect his individual rule and to demonstrate the continuity of the dynasty. Also like his father, Francesco wooed Petrarch to return to Padua.

During the early years of his rule, Francesco il Vecchio rekindled the Car- rara relationship with Petrarch. The poet spent time in Padua and at his home in nearby Arquà – built on land given to him by the Carrara – intermittently from the winter of 1358–1359 and more consistently from 1367.[74] In 1368, with Petrarch's connection to the court firmly re-established, Francesco urged the poet to complete *De viris illustribus*, his collection of moralising biographies of political leaders and military heroes, primarily from the Roman Monarchy, Republic and Empire.[75] Petrarch abandoned, returned to, and rewrote this work several times over the course of his life.[76] Ultimately, he left it unfinished at his death in 1374. Of the 36 biographies contained in the final, long version of the work, entitled *Quorundam virorum illustrium epithoma* (*Summary [of the Lives] of Certain Illustrious Men*), Petrarch completed 24. Lombardo della Seta (d. 1390), the poet's friend and the executor of his will, completed the remaining 12 biographies and presented the work to Francesco il Vecchio. Dated 1379 and written in Lombardo's hand, the presentation copy is now Paris, Bibliothèque nationale de France, lat. 6069 F.[77]

In his second preface to *De viris illustribus*, the so-called 'short' preface (1371– 1374), Petrarch acknowledged Francesco as an esteemed patron, identifying the

Carrara *signore* as the *vir illustris,* the noble lord, at whose request he completed his work. He wrote:[78]

> At your request, noble Carrara lord, who wields the scepter solely and with very moderate force over the great city of Padua, I have decided to collect or rather almost to compress into one place, certain illustrious men who flourished in outstanding glory and whose memory has been handed down to us in diverse and widely scattered volumes through the skill of many learned men.

Earlier in Petrarch's career and in the history of writing *De viris illustribus,* Petrarch had renounced all modern rulers as incapable of attaining the glory of their ancient counterparts.[79] So, when he named Francesco il Vecchio an 'illustrious man', Petrarch paid the prince a great compliment and intimated the respect in which the poet held his benefactor.[80] Adding Francesco to the company of lauded ancient heroes, Petrarch suggested that the *signore* shared the heroes' virtues. This compliment became central to the future patronage of the Paduan prince. For the remainder of his seigniory, Francesco il Vecchio used his patronage to present himself as a true successor to the heroes Petrarch commemorated in *De viris illustribus.*

The Hall of Famous Men

In his own turn, borrowing from Petrarch's moralistic view of the ancient heroes, Francesco il Vecchio commissioned a monumental fresco cycle that gave physical form to Petrarch's illustrious men and their histories in his new great hall, the *Sala virorum illustrium.*[81] Little of the original cycle remains. Although sharing the subject of Francesco il Vecchio's hall, the current fresco cycle dates to around 1540 and is the work of Domenico Campagnola (1500–1564) and Stefano dall' Arzere (ca. 1515–ca. 1575). An inscription over the main entrance to the hall announces that Girolamo Corner (ca. 1480–1550) – *capitano* of Padua from 13 April 1539 to 24 July 1540 – sought 'to restore, in its full splendour, the hall which was near to collapse because of old age'.[82] If this indeed is the case, Campagnola and dall' Arzere repainted the *Sala virorum illustrium* in an effort of renewal rather than re-creation (Plate 6). This is not to say that they did not alter the original conception.[83] They did, and most modern scholarship on Francesco's great hall has sought to reconstruct the lost original fresco cycle and to explain the significance of the iconographical changes in the context of sixteenth-century Padua.[84] For my purposes here, though, let us accept that while Campagnola and dall' Arzere altered the list of characters portrayed in the hall, they preserved the general, compositional makeup of the portraits.

The original cycle dates to 1370–1379 and was likely the work of Altichiero (ca. 1330–ca. 1390) and his workshop.[85] In the *Sala virorum illustrium,* Altichiero represented Petrarch's heroes in full-length, over life-sized colour portraits framed by fictive architecture and placed above *grisaille* scenes of their respective great deeds and triumphs. The frieze adorned the long (north and south) walls of the room (18 portraits to each side). Petrarch and Lombardo della Seta were portrayed on the narrow west wall.[86] The poets' portraits may have faced a large fresco of the Triumph of Fame on the east wall, which completed the cycle.[87]

Contemporaneous sources document the calculated relationship between the portrait frieze and Petrarch's work. For instance, Lombardo della Seta described an immediate connection between Francesco's hall and Petrarch's *De viris illustribus* in his dedicatory preface (1379). He wrote:[88]

> As an ardent lover of the virtues, you [Francesco] have extended hospitality to these *viri illustres*, not only in your mind and soul, but also very magnificently in the most beautiful part of your palace. According to the custom of the ancients you have honoured them with gold and purple, and with images and inscriptions you have set them up for admiration.

Lombardo's comment tells us that Francesco's commission honoured the heroes and showed their importance to the prince's 'mind and soul'. Given the connection between the portrait cycle and Petrarch's text, which Lombardo described, the portrait series likely followed the order in which Petrarch presented the men in *De viris illustribus*.

Petrarch wrote the biographies in chronological order, beginning with Romulus and ending with Trajan. In his preface to the *De viris illustribus*, Lombardo remarked upon the placement of Trajan's portrait in Francesco's great hall, writing:[89]

> I know that you, gracious lord of Padua, are eagerly waiting for the conclusion of this work so that you can learn briefly and in the right order about the deeds of your famous heroes. For this reason, just as you have placed Trajan among the others in the extreme corner of your beautiful hall, so I, in this work, set out to treat him as the last one.

From this comment, scholars have speculated on the original placement of the frescoes, believing that the frieze began with the portrait of Romulus, in the northwest corner, and ended with the portrait of Trajan in the southwest corner.[90]

In addition to Lombardo's account of the portraits, Michele Savonarola described the defining features of the cycle in his *Libellus de magnificis ornamentis regie civitatis Padue* (ca. 1446). Savonarola attributed the frescoes to Altichiero and one of his followers, Ottaviano of Brescia (fl. 1376–1412), and located the room inside the Reggia in relation to the *Sala Thebarum*. He wrote:[91]

> When one ascends the principal staircase, one finds balconies, all decorated, on the upper floor around the loggia, with marble columns and magnificent windows overlooking both courtyards. On either side are two most spacious halls which are elaborately decorated with pictures. The first of these rooms

is called the Theban Room (*Sala Thebarum*), the other one, which is larger and more glorious than the first, is named the Room of the Generals (*Sala Imperatorum*). In this room are depicted the Roman generals (*Romani imperatores*), in *wonderful figures with their triumphs, painted with gold and the best colours*. The representation of these men was the work of the famous painters Ottaviano [of Brescia] and Altichiero. This is indeed an imperial palace and worthy of an emperor.

This passage places Francesco's great hall in direct relation to his father's, which stresses a perceived genealogical connection between the rooms. Emphasising the theme of succession and continuity, Savonarola noted that the *Sala virorum illustrium* exceeded the preceding hall of state in its grandeur. According to his account, the figures were executed in the 'best colours' and in gold ('auro optimoque cum colore depicti sunt'), attesting to the expense, quality and importance of the original cycle.

Contemporaneous chronicles also attest to the highly visible role of the *Sala virorum illustrium* in the events held at Francesco's court. Banquets, wedding festivities, meetings with foreign dignitaries and even the private family funeral for Francesco il Vecchio were held in this space. For instance, three chronicles record the wedding festivals of the daughters of the last two Carrara lords. In the *Cronaca carrarese*, Gatari described the festivities for the wedding of Caterina (d. 1389), eldest daughter of Francesco il Vecchio and Fina da Buzzacarini (ca. 1325–1378), to Stefan Frankapan (fl. late fourteenth/early fifteenth century), Count of Veglia, in 1372.[92] Here, the chronicler commented only on the more public aspects of the celebration – the dancing and jousting – and did not describe the location of the ceremony.[93] However, in his account of the marriage of Gigliola (ca. 1379–1416), daughter of Francesco Novello and Taddea d'Este (d. 1404), to Nicolò III d'Este (1383–1441) in 1397, Gatari noted that the ceremony was held in the great hall of the Reggia – the *Sala virorum illustrium*.[94] Further, an anonymous chronicle written in 1383 recorded the hall as the site for the wedding ceremony of Lieta (fl. late fourteenth/early fifteenth century), youngest daughter of Francesco il Vecchio, to Frederick, Count of Oettingen (fl. late fourteenth/early fifteenth century), in 1382.[95] Since the *Sala virorum illustrium* was the site for the wedding ceremonies of her sister and niece, Caterina likely wed in the great hall as well.

In a similar way, both Vergerio and Gatari describe the funeral rites and procession for Francesco il Vecchio in 1393, noting that the private family service was performed in the courtyard of the Reggia, specifically just outside of the *Sala virorum illustrium*.[96] Judging by the prominent role the great hall played in festivals and celebrations, it seems clear that the room was important to Francesco il Vecchio's sense of self as a ruler and served as an avenue to project this understanding visually. But what message did Francesco intend to send by commissioning a cycle of monumental portraits of Petrarch's famous men? What was the relationship between the portrait frieze and the *signore*, and how did it function in the atmosphere of the court?

Lombardo della Seta suggests an answer to these questions in his preface to the *De viris illustribus*. In addition to confirming the relationship between the fresco cycle and Petrarch's text, Lombardo likened the exemplary role of the biographies to the role of the portraits that adorn Francesco's hall. He noted:[97]

> To the *inward conception* of your keen mind you have given *outward expression* in the form of most excellent pictures, so that you may always keep in sight these men whom you are eager to love because of the greatness of their deeds.

In this passage, Lombardo built upon his earlier remarks, in which he said that the portraits of the *viri illustres* reflected Francesco's mind and soul ('mente et animo').[98] According to Lombardo, the portraits were more than reflections; they were signs, 'outward expressions' ('extrinsecus expressisti'), of Francesco's invisible inner state. Their very presence in Francesco's hall manifested the prince's virtuous character to his visitors. Lombardo, following Petrarch, suggested that by commemorating and honouring these men in his soul, Francesco participated in their greatness. By having portraits of them painted on the walls of his palace, Francesco appropriated their moral authority and so denoted the rightness of his rule. Moreover, by juxtaposing himself with these men, Francesco united their different virtues in his person and located them in contemporaneous Padua and the surrounding Carrara territories.

The addition of Petrarch's portrait to the cycle commemorated his personal role in the introduction of these heroes into Francesco's 'mind and soul'. Only fragments of the original fourteenth-century fresco remain (Figure 4.1).[99] The presence of his portrait honoured the poet and revealed the esteem in which Francesco held him. It also served to remind Francesco and – perhaps more importantly – his visitors of exactly how Francesco came to know these men: through Petrarch's work and his influence. On the west wall of the *Sala virorum illustrium*, Altichiero and Ottaviano portrayed the poet in his *studiolo*, his study or personal library. He sits at his desk, which is strewn with the books and writing instruments of his vocation. The setting stresses the importance of the study as the place of quiet retreat in which Petrarch contemplated, read and wrote about his *viri illustres*.[100]

Petrarch's portrait emphasises the original literary context of the heroes and juxtaposes the heroes with their biographer – the keeper of their histories. Its presence in the frieze shows the viewer how to 'read' the images and connects the heroes to their illustrious histories. In effect, Petrarch's portrait encourages the viewer to map the narratives of the heroes' invisible lives onto their corresponding visible bodies, making their bodies a type of index for the entirety of their histories.[101] Furthermore, by having Petrarch portrayed among the Roman heroes, Francesco could claim the poet as an exemplar as well. The setting in which Petrarch works, however, demonstrates that he exemplified a different kind of virtuous life than that of the heroes his work describes: Petrarch epitomises the contemplative life of the scholar-historian rather than the active life of the political leader or soldier.

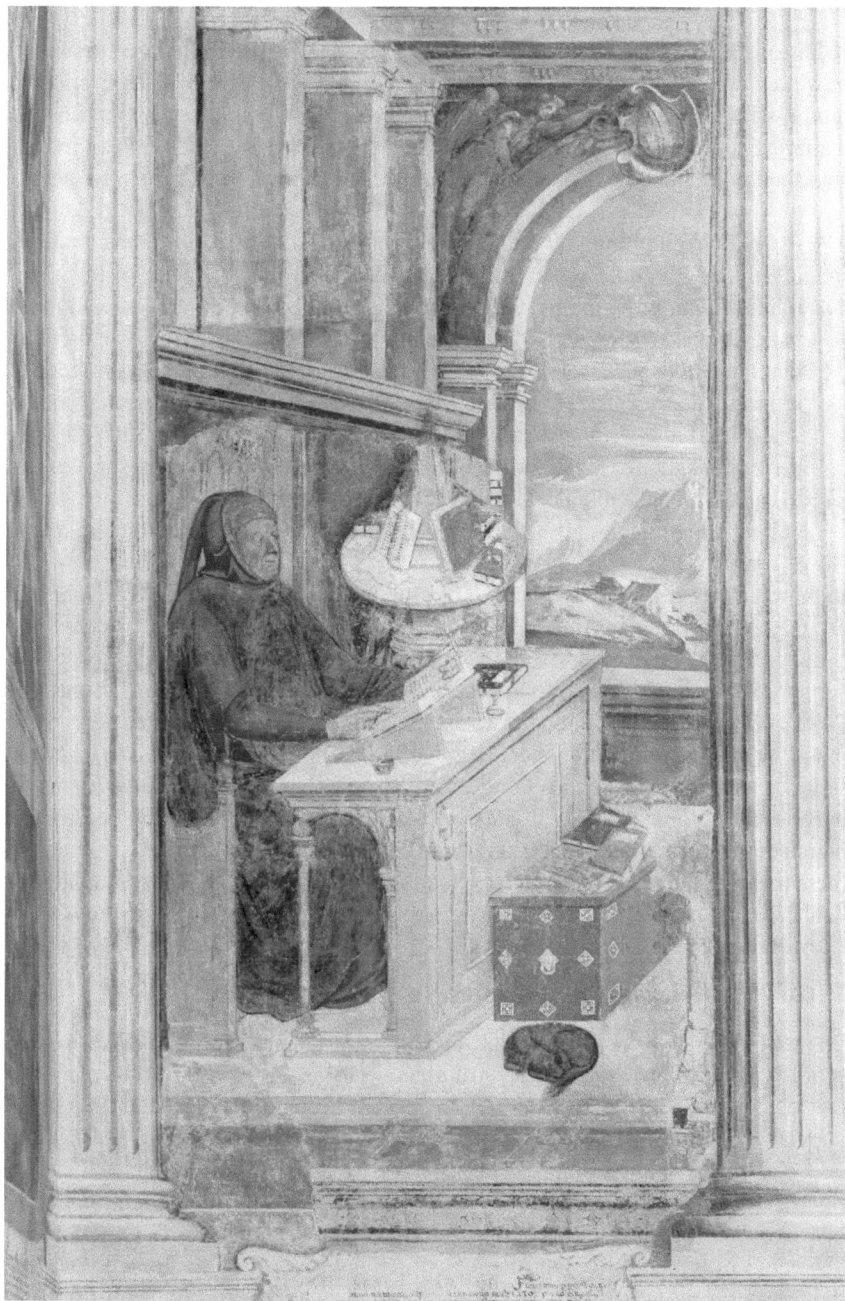

Figure 4.1 Altichiero (?), portrait of Petrarch (extensively repainted)

Sala dei Giganti (formerly *Sala virorum illustrium*)
Padua, University of Padua, Palazzo Liviano
Fresco, Padua, ca. 1374–1379

Su concessione dell'Università degli Studi di Padova – foto "Massimo Pistore © Università di Padova"

Late in his 'short' preface to *De viris illustribus* (1371–1374), Petrarch described how he viewed his role as an author and historian and how he wanted Francesco (and his future readers) to interpret his work. The poet explained his purpose in gathering together the scattered histories of '[these men] who flourished in outstanding glory and whose memory has been handed down to us'.[102] He wrote,[103]

> In my book, nothing is found except what leads to virtues or to the contraries of virtues. For, unless I am mistaken, this is the profitable goal for the historian: to point up to the readers those things that are to be followed and those to be avoided. Whoever would presume to wander outside this boundary, let him know that he is wandering on foreign territory and let him be reminded to return to the path, *except perhaps when he will be seeking to please his readers with amusing anecdotes*. And I myself cannot deny that I have often for long periods abandoned myself to such distracting digressions, when it was pleasant to call to mind the manner and domestic life of illustrious men, and their words neither stinging nor grave, their bodily stature, genealogy, or manner of death.

In this passage, Petrarch stressed two central themes of the *De viris illustribus* that are relevant to the pattern of patronage established by Francesco il Vecchio and his son: first, the exemplary role of biographies of famous men and, second, the supporting role that pleasure plays in the reception of the moralising lessons. For Petrarch, as for Horace long before him, the author binds edification to pleasure to make the process of learning more memorable.[104] The profitable goal is to teach the virtuous life-path to the reader. For Petrarch, the pleasurable digressions (his 'amusing anecdotes') are the details of the heroes' lives – their bodily stature, ancestry, the nature of their deaths and their triumphs. Altichiero and Ottaviano pictured many of these pleasing details in the fresco cycle of the *Sala virorum illustrium*, making the hall a space designed both for the profit and for the pleasure of the viewer.

Petrarch on pleasure and profit

Petrarch expanded upon the theme of striking a balance between pleasure and profit as a reader and explained how this balance helped to shape the reader's virtuous behaviour. In a lengthy letter to Francesco il Vecchio, written according to the conventions of the *Speculum principis* genre and dated 28 November 1373,[105] the poet elaborated on the role of history's *viri illustres* in the development of a good ruler's character and the important role of vision in this development. Peppering his narrative with positive and negative examples drawn from the actions and behaviour of Imperial Roman rulers, Petrarch promised to show Francesco 'what the ruler of a country should be' ('qualis esse debeat qui rempublicam regit') in order that[106]

> by looking at this [account] *as though looking at yourself in the mirror*, whenever you see yourself in what I describe . . . you may *enjoy* it and daily become more faithful and more obedient to [God] the Dispenser of all virtue

and good, and with a huge effort rise through the barriers of hardship to that level where you cannot rise any further.

In this passage, Petrarch describes the double goal of his letter: he aims to mould Francesco into a moral leader and to teach the *signore* how best to read history. Petrarch instructed Francesco to seek out his reflection in the historical examples of good leadership that he was about to recount. Moreover, the poet encouraged Francesco to enjoy seeing himself reflected in the lives of these *viri illustres*, a pleasure that – in turn – would help the prince to perfect his moral identity. The role of the text as a mirror for Francesco held up by Petrarch himself points to the dynamic relationship between reader, author, and text and emphasises the role of pleasurable (imaginary) vision as a tool for moral instruction in Petrarch's teaching practices.[107]

Bringing Petrarch's mirror metaphor into the physical realm provides an avenue of interpretation for the portraits in the *Sala virorum illustrium* and reveals how the portraits' role echoed that of the textual histories for Francesco il Vecchio. As Lombardo's preface to *De viris illustribus* makes clear, Francesco placed the portraits in his hall to 'set up [the great men] for admiration'.[108] The frieze denoted Francesco's respect for these men and their values. However, by keeping company with the heroes physically as well as mentally and by looking to them as though to a mirror, Francesco sought to approximate the *viri illustres* – or at least to convince his visitors that he did. By upholding himself as a contemporary reflection of ancient heroes and of their greatness, Francesco cultivated the admiration of literate citizens and visitors and consolidated his power by way of the heroes' moral authority. Furthermore, this moral authority was doubly powerful for Petrarch's deliverance of it.

The representation of Petrarch in the *Sala virorum illustrium* emphasises Francesco's connection not only to the poet as the author of *De viris illustribus* but also to his pursuit of the contemplative life and to his reverence for ancient texts. While the portraits of great men and their triumphs served as mirrors of a virtuous *active* life, the portrait of the poet was a mirror of its complement: the virtues of a *contemplative* life, a life that Petrarch encouraged Francesco to pursue when he counselled the *signore* to study the deeds of history's great men. The site of the poet's pursuit was his *studiolo*, and so the artists portrayed Petrarch in his library surrounded by his notable book collection – a collection that Francesco inherited upon the poet's death in 1374. While Francesco sold a number of the poet's volumes, he kept the majority of the collection for his own library.[109] He also inherited a portrait of the Madonna and Child by Giotto of which Petrarch was particularly fond – another sign of the high esteem in which the poet held the Carrara *signore*.[110]

Petrarch and the Carrara library

The volumes assumed into Francesco il Vecchio's collection from Petrarch's personal library were expansive. The poet prepared an inventory of the most prized books from his collection at Vaucluse, likely prior to his voyage to Rome to receive the laurel crown in 1337, which provides some insight into the general shape of his library.[111] In this inventory, Petrarch divided his books into four primary categories, reflecting themes that would continue to inform his pattern of book collection throughout his life. These four principal categories were ethics and rhetoric, history, poetry and grammar, and theology. Following Petrarch's list,[112] the philosophers and rhetoricians represented in Petrarch's book collection were Aristotle (ca. 384–322 BCE), Cicero (106–43 BCE), Seneca (4 BCE–65 CE) and Boethius (480–524 CE). The historians: Valerius Maximus (fl. 30 CE), Livy (59 BCE–17 CE), Justinus (fl. third century CE), Lucius Annaeus Florus (ca. 74 CE–ca. 130 CE), Sallust (86–ca. 35 BCE), Suetonius (70–130 CE), Sextus Festus (fl. late fourth century CE), Eutropius (fl. mid-late fourth century CE), Macrobius (fl. early fifth century CE) and Aulus Gellius (130–180 CE). The poets: Virgil (70–19 BCE), Lucan (39–65 CE), Statius (45–96 CE), Horace (65–8 BCE), Ovid (43 BCE–8 CE) and Juvenal (fl. late first–early second century CE); and the grammarians: Priscian (fl. 500 CE), and perhaps Marcus Valerius Probus (ca. 30–105 CE) and Papias (fl. 1040s–60s). Augustine (354–430 CE) was the theologian.[113]

The inventory is a panoply of some of the greatest minds of antiquity. Besides documenting Petrarch's admiration for Aristotle and Augustine, the list also shows the poet's love of ancient Roman history and culture, its heroes and ideals, and attests to his proficiency in their study from early in his career.[114] Petrarch's library grew richer during his travels prior to settling in Arquà in the 1360s. The 1426 inventory of the Visconti-Sforza library, the library into which Petrarch's collection was assumed after the fall of Francesco il Vecchio, adds information to Petrarch's early list.[115] Among other volumes, Petrarch's collection included copies of Plato's cosmology, the *Timaeus*, bound with the allegory of learning and the liberal arts, *De Nuptiis Philologiae et Mercurii* (*On the Marriage of Philology and Mercury*), by Martianus Capella (fl. fifth century CE), both of which were influential in medieval mythography.[116] He also owned copies of Homer's *Iliad* and *Odyssey*, poetry by Claudianus (ca. 370–404 CE) and the rhetorical handbook *Institutio oratoria*, by Quintilian (35–100 CE). Religious works in his collection included those by Cassiodorus (ca. 490–ca. 583 CE), Augustine, and other Doctors of the Church – Ambrose (ca. 340–397 CE) and Gregory the Great (ca. 540–604 CE).[117] Petrarch urged Francesco to study many of these texts for moral guidance, and he drew upon them repeatedly in his correspondence with the prince and in the *De viris illustribus*.[118] If works by these and other authors were represented in Francesco il Vecchio's collection, along with those written by Petrarch himself, the Carrara library would have been very grand indeed.

The inheritance of Petrarch's books cemented the Carrara library's prestige across the Veneto. It also enabled the library to become another locus for the cultivation of the lord's image as an illustrious man and leader. Like the *Sala virorum illustrium*, Francesco's library served as a physical and conceptual space.

It was a physical space that housed real books, which were Petrarch's sources for information on Roman history and values that he used in his biographies. But it was also a conceptual space in which Francesco il Vecchio's relationship with the characters in the *De viris illustribus* was mobilised. As Lombardo della Seta noted in his preface to *De viris illustribus*, Francesco sought to '[extend] hospitality to these *viri illustres* . . . in [his] mind and soul'.[119] The books were tangible signs of his mind's hospitality. Francesco's mind became the conceptual counterpart to the physical space of the library. The link between the physical and the conceptual spaces was, of course, Francesco il Vecchio himself, as the owner and principal reader of the books.

Francesco il Vecchio integrated his self-image as a public, active leader in the tradition of the great Romans (established in the portraits in the *Sala virorum illustrium*) with that of an enlightened and contemplative scholar (established in his library and book collection). He actualised the latter image by building up his book collection and emphasised the former through its content.[120] This confluence of ideals and objects served Francesco il Vecchio's purpose well. He was celebrated during his life and remembered in his death both as a good soldier and leader (practitioner of the active life) and as a wise and studious scholar (upholder of the moral values associated with the contemplative life).[121] Francesco Novello reinvented this confluence in his own book collection; however, he directed it to different ends.

*

When Francesco Novello became *signore* of Padua in 1390, he concentrated his artistic patronage on book collection, striving to reacquire and rebuild the Carrara library after the Visconti conquest. The younger Francesco's focus on book collection tells us that his father's relationship with the library and its books held similar value for the new lord. In his activities as a book collector, Francesco Novello sought to continue and surpass those of his father, as his ancestors had long sought both to preserve and to outdo each other's patronage. The books in Francesco Novello's collection in general, and the *Carrara Herbal* and other illustrated books in particular, were manifestations of the balance between competition and continuity within the family's patronage and between the pleasures and utilities afforded by the reading of them. Certainly, these books were attributes that pointed to Francesco's role as his father's successor. Their significance to the development of Francesco Novello's self-image as the new prince of Padua depended, in part, upon the ideal relationship between book collection, Petrarchan teaching practices, and the princely identities established by his ancestors in their portraits and other artistic commissions. Francesco Novello acknowledged the primacy of this relationship by incorporating textual and visual references to his father's rule and to his family's various uses of portraiture into his personal library, conflating their significance for his forebears with his own articulation of self as the 'physician prince' of Padua.

Notes

1 On the Commune of Padua, see Hyde (1966b: 193–251). Kohl (1998: 35–7) argues that during this era of relative peace and prosperity, the influence and power of the Carrara family grew in no small part because they cultivated ties through marriage with leading local and international families.

2 On the relationship between 'ideal' Carrara history and 'real' Carrara history in the chronicles and biographies produced under the elder and younger Francescos, see Kohl (2007).

3 In his chronicle, da Nono sorted over one hundred aristocratic Paduan families into four hierarchical categories, or degrees, of nobility. The categories ranged from the most powerful magnate families to the least. He described each family's origin, principal family members during his time, coats of arms, major houses in the city and their relative wealth (Hyde 1966b: 57 and 1993: 21–2 and 34–8). Currently, no complete edition of *De generatione* is available. For excerpts and discussion of da Nono's treatise, see Rajna (1875); Fabris (1932–1933); and Hyde (1966a).

4 Despite this lower ranking, da Nono did not doubt the family's claim to nobility. According to the chronicle, the Carrara descended from a noble family of German knights, the da Montagnone, who had taken up residence in Carrara, a small town in the southern Padovano, during the tenth century (Kohl 1998: 35). On the da Montagnone, see Hyde (1966b: 82).

5 Da Nono seems to defend his view of the family's nobility. He wrote, 'but I pass over what [the people] say, because today [the Carrara] are noble and powerful citizens of Padua' (tr. Hyde 1966b: 82, from *De generatione*, Padua, Biblioteca del Seminario, MS 11, ff. 37v–38r).

6 Hyde (1966b: 82–3) suggests that the discrepancy between public opinion and public records may be due to the relative obscurity and poverty of some members of the large, extended Carrara family at the time.

7 Mussato, *De traditione* (in *De gestis Italicorum post Henricum VII Caesarem*, XII.1 [ed. Muratori 1727: col. 725]). Mussato composed *De traditione* while in exile at Chioggia during the final years of his life (Witt 2000: 146). This work's history of publication is complex. Although not intended by Mussato to be part of his earlier *De gestis Italicorum post Henricum VII Caesarem* (*Concerning the Deeds of the Italians After Emperor Henry VII*), a chronicle of Italy after the Holy Roman Emperor's death in 1313, Lorenzo Pignoria (1571–1631), editor of the first edition of Mussato's collected works (*Opera Albertini Mussati* [Venetiis: Ex Typographia Ducali Pinelliana, 1636]), grouped *De traditione* together with Books I–VII and the fragment of Book IX then known from *De gestis*. Pignoria combined these Books with Mussato's epic poem *De obsidione Domini Canis Grandis de Verona circa moenia paduanae civitatis et conflictu ejus (Of Cangrande's Besieging the Walls of the City of Padua and of Its Fight)*, which he included as Books IX–XI of *De gestis*, adding *De traditione* as Book XII. Ludovico Muratori (1672–1750), historian and compiler of the *Rerum Italicarum Scriptores* series, repeated the earlier grouping, so scholars regularly have cited *De traditione* as Book XII of *De gestis*. Luigi Padrin (1838–1899) discovered the remaining seven books of *De gestis* in the late nineteenth century and published them separately (*Sette libri inediti del De gestis italicorum post Henricum VII* [Venice: A spese della Società, 1903]). For the history of publication of Mussato's works, see Witt (2000: 131n40 and n41).

8 Hyde (1966b and 1993) and Kohl (1998) have discussed the realities of the Carrara seigniory in detail. These scholars present an account of the city as it was ruled by the Carrara, and the portrait of the Carrara it conveys is quite different from the one that the Carrara lords presented of themselves.

9 Today, little remains of the once-extensive palace complex. It was heavily damaged by Austrian occupation in the eighteenth century and largely demolished by 1880 to make room for a school, the Scuola elementare 'Reggia Carrarese'. Between the decision to demolish the Reggia in 1873 and the erection of the school in 1880, Andrea Gloria (1821–1911), then director of the Museo Civico in Padua, unearthed and published as

much archival evidence on the Reggia's decoration as he could find to demonstrate its cultural and historical importance to Padua. Any examination of the Carrara palace is indebted to his comprehensive study of the extant documentation. See Gloria (1878).

10 On the Reggia Carrarese and other Carrara strongholds in the Padovano, see Gasparotto (1966–1967 and 1968–1969); Lorenzoni (1977); and Richards (2000 and 2007).

11 For the critical editions of Petrarch's *De viris illustribus* and the chronology of the work's development, see n75 and n76 in this chapter.

12 Ubertino da Carrara was the son of Giacomino da Carrara (d. 1319). He was Francesco il Vecchio's first cousin once removed.

13 For the wording of the statute, see Chapter 3, p. 107n20.

14 Kohl (1998: 3–99).

15 For an introduction to Marsilio 'il Grande', see Ganguzza Billanovich (1977g).

16 For an introduction to Niccolò, see Ganguzza Billanovich (1977h).

17 For an introduction to Marsilio I, see Ganguzza Billanovich (1977f).

18 Gasparotto (1966–1967: 1.80). For a more detailed account of the Reggia's architecture and placement within Padua, see Richards (2007: 17–23). My discussion of the Reggia's layout and its rooms' locations within the complex follows Richards' analysis.

19 'Porticum quadratam altissimis columnis in aedibus struxit, [ubi Canis grandis habere primus regiam coeperat], eamque duplicem esse voluit, ut et humi et in sublime deambulare liceret, ab imbre tectos. Aliam quoque in interiori domo, pari altitudine et intercolumniorum distantia, perfecit, quam duobus tantum lateribus constare jussit in septemtrionem occasumque spectantibus, ut esset prospectus in eas caeli plagas liber' (Vergerio, *Liber de principibus*, IV, 'De Ubertino de Carraria, tertio ex ea Familia Principe Paduae', §105 [ed. Gnesotto 1924: 431; tr. Richards 2007: 19]). Michele Savonarola and Angelo Portenari also describe the palace. See Savonarola's *Libellus*, II, 'De Temporalibus et Mundanis' (ed. Segarizzi 1902: 49) and Portenari's *Della felicità di Padova*, 3.8 (1623: 104).

20 See Chapter 3, pp. 92 and 108n25.

21 As noted earlier in this chapter (pp. 118–19), Marsilio's rule of Padua encompassed both his appointment by Cangrande della Scala as vicar of the city (1328–1337) and his independent rule as *signore* after ousting Alberto II della Scala in 1337.

22 This style of ornamentation was visible at the della Scala's palace, the so-called Castelvecchio, in Verona, as well as on the walls of a courtyard at the Visconti stronghold at Pandino and in a few of the apartments in the Carrara castle at Monselice (Richards 2007: 24). On the frescoes of the Castelvecchio, see Richards (2000: 35–75).

23 On account of the regional preference for this type of ornamentation, Richards (2007: 25) argues that the message conveyed through the decoration would have been familiar to courtiers accustomed to life under seigniorial rule.

24 The notice in the notaries guild's records from 30 September 1337 reads: 'dicti gastaldiones fecerunt depingi in ecclesia palacii et portas palaciis et dicto palacio signa et armatures communium Veneciarum, Florencie, Padue et magnifici domini Marsilii de Carraria' (*Reformationes frataleae notariorum Padua*, Padua, Biblioteca Civica, B.P. 825, f. 15r [ed. Cessi 1985: 1.145n19]). Cited and further discussed by Kohl (1998: 68).

25 Perhaps Francesco Novello used these rooms in a similar way. During his tenure as *signore*, the *Camera dei Carri* may have served as an antechamber in which Francesco's guests assembled and waited prior to meeting with the *signore* in the *Camera Lucretie* nearby (Gasparotto 1966–1967: 1.114, and Richards 2007: 24).

26 The *Sala delle Bestie*, which may have been frescoed by Guariento (1310–1370), was located directly below the *Sala Thebarum* and probably contained hunting scenes, a common theme in the decoration of northern courts during this period. The private chapel likely was located on the upper floor of the *Palazzo di Ponente* at the western end. Likely between 1349 and 1354, Guariento decorated the chapel with Old Testament

scenes (Richards 2007: 30–3). Only fragments of the frescoes commissioned by Giacomo II survive, including an image of the Angelic Orders with which Guariento adorned the ceiling of the chapel. The fragments are held at the Museo Civico in Padua.

27 Gasparotto (1966–1967: 1.25). Following a note in Guglielmo Cortusi's *Chronica* (9.10, 'De domina Isabella' [ed. Pagnin 1941: 117]), Kohl (1998: 92) and Richards (2007: 28) suggest that the *Sala Thebarum* likely was completed by the time Isabella del Fiesco (fl. mid-fourteenth century), wife of Luchino Visconti (1287–1349), the lord of Milan, came to visit Padua in March 1347.

28 The document is now Padua, Archivio di Stato, Archivio Corona, Busta 149, 2314 n.g. 7787.

29 My translation. Gloria (1878: 35) and Gasparotto (1966–1967: 1.95) further discuss the significance of this document. In addition, Michele Savonarola mentioned this room in the *Libellus* (II, 'De Temporalibus et Mundanis' [ed. Segarizzi 1902: 49]). However, he did not provide a detailed description of it, either. Savonarola noted the popular title of the room, which suggests the subject of its decoration, and addressed the placement of Giacomo's hall in direct relation to his son's *sala curiale,* the *Sala virorum illustrium.* Norman (1995c: 1.165) and Richards (2007: 28) further discuss Savonarola's comments.

30 Richards (2007: 30). At the time of the *Sala Thebarum*'s construction, there were two possible sources for a 'history of Thebes': Statius' *Thebaid* or a chivalric retelling of the story popular in twelfth-century French romances. Richards persuasively argues that the frescoes' narrative was based on Statius' version. He uses Giacomo's friendship with Petrarch and their shared love of Roman literature as evidence to support his view.

31 The manuscript is now Dublin, Chester-Beatty Library, MS 76. Mellini (1965: 102), Gasparotto (1966–1967: 1.95) and Richards (2007: 31–2) argue that this illustrated manuscript of the *Thebaid* may reveal some of the original frescoes' traits. Regardless of the exactness of the relationship between the manuscript illustrations and the frescoes, it seems probable that the Chester-Beatty *Thebaid* records aspects of the *Sala Thebarum.* There was a fashion for this type of copying in Padua at the close of the fourteenth century: other contemporaneous illustrated manuscripts record the Reggia's lost frescoes. For instance, six *grisaille* (grey-scale) portraits of the Carrara lords in Vergerio's *Liber de principibus Carrariensibus* (now Padua, Biblioteca Civica, B.P. 158) likely replicate frescoes from the entrance loggia of the Reggia, a point to which I will return in Chapter 6. In addition, a copy of Petrarch's *De viris illustribus* (now Darmstadt, Hessische Landes- und Hochschulbibliothek, Ital. 101) includes several *grisaille* illustrations that may record aspects of the monumental portrait series in the *Sala virorum illustrium* (see Mommsen 1952, and, on other late fifteenth-century illustrated copies of *De viris illustribus* that may reflect the frescoes, Armstrong 1999). Given this tendency to record fresco imagery in illustrated books, it is not unlikely that an illustrated version of Statius' *Thebaid* would copy a contemporaneous fresco cycle, at least in part.

32 Richards (2007: 31–2).

33 See n26 in this chapter for a brief outline of Guariento's work at the Reggia Carrarese.

34 For an introduction to Marsiglietto, see Ganguzza Billanovich (1977e).

35 The Papafava branch of the Carrara family descends from Giacomino da Carrara (d. 1289), nephew of Giacomo da Carrara (d. 1240), who was the father of Marsilio I (d. 1292). For a genealogical table, see Hyde (1966b: 83–4). Giacomino's nickname was 'Papafava', and it became the second surname of his descendants. This branch of the family was less politically prominent than the other two and sided with Marsilio il Grande and Ubertino against Niccolò da Carrara in the factional violence during the 1320s (Kohl 1998: 54).

36 Niccolò was deemed a traitor to the family and to Padua when he joined the della Scala forces and besieged Padua. In the summer of 1327, he secretly allied with the

della Scala and, that fall, joined in the della Scala attempt to seize Padua, a choice that alienated him not only from Marsilio il Grande but also from Ubertino, who supported Marsilio as head of the family. Rallying against Niccolò, Marsilio, along with the members of the Papafava branch of the Carrara family and other noble families of Padua, repulsed Niccolò and the della Scala forces with the help of a contingent of German knights. Niccolò was exiled to Chioggia for the remainder of his life. Despite his absence from Paduan politics, it was from Niccolò's line that the last three Carrara lords descended (Kohl 1998: 55–7).

37 Kohl (1998: 87).

38 Kohl (1998: 87–9).

39 Cortusi, *Chronica*, 9.1, 'De morte Magni Ubertini et ejus successoris' (ed. Pagnin 1941: 111–13). Kohl (1998: 89) further discusses Cortusi's account of the murder. Writing mid-century as a supporter of Francesco il Vecchio, Cortusi gives a pro-Carrara account of Paduan politics between 1311 and 1368. The later Gatari chronicle (also pro-Carrara) does not mention Giacomo II's bribery, preferring to attribute the choice to leave the doors unlocked to Marsiglietto himself, who 'thought himself well loved' ('[Marsiglietto] il predetto con benigno muodo, fidandosi d'ognuna persona: per che, credendo cosí lui eser amato, come lui amava altri, non soervava in sé tropo stretta guardi . . .') (Gatari, *Cronaca*, 'Come quelli da Carrara portano per arma il lione rampante in campo bianco; e come fu morto ser Marsilio Papafava da Carrara Signore, e poi fu messer Giacomo Signore', aprile 1345 [eds Medin and Tolomei 1931: 26; tr. Symes 1830: xxxii]).

40 While Giacomo II chased Marsiglietto's heirs and supporters into exile and murdered Marsiglietto's most trusted advisors, he also chased the favour of powerful families by giving them elaborate gifts of clothing, gold, arms, houses, horses and lands to atone for his crimes. Further, Giacomo recalled enemies of Ubertino from exile, granted amnesty to many citizens who had been imprisoned and obtained an oath of loyalty from all knights in the Carrara palaces. The day following the assassination, Giacomo II advantageously married his son and heir, Francesco I da Carrara, to Fina da Buzzacarini (ca. 1325–1378), the daughter of long-time Carrara family supporter and magistrate Pataro di Dusio (d. 1361). In the ensuing months, Giacomo II ratified his rule with the Venetians through a series of negotiations with the Doge, Andrea Dandolo (1306–1354), and effectively transitioned to his role as lord of Padua. For specific details of the treatise, especially regarding economics and exchange of prisoners, see Cortusi, *Chronica*, 9.1–2 (ed. Pagnin 1941: 111–12) and, for additional commentary, Kohl (1998: 89–90).

41 My references to the text of the *Gesta magnifica* correspond to the Latin version in the manuscript now Venice, Biblioteca Nazionale Marciana, lat. X, 381 (coll. 2802), a manuscript that likely belonged to Francesco Novello (see Lazzarini 1901–1902). Cessi's modern, critical edition (1942–1948) compares this redaction (redaction A) with several others – in both Latin and vernacular.

42 Vergerio and the author of the *Gesta magnifica* covered over Giacomo's murderous deed, rationalising that Marsiglietto eventually would see Giacomo as a threat to his power since Giacomo was the rightful claimant to the seigniory. Vergerio suggested that Giacomo pre-emptively acted against Marsiglietto out of necessity and because he was afraid for his life. He proceeded to parallel Giacomo's entrance into power with that of Julius Caesar, who similarly began his rule with a 'necessary' act of violence (Vergerio, *Liber de principibus*, VI, 'De Jacobo Minore de Carraria, qui quintus ex Carrariensibus Princeps fuit', §115–16 [ed. Gnesotto 1924: 441–2]). A similar account is presented in the *Gesta magnifica* (XX, 'Domini Ubertinus et Bonifacius Fratres', §91 [ed. Cessi 1942–1948: 31]), which parallels Giacomo II with his ancestor, Giacomo (d. 1240), who allegedly died a martyr for Padua. For an analysis of the *Gesta magnifica* account, see Richards (2007: 39). For details on Giacomo II's life and foreign policy, see Kohl (1998: 89–95).

43 Petrarch's letter to Boccaccio, *Rerum familiarium* XI.2 (discussed later in this chapter), is perhaps the most revealing example of the poet's sentiments.

44 Kirkham (2009b: 149). The excerpt from Petrarch's will is discussed in detail on pp. 123–4 in this volume.

45 Wilkins (1959: 4).

46 Cortusi's *Chronica* describes the assassination (10.4, 'De morte domini Jacobi de Carraria et nuptiis domini Bernabovis' [ed. Pagnin 1941: 127–8]). Kohl (1998: 95) and Richards (2007: 33) discuss Cortusi's account of the murder.

47 'questi Gulielmo non abiando Iddio ne la memoria, anzi il diavollo da lo 'nferno, e quello instigandolo a malfare, esendo una matina innel die di santo Tomio a dí XVIIII de dexembre il preditto Guielmo nel conspetto fil signore messer Iacomo, e di sotto tràtossi uno coltello e di quello dato nel ventre al suo signore, che voltava le spalle al fuogo e 'l viso contro il predetto e dimenando il 'detto coltello per lo ventre, tagliò molti degl'interiori: per la qualle ferita, subito chade morto, né altro non disse, se non – pigliatelo! – . Il predetto Guielmo non si mosse de quela parte, che tuto fu taglato a peze, e gitate le soe carne in qua e in làper la corte. E di presente tolto Marsilio da Cararam piccolo figliuolo del signor misser Iacomo, e quello aportato suso un cavallo in piaza, e dàtolli la signoria di la terre. E questo fu fato per lo meio, perché [né] misser Iacomino, fradello del signore, né Francesco da Carara suo figliuolo nin era in la città, anzi erano andati a Chanpo San Piero per chaziare a' gienghiari per la festa di Nadalle' (Gatari, *Cronaca*, 'Come messer Iacomo da Carrara fu fato Signor e morto', decembre 1350 [eds Medin and Tolomei 1931: 28–9; tr. Symes 1830: xxxii–xxxiii]). For additional accounts, see Vergerio, *Liber de principibus* (VI, 'De Jacobo Minore de Carraria, qui quintus ex Carrariensibus Pinceps fuit', §123 [ed. Gnesotto 1924: 449]), and the *Gesta magnifica* (XXIV, 'Dominus Marsilius Grandis', §182 [ed. Cessi 1942–1948: 61]).

48 *Rerum familiarium* XI.2 (eds Rossi and Bosco 1933–1942: 2.324–6).

49 'amantissimus studiorum et ingeniorum cultor extimatorque iustissimus' (Petrarch, *Rerum familiarium* XI.2, ll. 39–40 [eds Rossi and Bosco 1933–1942: 2.326; tr. Bernardo 2005: 2.88]). Richards (2007: 47) further discusses this passage and its significance. Vergerio, following Petrarch, later praised Giacomo as 'a prudent man and a generous prince' ('prudens vir et princeps magnanimus') in his educational treatise *De ingenuis moribus* ('Excellens studium tractat, armorum scilicet et litterarum', §31 [ed. and tr. Kallendorf 2002: 38–9]). In addition, Vergerio noted that although Giacomo 'held that this one thing had been lacking in his good fortune, that he was not educated to the extent that a modest man might wish to be', Giacomo 'nevertheless cultivated learned men wondrously' and welcomed and supported their community in Padua ('Iacobus de Carraria . . . ipse quidem non magnopere doctus, mirum tamen in modum doctos coluit, ut id unum fortunae suae defuisse iudicaret, quod non esset, quantum modestum hominem optare liceat, eruditus') (Vergerio, *De ingenuis moribus*, 'Excellens studium tractat, armorum scilicet et litterarum', §31 [ed. and tr. Kallendorf 2002: 38–9]). Francesco il Vecchio later emulated his father in this regard and so earned similar praise from both Petrarch and Vergerio.

50 'carissimum atque dulcissimum solamen . . . virum omni laude sed precipua quadam et angelica morum suavitate conspicuum' (Petrarch, *Rerum familiarium* XI.2, ll. 31–4 [eds Rossi and Bosco 1933–1942: 2.325; tr. Bernardo 2005: 2.87]).

51 'viri optimi optimeque de nobis meriti . . . verissimus patrie pater fuit' (Petrarch, *Rerum familiarium* XI.3, ll. 2–5 [eds Rossi and Bosco 1933–1942: 2.326; tr. Bernardo 2005: 2.89, with slight revisions to Bernardo's translation]).

52 Mommsen edited and translated Petrarch's last will (dated 4 April 1370) based on his consultation of the extant manuscripts and earliest printed editions. For a list of these sources, see Mommsen (1957: 65). In his introductory essay, Mommsen (1957: 51–64) discusses the complex history of the text's transmission. He notes that the

original document is lost. The earliest extant manuscript copy dates to the fifteenth century (Trieste, Biblioteca Civica, MS I. 8) and claims to have been made from the original 'ex archetypo' (Mommsen 1957: 51–2). Mommsen (1957: 55) further notes that the first printed editions of the will, published in Venice by Bernardino de' Vitali (fl. 1495–1539) (which he calls edition *b*) and by Andrea Torresano da Asola (1452–1528) (which he calls edition *t*) in 1499/1500 and 1501, respectively, derive from different manuscript sources. The *Opera omnia* published in Venice in 1501 and 1503, and in Basel in 1554 and 1581, contains the Torresano edition. Aldo Manuzio the younger (1547–1597) preferred the de' Vitali version and included it in his 1581 edition of Cicero's *De officiis* (with commentary), along with other last wills, including Boccaccio's. At the outset of his translation, Mommsen (1957: vii–viii) notes that he has attempted to put these different editions into conversation in his work to produce what he calls 'as good a text as can be given'.

53   'Si Padue, ubi nunc sum, moriar, in ecclesia Sancti Augustini quam fratres predicatores tenent, quias et locus animo meo gratus est et iacet illic is, qui me plurimum dilexit inque has terras piis precibus attraxit, preclarissime memorie Iacobus de Carraria, tunc Padue dominus' (Petrarch, *Testamentum*, §6a [ed. and tr. Mommsen 1957: 72]).

54   Richards (2007: 14 and 53) argues that, because Petrarch arrived in Padua so late in Giacomo's reign, it is more likely the poet influenced Giacomo's choices and was not involved directly in the design.

55   For instance, the only non-Virgilian Latin epics in Petrarch's library were by Statius and Lucan (de Nolhac 1907: 1.193). Petrarch's book collection also included Statius' commentary on Virgil (the poet upon whom Petrarch modelled himself), which was highly prized by Petrarch and adorned with a frontispiece by Simone Martini. Yet, in *De remediis utriusque fortunae* (*On the Remedies for Different Fortunes*, 1354–1360), Petrarch criticised Statius because of his association with the tyrannical Emperor Domitian (51–96 CE) (Richards 2007: 40). Earlier in the century, Statius had figured prominently in Dante's *Purgatorio* (XXI and XXII) as one of the few saved pagan souls in the *Commedia*.

56   Statius, *Thebaid* (ed. and tr. Shackleton 2003).

57   Anon., *Thebaid* (ed. and tr. West 2003: 42–57).

58   Ed. and tr. Sommerstein (2009: 152–275).

59   Richards (2007: 41).

60   Richards (2007: 37–8 and 40–1).

61   Richards (2007: 35–6).

62   Richards (2007: 41).

63   Richards (2007: 41).

64   *Gesta magnifica*, XXIV, 'Dominus Marsilius Grandis', §139 (ed. Cessi 1942–1948: 47). For further analysis of this passage and its relationship to the iconography of the *Sala Thebarum*, see Richards (2007: 41).

65   *Gesta magnifica*, XXIV, 'Dominus Marsilius Grandis', §139 (ed. Cessi 1942–1948: 47).

66   For an introduction to the first Giacomo da Carrara, see Ganguzza Billanovich (1977b).

67   Richards (2007: 38).

68   *Gesta magnifica*, XX, 'Domini Ubertinus et Bonifacius Fratres', §91 (ed. Cessi 1942–1948: 31). Richards (2007: 38–9) concludes that this heroic precedent had great value for both Giacomo II (who buttressed his role with his ancestors' heroic 'crusades' on behalf of the Paduan people) and for Francesco Novello (who, as the inscriptions on the reverse of medals he commissioned in 1390 read, 'recuperavit Paduam' ['recovered Padua'] from the new tyrant, Giangaleazzo Visconti).

69   Gloria (1884: 2. no. 1154). Richards (2007: 33) further discusses this document.

70   Richards (2007: 42 and 51).

71   See Livy, *Ab urbe condita* XXVIII.9 (eds and tr. Foster et al. 1943: 8.36–43).

72   Petrarch, *De viris illustribus*, 'Claudius Nero – Livius Salinatore' (ed. Martellotti 1964: 137–55).

73   Francesco il Vecchio shared the rule of Padua with his uncle, Giacomino (d. 1373), for the first five years of his rule. During this time, Giacomino assumed the less glamorous administrative duties of ruling the city while Francesco distinguished himself as a gifted military strategist and knight. Allegedly, his uncle became jealous and plotted Francesco's death in order to secure the seigniory for himself and his son. When the plot was uncovered, Francesco confronted and arrested Giacomino. He imprisoned his uncle in the Rocca at Monselice, where Giacomino lived comfortably until his death, from natural causes, in 1373. From 1355 onward, Francesco ruled Padua as the sole *signore* (Kohl 1998: 97).

74   For a chronology of Petrarch's life, works, and many travels, see Kirkham (2009a). For a more detailed discussion of Petrarch's later years, see Wilkins (1959).

75   For modern critical editions of *De viris illustribus*, see Martellotti (1964) and, more recently, Ferrone, Malta and de Capua (2006–2012).

76   The scholarship surrounding the dating of the versions of the work, especially the classic analyses by de Nolhac (1891), Calcaterra (1939) and Martellotti (1949), is summarised by Witt (2009: 105–10). Briefly, Petrarch began work on *De viris illustribus* in 1338 or 1339, focussing on Romans and other ancient heroes, and completed a draft in 1343. He revisited the work in 1351–1353, at that time intending to include biblical and mythological heroes (he did not produce this version). At the behest of the Carrara lord in summer of 1368, Petrarch returned to the work, and focussed again, primarily, on Romans, with select other ancient heroes. Among his non-Roman heroes, Petrarch included three foreigners, likely because of their great influence on Roman history: the Greeks Alexander the Great (356–323 BCE) and Pyrrhus (319–272 BCE) and the Carthaginian Hannibal (247–ca. 181 BCE) (Witt 2009: 106).

77   For descriptions of this manuscript, see de Nolhac (1891: 70–5); Pellegrin (1955: 109); and Martellotti (1964: xii). While Petrarch was completing the *Quorundam virorum illustrium epithoma*, Francesco asked him to provide a further condensed version, known as the *Compendium*, the presentation copy of which is housed in Paris, Bibliothèque nationale de France (lat. 6069 G). Stretched between the two projects, Petrarch completed neither: he had written 14 of the abbreviated biographies for the *Compendium* at the time of his death (de Nolhac 1891: 65). Lombardo finished both works and presented them to Francesco in 1379. The abridged version was likely a *vade mecum*, or a 'little manual' (as Mommsen called it), which Francesco could carry with him as a guide to his *Sala virorum illustrium* (Mommsen 1952: 106). Lombardo della Seta's preface to the *Compendium* confirms Francesco's request for it. The preface reads 'Iussisti enim multa et maxima quorundam virorum facta prius quodam epithomate neque prolixo neque artato, sed mediocri stilo declarari' (*Compendium*, Paris, Bibliothèque nationale de France, lat. 6069 G, f. 9v.). Mommsen (1952: 97–8) further analyses Lombardo's prefatory remarks.

78   'Illustres quosdam viros quos excellenti gloria floruisse doctissimorum hominum ingenia memorie tradiderunt, in diversis voluminibus tanquam sparsos ac disseminatos, rogatu tuo, plaustrifer insignis qui modestissimo nutu inclite urbis Patavine sceptra unice geris, locum in unum colligere et quasi quodammodo stipare arbitratus sum' (Petrarch, *De viris illustribus*, 'Prohemium' [ed. Martellotti 1964: 3, §1; tr. Kohl 1974: 142]).

79   See especially Petrarch's letter to Pierre de Poitiers (fl. mid-fourteenth century), Prior of St. Éloi, Paris, dated 27 February 1361 (*Rerum familiarium* XXII.14 [eds Rossi and Bosco 1933–1942: 4.138–52; tr. Bernardo 2005: 3.242–53]).

80   The year before his death, when unwell and frail, Petrarch paid a diplomatic visit to Venice with Francesco Novello on Francesco il Vecchio's behalf. He made a public

oration on 2 October 1373, *Orazione per la seconda ambasceria veneziana* (*Oration for the Second Venetian Embassy*), in an effort to reconcile the Carrara and Venice (Kirkham 2009b: 141). That the poet would risk his health for his benefactor suggests more than words the positive view in which he held Francesco il Vecchio. On the diplomatic mission in 1373, see Kohl (1998: 126–8). For details of the oration, see Kirkham (2009b).

81　The *Sala virorum illustrium* was not the only painted hall commissioned by Francesco il Vecchio. However, it is the most-studied hall and the hall for which we have direct evidence of Petrarch's involvement. We have records that testify to the existence of other rooms, but they do not describe the rooms' decoration. The rooms' names suggest Classical subjects or narratives of Carrara victories and, from these names, scholars have posited likely illustrative schemes: the *Camera Camilli* illustrated the life of the fourth-century BCE statesman and general, Camillus. The *Camera Herculis* celebrated the heroic deeds of Hercules. The *Camera Lucretie* illustrated the life of the virtuous Roman heroine. The *Sala nova virorum illustrium* likely illustrated the military victories of the Carrara and other contemporary allies, the 'new' illustrious men. The *Camera virtutum,* part of the *Palazzo di Levante* where Fina da Buzzacarini held court, likely portrayed the four cardinal virtues (Kohl 1998: 152). For an analysis of possible sources of imagery and Petrarchan influence in these rooms, see Richards (2007: 63–75).

82　The inscription reads: 'Hier[onymus] Cornel[ius] G[eorgii] F[ilius] Praef[ectus] Optimus / de hac urbe Benemeritus h[a]nc / aulam vetustate pene collapsam in hunc eregrium nitorem restituit / interior cubicula iam destinata / successoribus / angustia temporis / consumanda reliquit' (ed. Bodon 2009: 36; tr. Mommsen 1952: 102–3). Another inscription on the architrave of the same wall reinforces Corner's effort to 'renovate' rather than create the hall anew. It reads, in part, 'Hie / romini Cornellii Praefecti ex / composito has herorum imagines / una cum gestis ex historia / sumptis instaurari curarunt' (ed. Bodon 2009: 36). Bodon (2009: 36–7) speculates that the use of the verb 'instaurare' (to renew or repeat) suggests that the room's design meant to capitalise upon the original cycle's connection to Petrarch. For a more detailed interpretation of Corner's motives for 'restoring' the hall, see Bodon (2009: 34–7).

83　Despite the sentiment toward 'restoration', the new cycle included historical figures not mentioned in *De viris illustribus,* like Cicero. The hall is now an assembly room for the University of Padua. It is called the *Sala dei Giganti* because of its over life-sized figures, a name it acquired immediately after the repainting campaign in the sixteenth century (Mommsen 1952: 102–3).

84　See, most recently, Bodon's comprehensive study of the hall, both before and after the sixteenth-century restorations (2009). For the classic scholarship on the *Sala virorum illustrium*, see Schlosser (1895); Mommsen (1952); Gasparotto (1966–1967); Lorenzoni (1977); and more recently, Plant (1987); Armstrong (1999); Richards (2000: 104–34 and 2007: 75–95); and Dunlop (2009: 115–18).

85　Modern scholarship on the lost frescoes has focussed on the reconstruction of the original cycle's appearance, mostly by analogy to an illustrated copy of a translation of *De viris illustribus* produced in Padua around 1400 by Donato degli Albanzani (1328–1411) for the Papafava branch of the Carrara family (now Darmstadt, Hessische Landes- und Hochschulbibliothek, Ital. 101) and to a series of early illustrated printed versions of Albanzani's translation (see Armstrong 1999). With respect to this tradition of scholarship, for my purposes here, I am not concerned with the degree of similarity between the current frescoes and the originals or to what degree of fidelity the original cycle may have been copied in the Darmstadt illustrations. Rather than focussing on a reconstruction of the cycle, I am interested in how the room may have been perceived by Francesco il Vecchio and fit into the context of his family's patronage and what the representations of famous men may have contributed to that perception. From the scholarship on the *Sala virorum illustrium*, I accept that the original frescoes were likely Altichieresque – a style clearly valued at the Carrara court – and that the portraits and accompanying narrative scenes in the Darmstadt codex generally record the original appearance of the hall's portrait- and *dado* friezes. The panels likely included *grisaille* narrative scenes beneath the colour portraits, a design that accords with the eyewitness accounts of Michele Savonarola and Lombardo della Seta (and that is repeated in the frescoes by Campagnola and dall' Arzere as well). For formal comparisons between extant Altichiero works (especially of figures and fictive architecture) and the illustrations in the Darmstadt codex, see Richards (2000: 114). He concludes that while the codex's illustrations are similar, they are not quite Altichiero's style. Most likely, a follower executed them.

86 Lombardo's portrait likely was added between 1380–1388, after Lombardo completed Petrarch's work and gave it to Francesco (Mommsen 1952: 100, and Richards 2000: 120).

87 Norman (1995b: 1.168n35). Following long historiographic precedent, Norman suggests that the renditions of Triumph of Fame scenes in the illustrated copies of Petrarch's *De viris illustribus* reflect the presence of a Triumph of Fame opposite the portraits of Petrarch and Lombardo in the original fresco cycle. Richards (2000: 130–1) disagrees with her because of a lack of contemporary documentation about such a fresco. He suggests instead that the Triumph imagery in the manuscripts developed after Petrarch's death as a monument to the poet and to the patron's association with him.

88 'Hos non modo mente et animo ut uirtutum amantissimus hospes digne suscepisti, sed et aule tue pulcerrima parte magnifice collocasti et more maiorum hospitaliter honoratos auro et purpura cultos ymaginibus et titulis admirandos ornatissime tua prestitit magni animi gloriosa conceptio, que cum similes sui ut sopra dictum est reddat effectus' (Lombardo della Seta, *De viris illustribus*, 'Praefatio', Paris, Bibliothèque nationale de France, lat. 6069 F, f. 144r [ed. and tr. Mommsen 1952: 96, with minor revisions to Mommsen's translation]).

89 'Scio enim te, urbis Patavi inclite rector, tuorum clarissimorum heroum gradatim ut breviter acta cognoscas, huiusce opusculi avide finem exposcere. Ideoque ut in ultimo angulo tue venustissime aule Trayanum inter ceteros collocasti, ita et in hoc opera novissimum tradere perquiro') (Lombardo della Seta, *De viris illustribus*, 'Praefatio', Paris, Bibliothèque nationale de France, lat. 6069 F, f. 194r [ed. and tr. Mommsen 1952: 99]).

90 For interpretation of Lombardo's comments and possible organisation of the original frescoes, see Mommsen (1952: 99), and Armstrong (2003: 186).

91 'Cumque honoratas scalas ascendis, podiola lodiam parte in superiori circuentia, columpnis marmoreis ac magnificis fenestris, que ad utramque curiam aspectum habent, etiam ornate invenis. Stantque due amplissime et picturis ornatissime sale ad latera horum situate, quarum prima Thebarum nuncapatur, altera Imperatorum nominatur prima maior atque gloriosior, in qua Romani imperatore miris cum figures cumque triumphis, auro optimoque cum colore depicti sunt. Quos gloriose manus illustrium pictorum Octaviano et Alticherii configurarunt' (Savonarola, *Libellus*, II, 'De Temporalibus et Mundanis' [ed. Segarizzi 1902: 49, ll. 27–32; tr. Mommsen 1952: 101. Emphasis and slight revisions to Mommsen's translation are mine]). Savonarola goes on to praise the magnificence of the palace in superlative terms and to state that no other palace in Italy is as magnificent: 'Et ut uno verbo, pace aliarum civitatum, dicam, nullum in Italia ita magnificum, nullumque ita superbum invenitur'.

92 Gatari, *Cronaca*, 'Come Madonna Caterina da Carrara andò a marido a Segna', 10–12 giugno 1372 (eds Medin and Tolomei 1931: 59; tr. Symes 1830: 59–60).

93 On this passage of Gatari's account, see Norman (1995b: 1.158). The anonymous *Ystoria de mesier Francesco Zovene* records the events similarly (XXI, 'El mariazo de madona Katherina, fighiula del magnifico signor veyo da Carara' [ed. Cessi 1964: 182]).

94 Gatari, *Cronaca*, 'Quando Madona Ziliuolla da Carrara andò a marido nel Marchese da Ferrara a dí III zugno', giugno 1397 (eds Medin and Tolomei 1931: 453–4). On Gigliola's wedding, see also the anonymous *Ystoria de mesier Francesco Zovene* (II, 'Questo è el mariazo della nobele dona madona Ziliola, prima figliula del magnifico et excelso signor messire Francesco veghio da Carara' [ed. Cessi 1964: 177]), and Olivi (1888).

95 *Guerra da Trivixo*, CII, 'Como madona Lieta, fiiuola del magnifico segnore veyo da Carara, fo dà per moyere al conte de Otim' (ed. Cessi 1964: 264).

96 Gatari, *Cronaca*, 'Come il Signore fe' aportare el corpo de suo padre e l'onore che li fu fato, che fu a dí XVIII de novenbre 1393', 18–20 novembre 1393 (eds Medin and Tolomei 1931: 441–4). Also, Vergerio noted that Francesco Novello returned to the cathedral (where public ceremonies were held) after an oration on Francesco il Vecchio's merits was given at the palazzo (*De dignissimo funebri apparatu* [ed. Muratori 1730: 192C–93C, especially 193A]). For descriptions of the funeral rites and discussions of the eyewitness accounts, see also Cittadella (1842: 2.248–54); Norman (1995b: 1.156); and McManamon (1996: 43).

97 'nec tui nec innate uirtutis oblitus in forma excellentissime picture extrinsecus expressisti, quod intus ab arduo erat conceptum ingenio, ut assidue in conspectus haberes, quos diligere ob magnitudinem rerum studueras (Lombardo della Seta, *De viris illustribus*, 'Praefatio', Paris, Bibliothèque nationale de France, lat. 6069 F, f. 144r [ed. and tr. Mommsen 1952: 96. My emphasis]).

98 See pp. 128 and 144n88 in this volume.

99 The fire that destroyed the remainder of the original cycle at the end of the fifteenth century spared the portrait of Petrarch in his study. It is considered one of the earliest renditions of the poet and has highly influenced how scholars conceive of Petrarch's appearance. Although the portrait survived, it has since been overpainted, especially the landscape scene shown through the fictive window in the portrait. On the portraits of Petrarch in Padua, including the one in the *Sala virorum illustrium*, see Mardersteig (1974); Plant (1987: especially 179–82); Armstrong (1999); and Richards (2007: 117–23).

100 The artist who painted the illuminated initial in the *Carrara Herbal* would mimic this composition.

101 Fittingly, this shift of emphasis from reading a literary portrait to seeing a painted portrait aided Francesco's insertion of himself into the narrative of great men. Like the portraits of the *viri illustres*, Francesco's body became a sign of his heroic deeds, moral life and glorious history. I will return to this idea in the next chapters.

102 '[i]llustres quosdam viros quos excellenti gloria floruisse doctissimorum hominum ingenia memoriae tradiderunt, in diversis voluminibus tanquam sparsos ac disseminatos . . .' (Petrarch, *De viris illustribus*, 'Prohemium' [ed. Martellotti 1964: 3, §1; tr. Kohl 1974: 142]).

103 'hic enim, nisi fallor, fructuosus historicorum finis est, illa prosequi que vel sectanda legentibus vel fugienda sunt; quisquis extra hos terminos evagari presumpserit, sciat se alienis finibus errare memineritque e vestigio redeundum, nisi forte oblectandi gratia diversoria legentibus interdum grata quesierit. Neque enim inficior me talia meditantem sepe distractum ab incepto longius abscessisse, dum virorum illustrium mores vitamque domesticam et verba nunc peracuta nunc gravia et corporis staturam et orlglnem, genusque mortis meminisse aliis dulce fuit' (Petrarch, *De viris illustribus*, 'Prohemium' [ed. Martellotti 1964: 3, §6–7; tr. Kohl 1974: 143. Emphasis and slight modifications to Kohl's translation are mine]).

104 Petrarch had read Horace. An early self-inventory of his library lists the *Odes* among other works of Classical poetry in his possession (see pp. 133–4 and 146n111 for a discussion of the inventory). Also, Petrarch made direct reference to *Ars poetica* (*The Art of Poetry*, ca. 19 BCE) in the 1351–1353 preface to the *De viris illustribus* (the so-called 'long' preface), attesting to his familiarity with Horace's adage that the purpose of poetry is to teach and delight (*Ars poetica*, ll. 333–4). The 'long' preface precedes the edition of *De viris* included in Petrarch's collected *Prose* (ed. Martellotti 1955); for the reference to *Ars poetica*, see ed. Martellotti (1955: 222); tr. Kohl (1974: 140).

105 *Rerum senilium* XIV.1 (eds Nota and Dotti 2002–2013: 4.228–307).

106 'ut hoc velut in speculo tete intuens, ubi te talem videris qualem dico, quod persepe facies, gaudeas, et virtutum bonorumque omnium largitori devotior fias atque in dies obsequentior, et ingenti nisu per difficultatum obices assurgas usque ad illum gradum quo ire altius iam non possis' (Petrarch, *Rerum senilium* XIV.1, ll. 176–81 [eds Nota and Dotti 2002–2013: 4.241; tr. Bernardo et al. 1992: 2.525; my emphasis]).

107 For Petrarch, the worthiness of what was being seen – i.e.: the histories of the great men – demarcated the pleasures of vision. On Petrarch's selective history, see Kahn (1989: 145–6). The digressions of imagination serve to help the reader better envision the heroes so as better to emulate them. These digressions are connected to vision, especially inner vision, and are considered virtuous pleasures that cement the more nebulous biographical details into the reader's mind.

108 See pp. 128 and 144n88 in this volume.

109 As we will see, although no complete inventory for Francesco il Vecchio's library exists, it is possible to deduce an approximation of its scope from Petrarch's autograph 1337 inventory of his book collection and from the 1426 inventory of the Visconti-Sforza library. The 1426 inventory provides information about volumes once belonging to Petrarch and describes several volumes bearing annotations or seals that denote their original possession in the Carrara library. Mariani Canova et al. (1999) have traced the histories and whereabouts of several illustrated manuscripts that originally belonged to the Carrara.

110 Petrarch, *Testamentum*, §12 (ed. and tr. Mommsen 1957: 78–9).

111 The inventory is recorded on the final folio (58v) of the manuscript now Paris, Bibliothèque nationale de France, lat. 2201. The manuscript itself dates to the twelfth century and contains copies of Cassiodorus' *De anima* (*On the Soul*) and Augustine's *De vera religione* (*On True Religion*), along with three prayers written in Petrarch's hand (dated 1 June 1335 and 10 July 1338). For details on the manuscript, see Delisle (1896), and de Nolhac (1907: 2.293–6). Based on a reevaluation of the header that precedes the inventory, which he reads as 'libri mei Peculiares. ad reliquos n(on) tra(n)sfuga sed explorator tra(n)sire soleo' ('My specially prized books. To the others I usually resort not as a deserter but as a scout'), Ullman (1923: 22–3) argues that this inventory likely refers only to Petrarch's favoured books and does not account for the entirety of his collection.

112 De Nolhac (1907: 2.293–4) recreated Petrarch's diagrammatic list of authors, the ordering of which I follow here.

113 For a more detailed discussion of the inventory and its authors, see de Nolhac (1907: 1.42–3 and 2.293–4).

114 Augustine is *a propos* as the principal theologian for Petrarch's collection: he was the Doctor of the Church who most struggled with his love for Roman sources. See Augustine's *Confessiones*, especially Books III, IV and VII (ed. and tr. O'Donnell 1992).

115 The inventory (*consignatio*), taken 4–8 January 1426, is now Milan, Biblioteca Braidense AD XV 18.4. In the 1870s, historian Girolamo d'Adda (1815–1881) published the 1426 inventory, along with those taken in 1459 and 1469. While d'Adda began

to trace the volumes on the inventories to their homes in various European libraries, especially to the Bibliothèque nationale de France, the work remained incomplete at his death. Several scholars continued d'Adda's efforts, often focussing on particular categories of manuscripts from the inventories (for instance, volumes that belonged to Petrarch, or volumes written in Italian or French). Pellegrin (1955: 5–9) summarises the scholarly literature up to 1955 in the initial volume of her invaluable study on the Visconti-Sforza library. The classic works on the identification of volumes from the Visconti-Sforza library, especially from the 1426 inventory, are: Delisle (1884 and 1896); Mazzatini (1886a and 1886b); de Nolhac (1907); and Thomas (1911 and 1912). Notably, Leopold Delisle (1826–1881) began to document and identify volumes at the Bibliothèque nationale de France believed to be from the Visconti-Sforza collection prior to d'Adda's publication of the inventories. Delisle's later publications correct and supplement his original identifications.

116 On Plato and Martianus Capella in Latin mythography and their importance during the late Middle Ages, see Wetherbee (2012).

117 De Nolhac (1907: 1.103–4) identified these volumes and noted their titles and descriptions as recorded in the 1426 inventory. From the 988 articles recorded on the inventory, de Nolhac (1907), Minio-Paluello (1949) and Pellegrin (1951, 1955 and 1969) have identified over 50 manuscripts that once belonged to Petrarch. Of these, 38 are housed at the Bibliothèque nationale de France, which became home to the Visconti-Sforza collection. After his conquest of the Sforza in 1499, Louis XII of France (1462–1515, r. 1498–1515) moved many of the volumes from the Visconti-Sforza collection to his library at Blois. From Blois, these books eventually passed into the national library's collection. De Nolhac (1907: 1.103–4) identified 27 of Petrarch's manuscripts at the Bibliothèque nationale de France, Minio-Paluello (1949) added Petrarch's copy of Plato's *Phaedo*, and Pellegrin (1951) another ten volumes. In addition, de Nolhac (1907: 1.113–14) traced several volumes that once belonged to Petrarch to other libraries in Europe, including seven volumes at Rome, Biblioteca Apostolica Vaticana; Petrarch's *Virgil* at Milan, Biblioteca Ambrosiana (A 79 *Inf.*); his *Horace* at Florence, Biblioteca Laurenziana (plut. 34.1); his *Cicero* at Troyes, Bibliothèque municipale (MS 552); and a copy of Augustine's *De Civitate Dei* at Padua, Biblioteca Universitaria (MS 1490). Billanovich (1951) identified Petrarch's *Livy* at London, British Library (Harley 2493). Notably, this list of Petrarch's manuscripts outside of the Bibliothèque nationale de France corroborates the suggestion of de Nolhac (1907: 1.105–6) and Pellegrin (1955: 9) that Louis XII was unable to remove all of the Sforza's books to Blois and that many were hidden and dispersed to various other collections, including that of the Aragonese kings of Naples.

118 For instance, in his letter to Francesco il Vecchio (*Rerum senilium* XIV.1), Petrarch refers to both Classical Greco-Roman and Judeo-Christian authors. From the Classical tradition, he references Aristotle, Cicero, Livy, Seneca, Martial (ca. 38–ca. 102 CE), Lucan, Valerius Maximus, Suetonius, Aelius Spartianus (fl. late third–early fourth century CE), Flavius Vopiscus (fl. fourth century CE), Eutropius, Claudianus and Macrobius. From the Bible, he references the books of Leviticus, Kings, Psalms, Proverbs and Jeremiah (from the Hebrew Bible), and the Gospel of Matthew, Book of Acts, Paul's letters, and Book of Hebrews (from the New Testament). He also refers to the Church father, Ambrose. From this list alone, Petrarch's project to synthesise Roman and Christian values is evident. He also encourages Francesco il Vecchio to emulate his 'worthy and magnanimous father' ('glorioso et magnanimo patre'), Giacomo II. In the same manner that Petrarch coaxed Giacomo II to be a good leader, the poet sought to coax Francesco by teaching him the virtues of the ancient heroes and by encouraging him to follow their example in his own life. He advised the elder Francesco that, to be a true *pater patriae*, Francesco needed to possess in his heart an 'inner spark' ('favilla interior') of virtue that would kindle into flame when coaxed

by the poet's breath ('quam flando excites et in flammam erigas') (Petrarch, *Rerum senilium* XIV.1, ll. 89 and 143–4 [eds Nota and Dotti 2002–2013: 4.235, 237 and 239). For further analysis of this passage, see Richards (2007: 44–5).

119 See pp. 128 and 144n88 in this volume.

120 As Hampton (1990: 3) notes, the commingling of texts as records of active deeds and their role (in books) as physical touchstones of the contemplative life complicates any strict separation of these two paths. Petrarch himself did not practice a life of isolated contemplation, either. While ambivalent about his involvement in the 'active' life of court politics, Petrarch served as a diplomat for Francesco il Vecchio on at least one occasion (see n80 in this chapter). For an argument against Petrarch's apparent preference for the contemplative life of solitude, see Blanchard (2001: 401–23).

121 Vergerio expressed this view of Francesco il Vecchio in the funeral eulogy written for the *signore*, *De dignissimo funebri apparatu*, and in the orations written for Francesco Novello, *Oratorio in funere Francisci Senioris de Carrarias* and *Ad Franciscum Juniorem* (all three works ed. Muratori 1730). Petrarch's letter to Francesco il Vecchio (*Rerum senilium* XIV.1 [eds Nota and Dotti 2002–2013: 4.228–307]) also upholds this view of the *signore*.

5 Physiognomy in late medieval Padua

In his *Speculum phisionomie* (*The Physiognomic Mirror*, 1442),[1] dedicated to Leonello d'Este (1407–1450), the *signore* of Ferrara (r. 1441–1450), Michele Savonarola defined physiognomy as a medical science that uses visible bodily signs to perceive and understand the invisible human psyche, or soul. He noted:[2]

> physiognomy is a science pertaining to natural passions of the soul, principally taking notice of the inventions [innate characteristics] and accidents [acquired characteristics] to which the body is conditioned. Hence, mutual change happens in both [body and soul].

Savonarola stressed that – like Aristotle's advice to Alexander[3] – knowledge of this science would help Leonello to understand the secret hearts of men and their characters, the temperaments and the diseases to which they are prone, the marvellous secrets of nature, and the ideal proportions of the human body.[4] With such knowledge, Savonarola argued, Leonello could better choose his associates and advisors while safeguarding his own health as well.

The study and practice of physiognomy had a long history in Padua (where Savonarola himself was trained), and the patronage of the Carrara and other members of the Paduan elite often reflected its wide-ranging applications.[5] Physiognomy, as studied and practiced in Carrara Padua, was hermeneutically rich – it brought together ideas about the body and soul, medicine and visual art, and politics and moral philosophy. Physicians, artists and humanists used physiognomy in different ways and to different ends. However, these communities shared an understanding of the visible, external body as a potential sign for the invisible, internal character.

In medicine, perceiving the relationship between the physical body and the invisible personality helped the physician to determine the best ways to treat a patient's illness. In humanistic and devotional literature and in art, mapping certain exemplary characteristics onto the physical body or associating them with heraldic imagery (as a metaphorical body) helped authors or artists to better instruct the individual readers or viewers about moral virtue. For Francesco Novello, the physiognomy implicit in portraiture became a way of connecting to his ancestors' patronage of humanists and artists while consolidating his identity as a good and moral prince educated in the most current scientific theories and medical practices. To understand how Francesco Novello mobilised physiognomy in his own patronage, however, we must first explore how it served as a nexus of medicine, art, moral philosophy and politics in Padua.

Physiognomy in medicine and art

Although the earliest documents to mention the official use of physiognomy in the medical curriculum are the 1405 statutes from the University of Bologna,[6] commentaries by Pietro d'Abano (1257–ca. 1315), Jean Buridan (1295–1358), and other masters at Paris attest that its study was common at universities from the 1290s onward.[7] However, the idea of a connection between the physical body, invisible personality or character, and behavioural patterns and illness is even older. It is indebted to the Pseudo-Aristotelian views of the body and soul expressed in the *Physiognomonica (Physiognomonics)*[8] and the *Secretum secretorum (The Secret of Secrets)*,[9] and in Aristotle's discussion of inference from signs in *Analytica priora (The Prior Analytics)*.[10] Galen also discussed physiognomic signs in *De complexionibus (On the Complexion)*[11] and *Ars medica (The Art of Medicine)*.[12] For example, in Book X of *Ars medica*, Galen noted a relationship between the heat of the heart and a restless or rash spirit. This characteristic, Galen further explained, often is associated with broad, hairy chests (especially hairy below the breastbone) and small heads.[13] The connection between bodily signs and moral or mental character also appears in later commentaries on Galen's work. It appears both in the Arabic tradition, in the commentary on the second part of Galen's *Tegni* by Ibn Riḍwān (988–ca. 1061), which became part of the so-called *Articella* handbook for the community of physicians at Salerno, and in the Latin tradition, for example, in the *Liber physionomie* (ca. 1230) by Michael Scot (1175–ca.1232).[14]

A physician considered visible bodily characteristics as clues that helped to determine the patient's temperament and its imbalances, which cause illness. The patient's temperament influenced both body and mind and was a starting point for determining the best path to health maintenance and disease cures. This is not to say that physicians or other students of physiognomy considered physiognomic signs as indications of predetermined, immutable personal characteristics or physical limitations;[15] rather, the signs disclosed by physiognomic analysis revealed an individual's predispositions, which could be overcome through the exercise of reason or through God's grace.[16] So, although the study of physiognomy was useful to the practice of medicine, it was also firmly within the purview of moral philosophers, theologians and humanists. Furthermore, it was part of the visual language used by artists, who employed physiognomic associations, especially in their portraits, to convey moral or political messages.

The work of physician Pietro d'Abano illuminates the close relationship between the medical uses of physiognomy and those in the visual arts during the fourteenth century. In his Latin translation and commentary on Aristotle's *Problemata (Problems)*,[17] Pietro advanced a theory of portraiture founded on the practice of physiognomy.[18] Completed while teaching at the University of Padua in 1310, Pietro's comments are the first of a long line of accounts on the relation-ship between the art of portraiture and physiognomy that developed during the Renaissance.[19] By this time, Pietro's ideas about physiognomy already circulated among the physicians and students at the universities in Paris, where he taught from around 1290 to 1305, and in Padua, where he began teaching in 1305.[20] In addition, he wrote a more formal treatise on the study of physiognomy, the *Compilatio physionomiae* (*Compilation of Physiognomy*, ca. 1295),[21] which he dedicated to Bardellone de Bonacossi, *signore* of Mantua (r. 1292–1299).[22] Yet, in his translation and commentary on Aristotle's *Problemata*, Pietro's ideas reached a new audience. Expensive illuminated copies of this work began to appear and circulate among patrons and artists at courts, suggesting the growing interest both in Pietro's interpretation of Aristotle and in his ideas about physiognomy – and about physiognomy in artistic practice.[23]

Near the end of the *Problemata*, in Book XXXVI.1, Aristotle posed the ques-tion 'Why do men make likenesses of the face?'[24] Pietro, glossing Aristotle, noted that for the Philosopher there were two possible answers to the question: men make images of the face '[e]ither because this (i.e. the face) shows what *kind of people they are*, or because these images allow us *to recognise them* best'.[25] Pietro further interpreted Aristotle's answers within a physiognomic framework. He posited that men make images of the face because it is through facial features that 'the kind of constitutional arrangement [*dispositio*] of that person [is repre-sented]', and it is through an understanding of the person's constitutional arrange-ment that we can best recognise the person portrayed were we to see him in the flesh.[26] Specifically, Pietro expanded upon why the face is the best reflection of a person's constitution, writing:[27]

> [Aristotle says] that one makes the image of the face for the reason that through this it happens more easily that the individual depicted is recognized because (the face) is most articulated and well defined, through which *char-acteristic difference is perceived* and regarded as familiar and disclosed. . . . That someone can be truly recognized through a well marked image [of his face] for what *kind of man he is not only insofar as the body but also the soul*, is shown by the story in the physiognomy in the Book *De regimine principum*, written for Alexander by Aristotle about the figure of Hippocrates on a parch-ment and shown to Philemon, the great Physiognomist.

Pietro's example of such a physiognomist comes from the *Secretum secretorum*.[28] 'Philemon', allegedly the first physiognomist, was able to determine Hippocrates' inner qualities simply by examining a portrait of him.[29] Yet Pietro's example of a painter capable of creating such a revealing portrait of a face, a portrait that he calls a 'likeness in all respects' ('cum fuerit depicta pictore sciente per omnia assimilare'), was not an acclaimed Greek artist – like Zeuxis (fl. fifth century BCE) or Apelles (fl. fourth century BCE) – celebrated in Pliny's *Naturalis his-toria* (Book XXXV). Rather, Pietro named as his example a painter currently practicing in Padua: Giotto di Bondone (ca. 1267–1337) ('puta Zoto [Zotus]' – for example, Giotto).[30]

According to Pietro, Giotto created portraits that enabled the viewer not only to identify the sitter but also to determine the 'kind of man' portrayed. The 'kind of man' refers to the patient's *dispositio*, his constitutional arrangement or temperament, an idea central to Galen's theory of medicine.[31] When Pietro discusses a person's *dispositio*, he means both the continuously changing physical qualities of a person over time (which he calls the 'actual disposition') and the unchanging, internal qualities of a person fixed at birth (which he calls the 'permanent disposition').[32] Pietro's view of the different aspects of a person's constitution – internal and external – and their relationship to one another can be complicated since he often used the term *dispositio* indiscriminately to refer to both invisible moral qualities and visible physical ones.[33] However, despite any confusion Pietro's pluralistic use of the term causes, it evidences his understanding of the relationship between a person's moral and physical constitution as a close one. It points to how Pietro, as a physician, was attuned to both aspects of a person's disposition – physical and moral qualities were considered part of an analysis of an individual's constitution.[34]

Thus, for Pietro, representations of the body – especially the face – had the potential to show a man's complete moral and physical constitution, and Giotto's portraits showed this relationship and so disclosed the 'characteristic differences' between people. Considered from Pietro's perspective, a portrait by Giotto was a figural portrait (a recognisable likeness) of the sitter and a metaphorical one (an imagined likeness) at once.

The physician and the artist collaborated on at least one occasion. They likely worked together on the iconography for the monumental fresco cycle at the Palazzo della Ragione, the town hall of Padua. The creation of the fresco cycle coincided chronologically with the completion of Pietro's commentary on the *Problemata*. The cycle translated into images the astrological dimension of Pietro's theory of medicine as expressed in his *Compilatio physionomiae* (1295) and *Conciliator differentiarum philosophorum et medicorum* (*Conciliator of the Differences Debated between Philosophers and Physicians*, ca. 1300–1307).[35] Pietro used astrology, in part, to elucidate the relationship between physical signs of the body and invisible character. By incorporating personal character and astrology into his view of medicine, Pietro connected morality, ethics and the cultivation of self with health and with the physician's role in treating disease.[36] Giotto visualised these connections.

Paduan chronicler Giovanni da Nono (1276–1347) first recorded Giotto's involvement in the creation of the fresco cycle for the upper walls of the Palazzo in his chronicle of the city under communal rule, *Visio Egidii Regis Patavie* (*A Vision of King Egidius of Padua*, ca. 1320).[37] He described the astrological iconography of the cycle, writing:[38]

> Twelve heavenly signs [of the Zodiac] and seven planets with their attributes will shine in this ceiling, wonderfully wrought by Giotto, the greatest of painters; and other golden stars with mirrors [?] and other compositions will equally shine below.

Later, in the mid-fifteenth century, Michele Savonarola described the Palazzo and commemorated its fresco cycle in his treatise on Padua's great sites and citizens, *Libellus de magnificis ornamentis regie civitatis Padue* (*Book of the Magnificent Ornaments of the Regal State of Padua*, ca. 1446). Savonarola praised the frescoes' uniqueness, calling them 'singular and extraordinary paintings in which the bodies of the planets, and the works to which men are most inclined by them, are shown through figures in a wonderful manner'.[39] Like da Nono, Savonarola described Pietro d'Abano's involvement in the creation of the cycle's iconography. He noted that the 'institutor of this order was our glorious Conciliator [Pietro d'Abano]'.[40] By describing Pietro as 'our [i.e.: Padua's] glorious Conciliator', Savonarola suggested that the fresco cycle was a direct result of the ideas in circulation in Padua at the time of the cycle's creation.

Savonarola also discussed Giotto's slightly earlier work in the Scrovegni Chapel (ca. 1305), which Giotto painted while Pietro d'Abano taught at the University of Padua. Savonarola described the 'great chapel' as 'most ornate with pictures by Giotto, prince of painters, which is sanctified by three priests daily on the hours'.[41] Further, he attributed the frescoes' magnificence to Giotto's ability to create truly lifelike images. Savonarola wrote,[42]

> Zotus Florentinus, who first fashioned modern figures from ancient and mosaic figures in a wonderful manner; . . . [t]his man painted the magnificent and spacious Chapel of the noble Scrovegni with his own fingers at great expense, where images of the Old and New Testaments appear as if alive, and he also decorated the Capitol [chapter house] of our [basilica dedicated to] Antonio in such a way that a great crowd of visiting artists came to see this place and the figures in it. And the dignity of the city so moved him that he spent the greatest part of his life in it and, since those glorious figures were left after him, he lived on ever after in that city.

If we consider Savonarola's comment on Giotto's ability to create figures that 'appear as if alive' through the lens of Pietro d'Abano's celebration of the artist's skill, Giotto's portraits in the Scrovegni Chapel reveal a figure in body and soul – the individual's true *dispositio*.

In the chapel, beneath running scenes from the life of the Virgin and the life of Christ arranged chronologically over three horizontal registers, Giotto portrayed 'portraits', personifications, of the virtues and vices. Using physiognomic associations perhaps drawn from his knowledge of Pietro d'Abano's work, Giotto created the most famous precedents for the personification of immaterial personal qualities. The 'portraits' adorn the lowest register of the chapel's fresco cycle, the *dado*, which runs along the north and south walls at eye level. Giotto depicted the virtues on the south side of the chapel (the side beneath Heaven in the *Last Judgement* on the west wall), and the vices on the north (the side beneath Hell in the *Last Judgement*). The virtues, reading from west to east, are *Spes* (*Hope*), *Caritas* (*Charity*), *Fides* (*Faith*), *Iustitia* (*Justice*), *Temperantia* (*Temperance*), *Fortitudo* (*Fortitude*) and *Prudentia* (*Prudence*). The corresponding vices are *Desperatio*

(*Despair*), *Invidia* (*Envy*), *Infidelitas* (*Idolatry*), *Iniustitia* (*Injustice*), *Ira* (*Anger*), *Inconstantia* (*Inconstancy*) and *Stultitia* (*Folly*).

In his depictions of the virtues and vices, Giotto used exaggerated and fantastical physical features – hyperbolic physiognomic caricatures – to convey the specific moral and immoral character traits. Perhaps in accord with Pietro's commentary on Aristotle, the personifications' facial features are often their most vividly portrayed physical attributes. For instance, in Giotto's portrait of *Invidia* (*Envy*), which is the most pronounced example in the *dado* of the use of physiognomic caricature to articulate a moral message, Giotto stretched the ears of the figure to grotesque proportions, exaggerating a physical trait linked to envious character in treatises on physiognomy (Figure 5.1).[43] Portraying envy in this way, Giotto also emphasised a corresponding religious message: those afflicted with this vice listen closely to the whispers of the devil, encouraging their sin. Furthermore, the figure's tongue has transformed into a snake, which not only suggests her corrupted speech but also extends from her mouth to circle back and blind her. Demonic horns escape from beneath the figure's headscarf and curve downward toward the back of her head, digging into the flesh behind her ears. The grotesque features realised by Giotto complement his physiognomic exaggerations and reveal how envy consumes its victims from the inside, even as the fires of hell will leap up to consume them from the outside.

Giotto's personifications were an immediate success. They conveyed memorable impressions of their corresponding moral characteristics and served as positive and negative *exempla* for their viewers. For instance, shortly after Giotto completed the frescoes in the Scrovegni Chapel, Francesco da Barberino (1264–1348), the Tuscan lawyer and author of the popular handbook of manners, *I documenti d'amore* (*The Lessons of Love*, ca. 1309–1313), singled out Giotto's *Invidia* for praise and defined the vice in accord with the artist's imagery.[44]

In addition to praising Giotto's work at the Scrovegni Chapel in his *Libellus*, Savonarola may have leveraged the popular appeal of the Chapel's personifications to help convey his understanding of physiognomy to a courtly audience in his *Speculum phisionomie* (1442).[45] While indebted to Pietro d'Abano's more formal work on the subject, *Compilatio physionomiae*,[46] the physiognomic correspondences described and discussed in Book I of Savonarola's *Speculum*[47] seem to echo and explicate those correspondences visualised (and popularised) in Giotto's 'lifelike' personifications. Savonarola, for instance, described a correspondence between long and narrow ears and people afflicted with envy.[48]

Giotto's personifications and their reception by physicians and humanists alike reveal the enduring currency in Padua of the idea of physiognomic correspondence. He established a precedent for how a portrait could be used to convey a moral message.[49] Furthermore, the artist's appeal to physiognomy in the Scrovegni Chapel – to portray specific characteristics as guides to living a Christian life – parallels the popular use of corporeal metaphors in the *Speculum principis* literary tradition and in the chronicles and biographies written during the Carrara rule. In such works, a healthy physical body served as an indication of virtue and as a metaphor for a healthy moral 'body'.

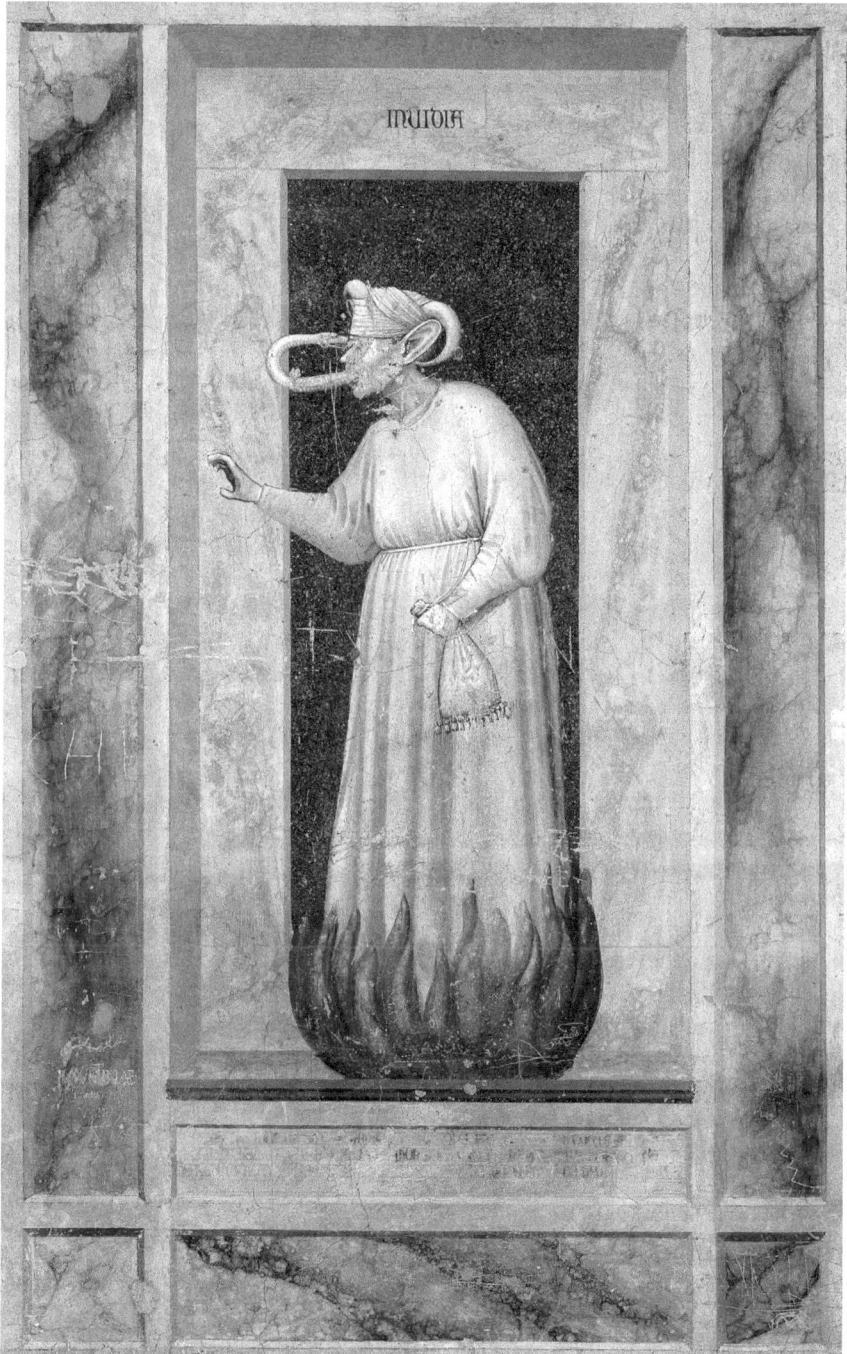

Figure 5.1 Giotto, *Invidia* (*Envy*)

Padua, Scrovegni Chapel
120 × 55 cm, fresco, Padua, ca. 1305

Photo: Mauro Magliani. Photo credit: Alinari / Art Resource, NY

Physiognomy in humanism and politics

Beginning with Petrarch, humanists and chroniclers working for the Carrara used corporeal metaphors and the terminology of sickness and health to describe invisible moral qualities (the psyche or soul) of the *signori*. In literary portraits, they described the princes' fit and noble bodies, which they used to illustrate the princes' morality and its role in preserving the moral health of Padua's citizens.[50] Unlike the physicians Pietro d'Abano or Michele Savonarola, these authors did not discuss the specific details of physiognomic associations (like narrow ears being a sign of an envious character, or hairy chests being a sign of rashness), nor did they focus exclusively on the importance of the physiognomy of the face in determining a person's *dispositio*. Rather, they incorporated a more general sense of physiognomy into their narratives, one that acknowledged the wide-ranging reception in Padua of physiognomy's fundamental premise – that the physical body can reveal the invisible soul.

The use of corporeal metaphor and medical terminology appears in several of Petrarch's works, including his letter to Francesco il Vecchio (r. 1350–1388)[51] and *De remediis utriusque fortunae* (*On the Remedies for Different Fortunes*).[52] Petrarch's humanist successors employed similar language in their works. Metaphors premised on physiognomic associations play a role in Pier Paolo Vergerio's *Liber de principibus Carrariensibus et gestis eorum* (*The Book of the Carrara Princes and Their Deeds*), a work to which I will return, and in the work of fellow court humanist Giovanni Conversini (1343–1408). Conversini's *De dilectione regnantium* (*On the Proper Love Due Princes*, dated 5 September 1399) is a moral treatise in letterform addressed to his friend Paolo Leone (fl. late fourteenth century), counsellor to Francesco Novello, in which Conversini mirrors ideals expressed in Petrarch's letter to the elder Francesco but in relation to the younger Francesco's government.[53]

Petrarch's use of allusions to bodily sickness and health conveyed a message about the importance of a prince's morality to his ability to govern justly. In his letter to Francesco il Vecchio, he cast the figure of the *signore* as the head of the civic body who must rule in the interest of this body's health and welfare. Petrarch likened the citizens of Padua to 'the limbs of [Francesco's] own body or the parts of [his] own soul', and instructed Francesco to love his citizens 'like sons' because 'the state [*res publica*] is but one body of which you are the head'. The complete passage reads:[54]

> I daresay, without prejudice to any truer opinion, that you must love if not each of the citizens, yet all the citizens together and the entire republic not only as much as a son or your parents, but as much as yourself. In the case of individual dear ones, we have a special feeling for each; but in the state you must love all: your citizens, then, are like your children, or rather, to put it a different way, like the limbs of your own body or the parts of your own soul, for the state is but one body of which you are the head.

Later in his letter, Petrarch used the language of sickness and health to argue the importance for a ruler to set a good example through his behaviour and bearing for his citizens to imitate. Petrarch wrote that a prince must beware the 'dangerous contagion of [ungoverned and unruly] imitation'.[55] He continued his letter by praising Francesco's modest dress, good manners and lack of ostentation because they set good examples for his citizens to follow. He explained further:[56]

> The people strive to imitate all the actions and mannerisms of their prince. It is thus very true that no one harms the state more than those who harm by example, for what the poet [Claudius Claudianus (ca. 370–404 C.E.)] says is true, 'The whole world follows the example of the king'. So it is, by heaven: the bad habits of rulers are harmful not only to themselves but to everyone.

To assure the health of Francesco's people, Petrarch advised the prince to curb his 'bad habits' (vices) and so resist spreading the 'dangerous contagion' of poor morals to his citizens.

As we have seen, Petrarch gave Francesco the tools to strengthen his morality (his virtues) when he advised Francesco to adhere to the examples of history's exemplary leaders.[57] Because '[he] would like to compare [Francesco] only to the good and illustrious', Petrarch urged the prince to 'imitate them and follow the examples of those who by deeds and words have earned loud praise for justice'.[58] Inspired by the poet's knowledge of history, the resulting moral stance of the prince would ensure the moral health of the community (the body of Padua) and garner the admiration of its citizens and the respect of foreign leaders.

Paduan chroniclers and artists similarly commemorated the princes and idealised their governments through descriptions – literary and visual – of the princes' noble bodies. In their chronicle of Padua under the Carrara, the *Cronaca Carrarese* (ca. 1355–1406), Galeazzo Gatari and his sons closed the chapters of each lord's life with an account of the manner of his death and a detailed description of his body and heraldic arms, followed by a list of his characteristic virtues. For instance, at the close of the final version of his treatise, penned after Francesco Novello's death, Andrea Gatari introduced a vivid account of the death, person and virtues of the last Carrara *signore*. In this literary portrait, Gatari associated Francesco's physical characteristics with what he considered Francesco's inner character and good governance.

According to Gatari, Francesco Novello was strangled (with great difficulty) in a Venetian prison as a traitor to *La Serenissima* (a martyr to Padua) on 17 January 1406, and the following day he was buried at the Church of Santo Stefano in Venice.[59] Gatari described Francesco's body as it lay in state before burial using heroic terms. He wrote:[60]

> [although] his face was quite bruised and battered . . . [Francesco's] body was clothed in his suit of Alexandrian velvet, with his gold sword girded

about his waist, and his golden spurs upon his heels. [He] was . . . of normal stature, heavy with strong limbs more so than other men. He was swarthy in complexion and rather proud in bearing, discerning in his speech, gracious and merciful to his people. Everyone thought him most wise and strong in body.

In this passage, Gatari memorialised Francesco's body, dressed according to conventions of nobility, in direct connection with his personal qualities that benefited the people of Padua: his careful judgement, grace and mercy.

In a similar way, corporeal metaphors informed the visual rhetoric of commemorative portraiture on the Carrara tomb chests (*arche*). The marble tombs of Ubertino (r. 1338–1345) and Giacomo II da Carrara (r. 1345–1350), commissioned during the 1350s from the workshop of the prolific and locally recognised sculptor Andriolo de' Santi (ca. 1320–1374), show the *signori* in exacting detail (Figures 5.2 and 5.3).[61] From the heavy fabric of their robes adorned with buttons and intricate girdles that falls across their limbs, to the wrinkles on their faces and the pronounced veins on their hands, the sculptures strongly convey the physical presence of the deceased. Their faces are dignified and calm in death and their

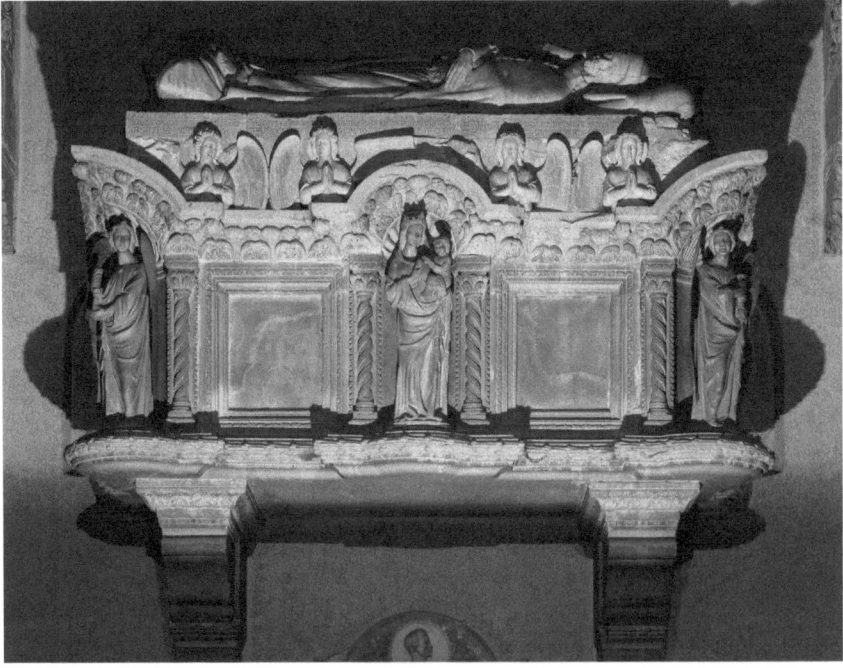

Figure 5.2 Andriolo de' Santi, tomb of Ubertino da Carrara

Padua, Church of the Eremitani
Marble, Padua, ca. 1345

Photo: A. De Gregorio © DeA Picture Library / Art Resource, NY

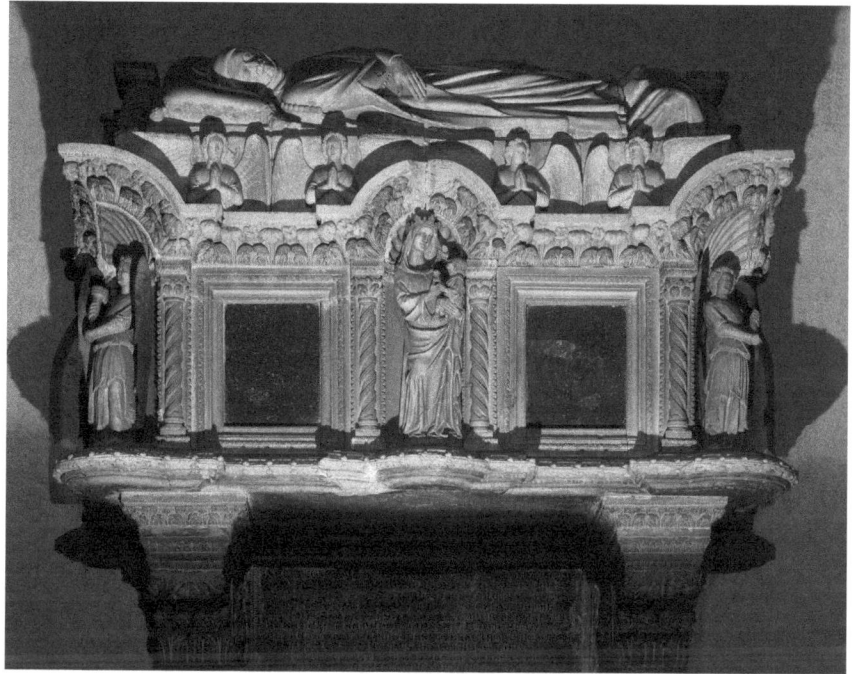

Figure 5.3 Andriolo de' Santi, tomb of Giacomo II da Carrara
Padua, Church of the Eremitani
Marble, Padua, ca. 1350

Photo: A. De Gregorio © DeA Picture Library / Art Resource, NY

clothing reveals them as influential, educated citizens who belonged to the class of scholars, lawyers and merchants in Padua.[62]

Originally elaborate constructions combining fresco, sculpture and architecture, the tombs consisted of colourful painted donor portraits of the living Carrara *signori* kneeling before an image of the Coronation of the Virgin above their sculptural effigies asleep in death (Figure 5.4).[63] In addition, each tomb included a type of commemorative attribute for the prince that connected his body to the health of the city. A miniature replica of the city of Padua lay at the foot of Ubertino's effigy, reminding its viewers of Ubertino's role in the successful governance of the city.[64] The sculptural representation of the city placed at Ubertino's feet bound the physical body of the city with the physical body of its former ruler (in perpetuity).[65] This juxtaposition of the body of the ruler with a representation of the 'body' of the city recalls Petrarch's description of the ideal relationship between the prince and his people: 'the state [*res publica*] is but one body of which you are the head'.[66] Here, on Ubertino's *arca*, the city rests beneath the lord's feet – he is literally the head of the city.

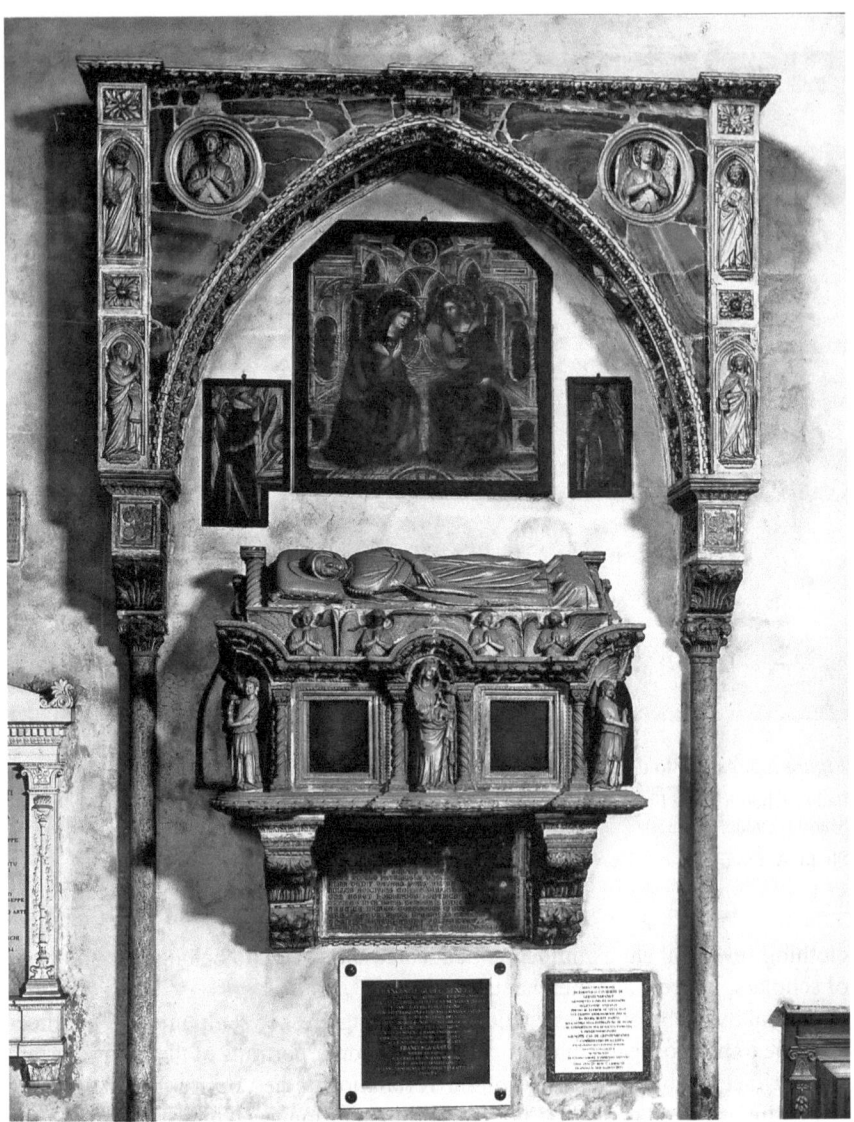

Figure 5.4 Pre–World War II photograph showing Andriolo de' Santi's tomb of Giacomo II
with donor portraits and fragments of *Coronation of the Virgin* fresco

Padua, Church of the Eremitani
Padua, ca. 1350

Photo credit: Alinari / Art Resource, NY

Taking a different tack but conveying a similar message, Giacomo's effigy rests above an inscription of an epitaph penned by Petrarch. Written in elegiac verses, the epitaph reads in part:[67]

> Alas! O abode so confined for so great a man! / Here, under a small marble slab, lies the father, the hope and salvation of his country. / Whoever you may be, O reader, who turns your eyes to this stone, / In reading about the public downfall [of the city] add prayers to your tears.

In the epitaph, Petrarch commemorates Giacomo and grieves for the good government of Padua that he believed was lost when Giacomo was assassinated. He commemorates Giacomo's positive relationship with the city in words just as the ideal city-model sculpted to accompany Ubertino's effigy does so in images. Words and images commemorating the apparently ideal, ordered government of the Carrara were connected to representations of their bodies.

*

Portraiture played significant roles in the artistic and literary patronage of Francesco Novello's ancestors. The Carrara princes commissioned portraits – in words and images – of family members and their heraldry to celebrate (and reinterpret) the family's past achievements, to advance specific idealised images of the lords and their histories, and to commemorate the *signori*. As we have seen, Ubertino consolidated an image of the family's strength and virtue by, among other things, adorning the family palace with Carrara heraldry – metaphorical portraits of the princes. Giacomo II and Francesco il Vecchio commissioned portraits of family members (in fresco and in stone) and also portraits of heroes drawn from ancient texts, which served as metaphorical portraits of their own characters in the tradition of Petrarchan *imitatio antiquorum*.

Considered in the context of the wide-ranging studies and practices of physiognomy in Padua, these representations of the lords conveyed not only their physical likenesses but their moral ones as well. As we will see in the next chapter, rather than commissioning new figural portraits of himself or his family members, Francesco Novello appropriated the historic portraits of Carrara family members and representations of their heraldry into his illustrated books. The physiognomic associations implied in his ancestors' portraits and described in the works of earlier humanists and chroniclers made the representations of Carrara bodies even more appropriate in a book collection dominated by works on the theory and practice of medicine. The plurality of physiognomy's uses in Padua allowed Francesco to appropriate his ancestors' very bodies as signs for his own virtues and the family's shared history.

Notes

1 Currently, there is no critical edition of Savonarola's *Speculum*; however, Gabriella Zuccolin is preparing such an edition, primarily from the manuscript now Leipzig, Universitätsbibliothek, 3472 (Haenel), ff. 2r–82v. She graciously shared her work with

me and enriched my understanding of this complex text. Additionally, Denieul-Cormier (1956) published an analysis and diagrammatic synthesis of Savonarola's physiognomic associations based on the manuscript now Paris, Bibliothèque nationale de France, lat. 7357, ff. 1r–67r.

2 'phisionomia est scientia ad naturales anime passiones cognoscens principaliter inuenta corporisque accidentia quibus habituatum est. Unde mutua in utrisque permutatio contingit' (*Speculum*, f. 1v, Paris, Bibliothèque nationale de France, lat. 7357 [ed. Ziegler 2007: 305n61; my translation]).

3 Savonarola specifically mentions Aristotle (and his advice to Alexander) and Pietro d'Abano as important authorities on the subject of physiognomy (*Speculum*, 'Prohemium', Leipzig, Universitätsbibliothek, 3472 [Haenel], f. 2ra [ed. Zuccolin: forthcoming]). For more detailed analyses of Savonarola's understanding of physiognomy, see, most recently, Ziegler (2007) and Zuccolin (2012).

4 This view of the value of physiognomy is indebted to the *Secretum secretorum*, which Savonarola references throughout his work (Zuccolin 2012: 875n7). It was an apt resource for his own treatise. In the long version of the *Secretum secretorum* (ca. 1230s), Philip of Tripoli gives advice about the prince's ideal character and health (Books I–II), along with advice on how to choose the best political advisors, ambassadors, soldiers and other members of court administration according to certain desired characteristics (Books IV–VIII) and how to wage war successfully (Book IX). He also explores the 'secrets of nature' and other occult and alchemical knowledge (Book X). For a detailed description of contents of the *Secretum*, especially Philip's influential Latin translation, see Williams (2003: 10–11). On the significance of the *Secretum secretorum* to the role of the court physician, in general, and to Savonarola in particular, see Chapter 3, pp. 96–100.

5 On physiognomy in late medieval medical and humanist discourse, see, as a starting point, Vescovini (1996 and 2001).

6 Statuti dell'Università di Medicina e di Arti del 1405, rubrica 78 'De lectura et ordine librorum legendorum' (ed. Malagola 1888: 274). The statute shows that, by the early fifteenth century, physiognomy played an especially strong role in the studies of first-year medical students. For further analysis of the statute, see Ziegler (2007: 292).

7 Ziegler (2007: 291–3) discusses the scholarship emerging from the University of Paris in the late thirteenth century and its relationship to physiognomy.

8 Eds Page et al.; tr. Hett 1936.

9 For Roger Bacon's Latin translation of the *Secretum secretorum*, see ed. Steele 1920.

10 *Analytica priora*, II.27 (70b7–70b40) (ed. and tr. Tredennick 1937: 527–53). For an introduction to physiognomy in *Analytica priora*, see Ziegler (2007: 290–1).

11 *De complexionibus* 2.6 (ed. Durling 1976: 84).

12 Ed. and Latin tr. Kühn (1821–1833); English tr. Singer (1997). For a brief analysis of Galen's use of physiognomy in *Ars medica*, see Ziegler (2007: 309). See also Nutton (2013: 274), who notes that Galen referenced physiognomy in several headings accompanying his commentary *In Hippocratis Epidemiarum* (*On the Epidemics of Hippocrates*).

13 Galen, *Ars medica* X (ed. and Latin tr. Kühn 1821–1833: 1.331–4; English tr. Singer 1997: 357–8). For another analysis of this passage, see Evan (1945: 290). While Galen cautioned against basing a diagnosis on a single sign, he nevertheless attempted to connect physiognomy with his theory of the humours (see *De complexionibus* 2.6 [ed. Durling 1976: 84], and, for further analysis of this passage, see Ziegler 2007: 289). On Galen and physiognomy more generally, see Evan's classic study (1945). For more recent analyses, see Barton (1994), and Knuuttila (2004: 87–102).

14 On the transmission and transformation of Aristotelian, Pseudo-Aristotelian and Galenic views of physiognomy, see Ziegler (2007: especially 289–93 and 305–6). On physiognomy in the work of Michael Scot, see Ziegler (2001: 177 and 2007: 287–8).

15 Ziegler (2001: 172–3) notes that medieval commentators on the physiognomy in the *Secretum secretorum* and the *Physiognomonica*, especially in versions intended for

pastoral audiences, alleged that since physiognomic signs were understood as only *potential* indicators, one must take into account people's actions (deeds) to truly judge their characters. Ziegler draws his example from an unknown scribe's comments that accompany a version of the *Secretum secretorum* included in a small, early fifteenth-century *miscellanea* of pastoral works, now Paris, Bibliothèque nationale de France, nouv. acq. lat. 711, f. 29r–v.

16 Ziegler (2001: 160–7) discusses how physiognomy coexisted with the Christian concept of free will: physiognomic signs only could indicate possibilities, inclinations or aptitudes. They could not denote 'inevitable destiny' (Ziegler 2001: 164). To clarify his point, Ziegler (2001: 162) quotes Albertus Magnus, who argued that while physiognomy showed 'inclinations' reflecting the quality of blood and spirits within an individual, these inclinations could be controlled by reason ('Est autem haec scientia non necessitatem imponens moribus hominum, sed inclinationes ex sanguine et spiritibus physicis ostendens, quae retineri possunt freno rationis') (*De animalibus libri XXVI*, I.2.2, 'De scientia physonomyae per habitudines membrorum hominis considerata in capitis partibus usque ad occulos', §127 [ed. Stadler 1916–1920: 1.46]).

17 Also known as *Commentarius in Problemata Aristotelis* or *Expositio problematum Aristotelis*. For an introduction to this encyclopaedic Aristotelian text and to Pietro's responses to it, see Siraisi (1970). In consultation with the original Greek, Pietro may have corrected an earlier Latin translation of the *Problemata* by Bartholomaeus of Messina (fl. 1258–1264) (Thomann 1991: 239). On Bartholomaeus, translator for Manfred, King of Sicily, see Kraye (2005: 423–4).

18 Thomann (1991: 240–1). Thomann discusses Pietro's theory in detail, especially focussing on how it relates to the art of Giotto. My interpretation of Pietro's theory and its significance to the artistic and humanistic milieu of Carrara Padua is indebted to Thomann's study.

19 Ziegler (2007: 302). Such theories are much more prevalent in the Quattrocento. See *Il libro dell'arte* (*The Craftsman's Handbook*) by the artist and writer Cennino Cennini (1370–1440) and *Della pittura* (*On Painting*) by the artist and architect Leon Battista Alberti (1404–1472) as principal early examples. Cennino described painting as an art 'for which it is necessary to have fantasy and skill of hand, to find things not seen, hiding in the shadow of natural ones, and to fix (or trace) them with the hand, thus demonstrating that that which is not, is' (tr. Thompson 1960: 1) – which seems an apt description for Pietro's understanding of physiognomy and its revelations about character and health. For a discussion of Cennino's comment and Giotto's frescoes, see Pardo (1997). Alberti's advice to painters is similar to Pietro's theory, as well. Alberti advocates the role of physiognomy in conveying a sense of character. He recommended many visual strategies to help painters convey the characters of their figures, which included not only facial features but posture and gestures as well (*Della pittura*, II [ed. and tr. Spencer 1956: 77, 81–5]). On the perpetuation of physiognomy in later Renaissance art, see Britton (2002). Additionally, Manca (2001: 54) cites passages from later treatises by Bartolomeo Fazio (1400–1457) and Antonio Filarete (1400–1469) that demonstrate the trend in portraiture to articulate morality and character with stance and facial expression.

20 The currency of Pietro's ideas about physiognomy in the medical community, especially, extended well into the Early Modern era. For examples of the influence of Pietro's views of physiognomy on later physicians, see Ziegler (2007: 305–12). One example points to the impact of Pietro's views into the sixteenth century: in *Chyromantie ac physionomie Anastasis* (*Chiromancy and Physiognomy of Anastasis*, 1504), the scholar and physiognomist Bartolomeo della Rocca – better known as Cocles (1467–1507) – copied Pietro d'Abano's definition of physiognomy verbatim and defended the discipline (Ziegler 2007: 310n76).

21 *Liber compilationis phisonomie* (Padua: Maufer, 1474). There is no modern critical edition of Pietro's treatise on physiognomy currently available. See Ziegler (2005: 400).

22 Ziegler (2001: 177) notes that all Early Modern contributions to the study of physiognomy were dedicated to rulers. He connects the changing concept of nobility – as a moral virtue rather than an inherited quality – with the circulation of physiognomic texts among rulers and princes in this era.

23 A copy illustrated by miniaturist Pietro da Pavia (fl. late-fourteenth century), now Paris, Bibliothèque nationale de France, lat. 6541, is listed on the 1426 inventory of the Visconti-Sforza library. The treatise bears the Visconti arms on the flyleaf, but Pasquino Capelli (d. 1398), Giangaleazzo Visconti's ('traitorous') chancellor, originally commissioned it (Sutton 1993: 90).

24 Aristotle, *Problemata*, XXXVI.1 (965b1–3) (ed. and tr. Hett 1937: 238–9).

25 'Utrum quia hec ostendit *quales quidam sunt* aut quia his *maxime cognoscuntur*' (Pietro d'Abano, *Expositio*, XXXVI.1, §1, Paris, Bibliothèque nationale de France, lat. 6540, f. 235vb [ed. and tr. Thomann 1991: 241–2; my emphasis]). Thomann's translation of Pietro's commentary draws upon three manuscripts, including the copy at Paris noted here. The other two manuscript copies are housed at Cesena, Biblioteca Malatestiana, under the shelfmark plut. XXIV. Dext. 2, f. 157rb–va (dated 1381) and plut. VI. Sin. 3, f. 193ra–rb (fourteenth century). Thomann indicates any discrepancies between these copies in his notes.

26 'causam esse quia per imagines faciei representatur qualis fuerit dispositio ipsius cuius est imago, et maxime cum fuerit depicta pictore sciente per omnia assimilare . . . ut ea deveniamus in cognitionem illius ita . . .' (Pietro d'Abano, *Expositio*, XXXVI.1, §3 [ed. and tr. Thomann 1991: 241–2]).

27 'dicens ideo facere faciei imaginem, quia per ipsam magis contingit cognosci eum cuius est, cum ea sit dearticulata et distincta potissime, quo *percipitur differentia*, distincta et conspicitur ut assueta et delecta . . . Quod autem quis imagines qualis sit recte cognoscatur expressa *non solum quantum ad ea que corporis, verum etiam anime* monstratur ex historia physionomie libri "de regimine principum" Alexandro ab Aristotele conscripti, de figura Hippocratis in pergameno depicta et Philomoni ingenti physionomo monstrata' (Pietro d'Abano, *Expositio*, XXXVI.1, §5–6 [ed. and tr. Thomann 1991: 241–2; my emphasis]).

28 The *Secretum* reads: 'Discipuli siquidem Ypocratis sapientis depinxerunt formam ejus in pergameno et portaverunt earn Philimoni dicentes: Considera hanc figuram et iudica nobis qualitates complexionis ejus' (Bacon IV.1 [ed. Steele 1920: 165]).

29 Thomann (1991: 243n10) observed that Pietro misremembered the story here, which he had recalled correctly in his earlier treatise, the *Compilatio physionomiae*, I.2.1 (Venice 1548, f. 2v). Rather than referring to Hippocrates, the original anecdote refers to a physiognomist known as Zopyros, who (allegedly) read Socrates' character from a portrait. Thomann remarked that in later exegeses on the story, Socrates became confused with Hippocrates because of the similarity between their names in Arabic (Buḵrāṭ [Hippocrates] and Suḵrāṭ [Socrates]). In addition, Thomann (1991: 241n22) noted that Pliny recounted a story of a physiognomist (*metoposcopos*) who was able to determine the length of a man's life by examining a portrait painted by Apelles (*Naturalis historia* 35.89 [ed. and tr. Jones 1956: 327]).

30 Pietro d'Abano, *Expositio*, XXXVI.1, §3 (ed. and tr. Thomann 1991: 241).

31 On Galen and Galenic medicine, see, as a starting point, Nutton (2004 and 2013: 222–53). For Galen (and subsequently for Pietro), each individual possessed a unique temperament influenced and fixed by the astrological signs and planets under which he or she was born. Each person's constitution reflected a combination of the four humoral complexions, and the dominant humour in the mix determined the category of temperament into which the individual was grouped. Each of the four complexions has a corresponding bodily fluid, quality, element, season, and planetary and astrological complement. Each also has behavioural tendencies – predispositions toward good and bad personal qualities – associated with it. On Pietro's medical philosophy and its relationship to Galenic medicine, see Alessio (1976); Siraisi (1985 [repr. 2001b: 79–99]); and Klemm and De Leemens (2005).

32 Pietro discusses these aspects of a man's *dispositio* in his *Conciliator differentiarum philosophorum et medicorum* (*Conciliator of the Differences Debated Between Philosophers and Physicians*, ca. 1300–1307). He writes: 'It should be said that there is a twofold inherence of *dispositio*: one permanent, and this remains for ever in its way and has a tendency toward its principles, as becomes obvious from the variability of the face in Hippocrates' *De aeris aquis locis* (i.e. ch. xii; the climatic types of men). The other is the actual, and this is continuously changing in consequence (of the fact) that the heat affects something moist now differently than before' ('dicendum, quod duplex est dispositionis inhaerentia: una quidem habitudinalis, et haec semper permanet suo modo, et inclinationem habet ad sua principia, ut apparet de permutatione faciei, in de aere, et aqua: alia vero actualis, et haec permutatur continue secundum quod calor aliter afficit humidum nunc, quam prius') (*Conciliator*, differentiae XIX.3 [Venice 1565, f. 30r–v]; tr. Thomann 1991: 243). On this interpretation of Pietro's *inhaerentia dispositionis*, see Thomann (1991: 243–4).

33 Pietro sometimes differentiated the invisible moral qualities from other aspects of a person's constitution by referring to moral disposition as *dispositio occulte* (See *Expositio*, X.10 [Venice 1501, f. 100rb]). For a discussion of Pietro's *dispositio occulte*, see Thomann (1991: 243–4). For a brief overview of Pietro's complementary view of morality and the physical body, see Klemm and De Leemens (2005).

34 This relationship between physical and moral characteristics was also central to Pietro's successors, the court physicians, and especially to Michele Savonarola. In Pietro's treatise on the subject, *Compilatio physionomiae* (1295), and in Savonarola's, *Speculum phisionomie* (1446), the authors demonstrate how the physiognomic associations drawn from the appearance of a patient's body and symptoms could be used to treat individual health concerns. See Denieul-Cormier (1956); and Vescovini (1996 and 2001).

35 On the iconography of the frescoes, see Barzon (1924); Grossato (1964); Ivanoff (1964); Mor (1964b); Vescovini (1986); Castellini (1993); Norman (1995a and 1995c: 1.141); and Frojmovič (1996), with their relevant bibliographies. On Pietro d'Abano's influence on the iconography of Giotto's earlier frescoes in the Scrovegni Chapel, and on the frescoes' relationship to both science and rhetoric, see Frojmovič (2007).

36 For a brief overview of Pietro's inclusive view of medicine, see Klemm and De Leemens (2005).

37 da Nono, *Visio*, 'De mutacione forme communis palacii urbis Padue' (ed. Fabris 1934–1939: 20). See Fabris (1932–1933 and 1977), and Frojmovič (1996: 27) for more detailed discussions of da Nono's commentary.

38 'Duodecim celestia signa et septem planete cumsuis proprietatibus in hac cohopertura fulgebunt, a Zotho summon pictorum mirifice laborata, et alia sidera aurea cum speculis et alie figurationes similiter fulgebunt inferius [interius]' (da Nono, *Visio*, 'De mutacione forme communis palacii urbis Padue' [ed. Fabris 1934–1939: 20, tr. Frojmovič 1996: 27]).

39 'singulares et egregie picture illud circuunt, quibus corpora planetarum, et ad que opera peragenda magis homines ab eis inclinantur, mirum in modum etiam per figuras demonstrantor' (Savonarola, *Libellus*, II, 'De Temporalibus et Mundanis' [ed. Segarizzi 1902: 48, ll. 1–3; tr. Burckhardt 2005: 71]).

40 'Huius autem ordinis [sic] institutor noster gloriosus Conciliator exstitit' (Savonarola, *Libellus*, II, 'De Temporalibus et Mundanis' [ed. Segarizzi 1902: 48, l. 3; tr. Burckhardt 2005: 71]).

41 'Cappella magna picturis Zoti [Giotto] pictorum principis ornatissima, que tribus sacerdotibus in dies et horas santificatur' (Savonarola, *Libellus*, II, 'De Temporalibus et Mundanis' [ed. Segarizzi 1902: 50, ll. 5–6]; unpublished tr. Margaret Musgrove; personal correspondence). For further interpretation of Savonarola's description of the Scrovegni Chapel, see Derbes and Sandona (2008: 28–9).

42 'Zotum Florentinum, qui primus ex antiquis et musaicis figuris modernas mirum in modum configuravit; . . . Hic magnificam amplamque nobilium de Scrovineis Cappellam suis cum digitis magno cum pretio pinxit, ubi novi et veteris Testamenti imagines velut viventes apparent, Capitulumque Antonii nostri etiam sic ornavit, ut ad hec loca

et visendas figuras pictorum advenarum non parvus sit confluxus. Et tantum dignitas civitatis eum commovit, ut maximam sue vite partem in ea consummaverit, et ut in sic post se relictis gloriosis figuris ea in civitate semper viverit' (Savonarola, *Libellus*, I.3, 'De viris illustribus non sacris' [ed. Segarizzi 1902: 44, ll. 25–32; unpublished tr. Margaret Musgrove; personal correspondence]).

43 See n48 in this chapter.

44 'unde Invidiosus invidia comburitur intus et extra hanc padue in arena optime pinsit Giottus' ('as where Envy is consumed with envy inside and out, this Giotto painted excellently in the Arena at Padua') (Barberino, *I documenti d'Amore*, Rome, Biblioteca Apostolica Vaticana, Barb. lat. 4076 [ed. Egidi 1905–1927: 2.165; tr. Gunzburg 2013: 415]). On Barberino's comments on *Envy*, see Murray (1953); Stubblebine (1969: 109); and Gardner (2011: 4 and 141n10). With thanks to Shelley MacLaren for alerting me to Francesco's comments in her paper for the College Art Association annual conference (2010) and for our subsequent conversations about *I documenti*.

45 See pp. 153 and 165n42 for Savonarola's comments on the Scrovegni Chapel in the *Libellus*.

46 On the relationship between Pietro d'Abano's physiognomic work and that of Savonarola, see Denieul-Cormier (1956: xliii), and Zuccolin (2012: 874).

47 Book I of the *Speculum phisionomie* comprises what Zuccolin (2012: 876n12) terms a 'traditional' physiognomic manual that charts correspondences between parts of the body and certain moral and psychological characteristics. Conversely, Book II primarily considers the influences of astrology upon human generation (Zuccolin 2012: 876n12).

48 'Aures autem oblonge et anguste invidie dixit esse signum' (Savonarola, *Speculum*, 4.14, 'De auribus', Leipzig, Universitätsbibliothek, 3472 [Haenel], f. 40rb [ed. Zuccolin: forthcoming]). Further, Zuccolin (2012: 883) notes that, in the section dedicated to the physiognomy of the ear (I.34, 'De phisionomia auris') in the version of the *Speculum* housed in Venice, Savonarola mentioned the long, pointed ears of Attila, King of the Huns (d. 453) (Venice, Biblioteca Nazionale Marciana, lat. VI, 156 [coll. 2672], 74rb–75va). Known as the scourge of God (*flagellum Dei*), Attila, in many ways, would have embodied the traits of cruelty and avarice for Savonarola's readers. Other potential correspondences between Giotto's personifications and Savonarola's physiognomy include small ears (as seen in *Folly*), which Savonarola (following the physician Loxus [third century, BCE]) associated with silliness of character (*Speculum*, 4.14, 'De auribus', Leipzig, Universitätsbibliothek, 3472 [Haenel], f. 40rb [ed. Zuccolin: forthcoming]; see also Denieul-Cormier 1956: 91), and a long and pointed chin (as seen in *Injustice*), which he associated with an excessively hot temperament and tendency toward violence (*Speculum*, 4.19, 'De mento', Leipzig, Universitätsbibliothek, 3472 [Haenel], f. 45rb [ed. Zuccolin: forthcoming]; see also Denieul-Cormier 1956: 93]).

49 Later in the century, around 1370, Giusto de' Menabuoi (1320–1391) depicted personifications of the virtues and vices in *grisaille* in a side chapel of the Church of the Eremitani for a member of the Carrara court, the jurist Tebaldo de' Cortellieri (fl. late fourteenth century). Although the cycle was largely destroyed during World War II, Marcantonio Michiel discussed it in his description of the chapel in the *Notizia d'opere del disegno* (1530) (*Notizia* I.9 'Alli Heremitani' [ed. Frizzoni 1884: 63–4; tr. Mussi 1903: 28]). Michiel noted that the virtues and vices mirrored one another across the central space of the chapel, much as they do in the Scrovegni Chapel. In Cortellieri's chapel, a smaller, more personal commemorative space than the Scrovegni chapel, the *grisaille* personifications were juxtaposed with portraits of exemplary Augustinians. Together with these portraits, the personifications of the virtues would have been perceived as even stronger exemplars, and the vices, in contrast to the monks' lives of good works, even greater negative exemplars. On the Cortellieri chapel, see Kohl (1989: 13–14 and 2001: 26).

50 As noted in the Introduction (pp. 10–11), fourteenth-century humanists drew their use of corporeal metaphor from Seneca's first-century *De clementia* (*On Mercy*) (ed. Hosius 1914; tr. Basore 1928: 1.357–447), in which the Roman philosopher described the

relationship between the emperor and his state using visceral corporeal imagery. As a product of Imperial Rome, Seneca recast the Republican virtues (most ardently articulated in Cicero's *De officiis*) as virtues of the Imperial prince: for Seneca, the righteous prince became the true and worthy successor to the *civis* (Stacey 2007: 10). This rhetoric naturally appealed to fourteenth- and fifteenth-century *signori*, like the Carrara and the Visconti, who usurped power from communal governments.

51 *Rerum senilium* XIV.1 (eds Nota and Dotti 2002–2013: 4.228–313; tr. Bernardo et al. 1992: 2.521–52).

52 Ed. Fenzi (2009); tr. Rawski (1991). On Petrarch's use of corporeal metaphor in *De remediis* and on the work's importance to Francesco Novello, see Kyle (2015).

53 On Conversini and his position at court, see Kohl (1983: 574–8). On the identity of Giovanni's addressee, see Pesenti Marangon (1976: 50–2).

54 'Audebo tamen dicere sine preiudicio verioris sententie: etsi non quemque civium, omnes tamen simul cives universamque rempublicam, non quantum filium modo vel parentes, sed quantum temet ipsum amare debes. In singulis enim caris capitibus singuli sunt affectus, in republica autem omnes. Amandi tibi sunt igitur cives tui ut filii, imo, ut sic dixerim, tanquam corporis tui membra sive anime tue partes: unum enim corpus est res publica cuius tu caput es' (Petrarch, *Rerum senilium* XIV.1, ll. 293–301 [eds Nota and Dotti 2002–2013: 4.249; tr. Bernardo et al. 1992: 2.528–9]).

55 The relevant passage reads, 'ut te dominum non vestis, non elatio, sed sola morum gravitas et frontis probet auctoritas. Bonum duplex ut, in contrario, duplex malum, et iactantia per se ipsam odiosa et imitationis periculosa contagio' (Petrarch, *Rerum senilium* XIV.1, ll. 1060–64 [eds Nota and Dotti 2002–2013: 4.297; tr. Bernardo et al. 1992: 2.548]).

56 'Populi enim omnes et actus principum et habitus imitari student. Ita sit verissimum nullos magis rei publice nocere quam qui exemplo nocent, quia verum est quod ait ille: *Componitur orbis Regis ad exemplum*. Sic est hercle: mali mores principum non eis tantum, sed omnibus sunt damnosi . . .' (Petrarch, *Rerum senilium* XIV.1, ll. 1064–71 [eds Nota and Dotti 2002–2013: 4.297; tr. Bernardo et al. 1992: 2.548]).

57 See Chapter 4, pp. 132–3.

58 'Proinde, quoniam te non nisi bonis et illustribus comparatum velim, hos imitare, obsecro, atque horum exempla complectere qui rebus ac verbis claram laudem iustitie meruerunt' (Petrarch, *Rerum senilium* XIV.1, ll. 668–70 [eds Nota and Dotti 2002–2013: 4.273; tr. Bernardo et al. 1992: 2.538]).

59 Gatari, *Cronaca*, 'La morte del signore misser Francesco da Carara e dî figliuoli misser Francesco Terzo e misser Iacomo da Carara', 17 gennaio 1406 (eds Medin and Tolomei 1931: 579–80; tr. Symes 1830: 237).

60 '[El corpo suo fu] dopieri ala cassa e vesititi d'una dele sue pelande de veluto alesandrino. Ed era nel vixo tutto infiatto e batuto, con una spada dorata cinta e due speroni dorati in piedi. Fu il deto signor misser Francesco da Carara di persona non tropo grande, ma di comune grandeza, e grosso e ben menbruto quanto niun altro, e bruno nel vixo e nela cierra sua alquanto fierra, ne suo parlare discretisimo, gracioxo, a suo puopollo misericordioxo, a tuti sapientisimo, e forte di sua persona' (Gatari, *Cronaca*, 'La morte del signore misser Francesco da Carara e dî figliuoli misser Francesco Terzo e misser Iacomo da Carara', 17 gennaio 1406 [eds Medin and Tolomei 1931: 580; tr. Symes 1830: 237]).

61 The contract for Giacomo's tomb survives. Dated 26 February 1351, it names Andriolo de' Santi as the designer and notes that two other unnamed sculptors executed the tomb. Wolters published the contract (1976: 1.169 [cat. no. 41]). Due to its stylistic similarities, the *arca* for Ubertino is believed to be an earlier work by the same sculptor. The marble tombs were originally located in the Church of San Agostino, the church in which elite Paduans were interred and in which Petrarch and Pietro d'Abano had wanted to be buried (see Petrarch's *Testamentum*, §6a [ed. and tr. Mommsen 1957: 73]. For Pietro's wishes, see Toffanin 1988: 25–8, and Norman 1995b: 1.157n14). Currently, the tombs mirror one another across the nave of the Church of the Eremitani as they once

mirrored each other in the Carrara family chapel at the Church of San Agostino, which was destroyed in 1819 (Norman 1995b: 1.157).

62 Norman (1995b: 1.157). Norman identifies the costumes on account of the headdress, which is also visible in fresco portraits of the Carrara lords and in the illustrations in the *Liber de principibus* and the *Gesta magnifica*. She further notes that the artists portrayed the Carrara as citizens, not as warrior-knights, which suggested their ability to govern fairly and to administer the city.

63 The use of multiple media in commemorative monuments was popular among the elite in Padua during the Trecento. Three fragments remain from the fresco programmes that accompanied the sculptural effigies of the Carrara lords. Attributed to Guariento, the fragments include an image of the *Coronation of the Virgin* and votive portraits of two Carrara men. The *arche* and their accompanying frescoes were damaged during the Allied bombings in 1944, which destroyed Mantegna's *Ovetari Chapel*. The bombings heavily damaged the architectural *baldacchino* above Ubertino's tomb, and its sculptural details have been reconstructed (Norman 1995b: 1.158). Photographs taken prior to World War II show the three fresco fragments in their original location above Giacomo's tomb. The fragments are now in the chancel of the Church of the Eremitani. The frescoes that once framed Ubertino's tomb have not been recovered.

64 The model of the city was moved prior to World War II to prevent damage. It has not been replaced. Giusto de' Menabuoi likely imitated the accurate topography of Andriolo's model-city in his representation of Padua included in the fresco of Saint Anthony appearing to the Blessed Luca Belludi (d. 1286), the saint's companion and disciple, which Giusto completed in 1383 for the Conti Chapel in 'Il Santo' (Norman 1995b: 1.158).

65 Norman (1995b: 1.158).

66 'unum enim corpus est res publica cuius tu caput es' (Petrarch, *Rerum senilium* XIV.1, ll. 300–1 [eds Nota and Dotti 2002–2013: 4.249; tr. Bernardo et al. 1992: 2.529]).

67 'Heu magno domus arcta viro sub marmore parvo / En pater hic patrie spesque salusque iacent. / Quisquis ad hoc saxum convertis lumina, lector, / Publica damna legens iunge preces lacrymis'. Petrarch appended the epitaph to his letter to Giovanni d'Arezzo (*Rerum familiarium* XI.3, dated 1351). The epitaph continues: 'Illum flere nefas, sua quem super ethera virtus / Sustulit, humano siqua fides merito; / Flere gravem patrie casum fractamque bonorum / Spem licet et subitis ingemuisse malis. / Quem populo patribusque ducem Carraria nuper / Alma dedit, Patavo mors inimica tulit. / Nullus amicitias coluit dulcedine tanta, / Cum foret horrendus hostibus ille suis; / Optimus inque bonis semper studiosus amandis, / Nescius invidie conspicuusque fide. / Ergo memor Iacobi speciosum credula nomen / Nominibus raris insere, posteritas' (Petrarch *Rerum familiarium* XI.3, ll. 117–28 [eds Rossi and Bosco 1933–1942: 2.330; tr. Bernardo 2005: 2.91–2, with slight edits to Bernardo's translation]).

6   Embodiments of virtue in Francesco Novello's library

Of the books listed on Francesco Zago's inventory of Francesco Novello's library, only six manuscripts – four richly illustrated and two ornamented but comparatively unillustrated – have been identified.[1] The *Carrara Herbal*, Zago's 'Serapiom in volgare', is the only medical codex firmly identified from the inventory. The other three identified illustrated manuscripts and the two identified unillustrated manuscripts represent the secondary focus of Francesco's collection: biographies and local chronicles. One of the unillustrated manuscripts is the *Cronica del Mussato per letra* (*The Chronicle of Mussato, in his own hand [?]*), likely the account of communal Padua's early history by Albertino Mussato (1261–1329), *De traditione Patavii ad Canem Grandem anno 1328 mense septembri et causis precedentibus* (*On the Tradition of Padua to [the Time of] Cangrande in September 1328 and its Preceding Causes*).[2] The Carrara family *stemma* (the *carro*) and the initials 'FF' appear on the lower margin of the manuscript's first folio. The other unillustrated manuscript is the *Libro del chataro* (*The Book by Gataro*), likely the *Cronaca Carrarese* (*The Chronicle of the Carrara*), an account of seigniorial Padua written by Galeazzo Gatari (d. 1405) and his sons.[3] A partially defaced *carro* appears on the lower margin of the first folio of this manuscript as well. Along with similar representations of the family's *stemma*, the four illustrated manuscripts contain portraits of the Carrara lords or representations of their individual heraldic arms that imitate, or directly copy, those in the fresco cycles commissioned by Francesco's ancestors and their court intimates.[4]

When Francesco Novello had the historic images of the *signori* and their heraldry translated into his illustrated books, he mobilised in a new way the physiognomic system of associations between healthy (and heroic) bodies and moral characteristics in circulation in Padua. The appropriation of his ancestors' imagery enabled their representations to become a type of heraldry for Francesco Novello – an index of his past and the 'great deeds' of his family. Moreover, in the context of Francesco's library, the relocated representations of the Carrara provide an interpretative infrastructure with which to experience – and understand – the *Carrara Herbal*. Considered in relationship to the illustrated biographies and chronicles, the *Herbal* becomes a materialisation of Francesco's role as the new, 'health-giving' Carrara leader of Padua. Its illustrations of plants become 'portraits' with medical, moral and political significance.

The *Liber cimeriorum dominorum de Carraria*

In Francesco Novello's illustrated chronicles and biographies, the textual content clarifies the significance of the figural portraits and heraldic devices of the Carrara as manifestations of their invisible virtues and great deeds. As we saw in Chapter 5, artists, chroniclers and humanists associated the physical body of the lord with his moral virtue and the health of the city and its citizens. Pictorial and literary representations of the lords' bodies accompany accounts of their actions – a juxtaposition visualised in the *Sala virorum illustrium* (*The Hall of Famous Men*) in relationship to the deeds of Petrarch's ancient heroes and described in earlier chronicles in relationship to the deeds of the Carrara. The content of one of Francesco Novello's illustrated books, in particular, teaches its readers how to interpret the representations of the Carrara lords' bodies and heraldry as signs of the lords' moral virtues and good governance and as embodiments of their 'great deeds'.

The book inventoried by Zago as the *Liber cimeriorum dominorum de Carraria* (*The Book of the Carrara Lords' Cimieri*), a small, luxury codex (27 × 20 cm) comprised of 20 parchment folios,[5] contains colourful, full-page illustrations of the personal heraldry (*cimiero*) of each *signore* enclosed in a quatrefoil frame. The illustrations' composition mimics the heraldry portrayed in the *Camera dei Carri* (*Room of the Carri*) and the *Anticamera dei Cimieri* (*Anteroom of the Cimieri*) commissioned by Ubertino in the early 1340s for the Carrara family palace (see Plate 5).[6] The text of the book, penned in gold ink, recounts an idealised history of the Carrara lords, in verse, by analogising each lord's life and character to his heraldic imagery.

Lazzaro de' Malrotondi da Conegliano (fl. 1376–1405), the grammarian and tutor to Francesco Novello's children, composed the verses in the *Liber cimeriorum*. De' Malrotondi borrowed the verses' content from the Gatari *Cronaca*, which, while analogising the lords' moral characteristics through descriptions of their physical ones,[7] similarly used family heraldry as metaphors for the lords' characters.[8] For instance, de' Malrotondi related Ubertino's *cimiero* – the fierce Moor with the golden-horns – to the *signore*, who, like his personal device, was regal, fierce and prepared to defend Padua against its enemies (Plate 7). The passage reads:[9]

> Ubertino, third Carrara lord of Padua, / Bore the horned Moor to drive out his enemies. / He had the bearing and habits of the palace. / At the same time, he increased the honors of the Carrara. / He laid traps for those whom he saw to be enemies / And killed them all fiercely.

In combination, the verses and imagery in the *Liber cimeriorum* teach the reader how to interpret the lords' heraldry as indices for their imagined selves. This skill is useful to the interpretation of Ubertino's fresco cycles, in which the *cimieri* originally appeared, and to the portraits of the Carrara lords in the family palace and in Francesco Novello's other books.

Given the large role metaphorical portraiture played in the elder Francesco's patronage and the younger Francesco's desire to imitate and outdo his father, it is perhaps unsurprising that an illustrated book once belonging to Francesco il Vecchio may have set a precedent for such use of the family's heraldry and inspired Francesco Novello's commission of the *Liber cimeriorum*. In *De currus Carrariensis moraliter descriptus* (*The Carrara Cart, Morally Described*),[10] written by the Franciscan teacher Francesco Caronelli (fl. 1373–1413) and dedicated to Francesco il Vecchio in 1376, the *carro* is used metaphorically to structure an account of the family's virtues and history. The manuscript includes an illustration of the *carro*, the parts of which are labelled with the cardinal virtues and their associated moral qualities. In conjunction with the text, the illustration instructs the reader on how to interpret the family's arms as a symbol of their virtues (Figure 6.1).[11] Likewise, the verses in the *Liber cimeriorum* present the accompanying personal heraldry of each lord as a metaphor for his individual virtues and history. In the other illustrated books commissioned by Francesco Novello, the figural portraits of the lords – often together with their heraldry – similarly 'embody' and personify the lords' histories and idealised personal characters.

The *Gesta magnifica* and the *Liber de principibus*

The book identified by Zago as the *Liber Jntroitus Magni. Dominj* (*The Book of the Entrance of the Magnificent Lord*) is likely the *Gesta magnifica domus Carrariensis* (*The Magnificent Deeds of the Carrara House*), an anonymously written pro-Carrara account of the family's history from the twelfth century to 1368.[12] Dedicated to Francesco Novello in the *proemio*, the *Gesta magnifica* records the family's history in neat textura script – penned in sepia ink and accented in red. The codex itself is very large (58.4 × 43.2 cm) and contains 45 parchment folios. The text is organised into two columns and includes 90 spaces for illustrations, usually at the base of the columns, only four of which were used.[13] An unknown artist painted four narrative scenes that depict the family's active, 'heroic' role in Padua. The scenes show the 'great deeds' of the Carrara in the manner of Petrarch's *viri illustres*. In their narrative format, they also allude to the many fresco cycles of saints' lives in Padua in which artists portrayed Carrara family members as pious witnesses.[14] In the *Gesta magnifica*, however, the Carrara become the focus of the narrative action and assume the 'salvific' role of the saints.

The scenes in the *Gesta magnifica* respond to a trend in portraiture in which detailed portraits of the Carrara family and members of their court were included in monumental religious fresco cycles across Padua ('hidden', as it were, in plain sight). The Carrara play only passive roles in the fresco cycles' complex visual narratives, which recount stories from the Bible or from saints' lives and serve as moral *exempla* or contemplative touchstones for their viewers. These multiple 'hidden' portraits of the Carrara and their court *famiglia*, primarily produced during Francesco il Vecchio's tenure as *signore*, have been discussed extensively by art historians, and debates about attribution and dating colour the scholarship on the fresco portraits.[15] I draw attention to the portraits here, however, not to

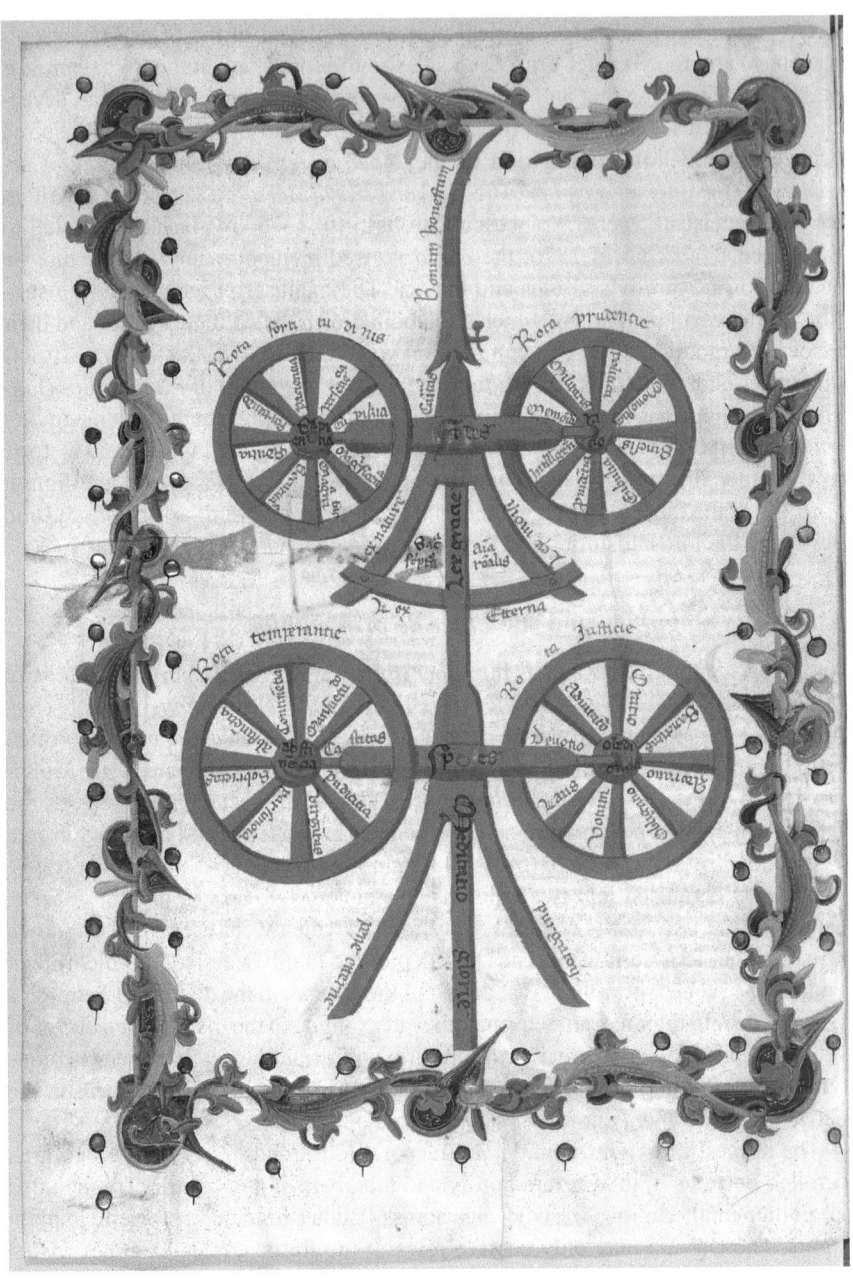

Figure 6.1 Diagram of the *carro* labelled with Cardinal virtues

De currus Carrariensis moraliter descriptus
Paris, Bibliothèque nationale de France, lat. 6468, f. 9v
Folio 35 × 25.5 cm, Padua, ca. 1376

Source: Bibliothèque nationale de France, Département des manuscrits, Latin 6468

engage with these debates but to establish the prominence and popularity among the Paduan elite of recognisable contemporary portraits in narratives of historic sacred scenes.

So, for instance, portraits by Altichiero of the elder and younger Francesco, accompanied by Petrarch and Lombardo della Seta, adorn the chapels of the Carrara retainers Bonifacio (1316–1390) and Raimondino Lupi (d. 1379) in the Chapel of San Giacomo (now Felice) in 'Il Santo' (ca. 1377–1379) and in the neighbouring Oratory of San Giorgio (ca. 1380–1384), respectively.[16] 'Il Santo', the great pilgrim-age church dedicated to Saint Anthony, is the spiritual heart of the city and, like the Baptistery, was very much a part of everyday life in late-medieval Padua. A large cross-section of Padua's citizens would have seen the fresco portraits in these areas.

In the Lupi Chapel at 'Il Santo', portraits of the Carrara lords and illustrious members of their court appear in scenes from the life of Saint James the Great.[17] The episodes derive from the *Legenda Aurea* (*The Golden Legend*) by Jacopus da Voragine (ca. 1230–1298) and from anonymous chivalric legends associated with Santiago de Compostela, which tell the story of the rediscovery of the saint's body in northern Spain and the subsequent miracles associated with his relics. In particular, the three central scenes in the chapel focus on episodes drawn from the Santiago stories. The first scene shows Asturian King Ramiro (ca. 790–850) receiving a vision of Saint James in which the saint urges the king to fight the Muslims in the northern Iberian Peninsula and promises him victory. The central scene – incorporating portraits of Francesco il Vecchio, hooded and bearded, and his son, heavy-set, bearded and wearing a cap, as well as portraits of Petrarch and Lombardo della Seta – shows King Ramiro recounting the vision to his council (Figure 6.2). The subsequent scene portrays the ensuing Battle of Clavigo (843 CE) and Ramiro's victory (allegedly) through Saint James' intervention. Scholars interpret these scenes as a political allegory in which King Ramiro rep-resents King Louis of Hungary (1326–1382) – the *fleurs-de-lis* of the House of Anjou adorn the king's surcoat in the battle scene and appear on the throne in the council scene. King Louis of Hungary, rival of the Venetians, became an ally to the Carrara when Francesco il Vecchio broke from his alliance with Venice in 1356.[18] The militaristic focus of the scene, however, also suited the chapel's patron, Boni-facio Lupi, who served the Carrara as a knight.[19]

Additional portraits of the elder and younger Francesco appear in Altichiero's frescoes in the Oratory of San Giorgio, located beside 'Il Santo'. Raimondino Lupi commissioned the oratory as another family chapel; however, his cousin, Boni-facio, commissioned the frescoes after Raimondino's death in 1379. The fresco cycle includes scenes from the lives of several saints, including Saint George, Saint Cath-erine of Alexandria and Saint Lucy, which accompany scenes from the life of Christ. Altichiero portrayed the Carrara lords in the scene in which Saint Lucy is condemned to death, and, in an episode from the life of Saint George, he portrayed Francesco il Vecchio with the poets watching the Baptism of King Sevio. Further, in the scene of Saint George's martyrdom, Francesco il Vecchio appears on horseback sporting his personal heraldry (the golden-horned Moor).[20] Portraits by the Carrara court painter Giusto de' Menabuoi (1320–1391) of Francesco il Vecchio, Fina da Buzzacarini

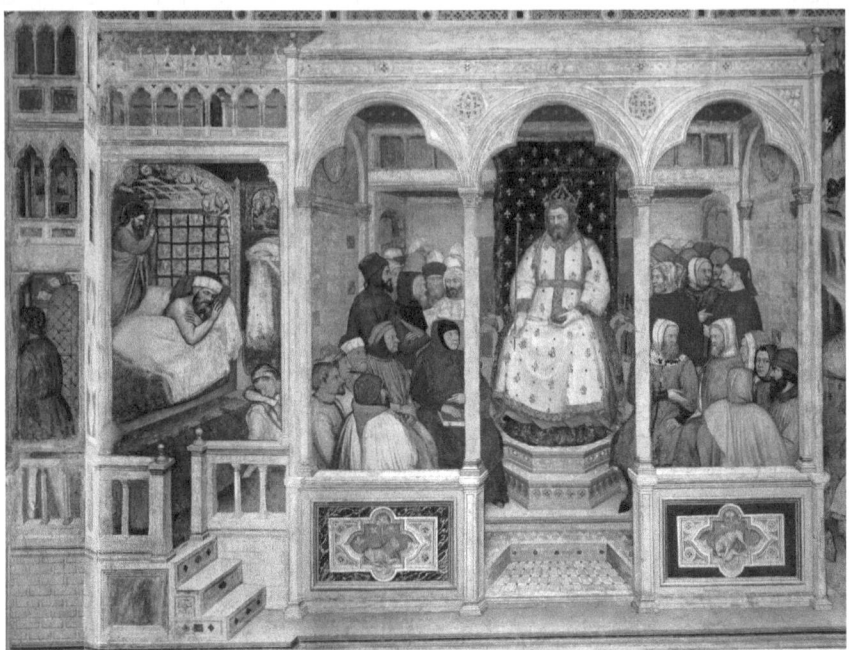

Figure 6.2 Altichiero, *The Council of King Ramiro*

Padua, Chapel of San Felice (formerly San Giacomo), Basilica of Sant'Antonio
Fresco, Padua, ca. 1373–1379

Photo credit: Alfredo Dagli Orti / Art Resource, NY

(ca. 1325–1378), and their daughters also adorn Padua's Baptistery (ca. 1370s), where Francesco and Fina originally were interred.[21] Francesco il Vecchio, Fina, Fina's sister Anna, and Petrarch observe the scene of Christ healing the sick, and Fina and her daughters witness the birth of the Virgin.[22]

The four scenes in Francesco Novello's copy of the *Gesta magnifica* are narrative, like the fresco cycles in the Lupi chapels and the Baptistery, and they may even compositionally relate to the cycles' scenes. However, the portraits of the Carrara in the *Gesta magnifica* differ from this local tradition. Rather than popping up in sacred stories only alluding to their civic lives and moral virtues, in the *Gesta magnifica* the Carrara lords directly appear in narratives of Padua's history, aligning representations of their bodies with idealised accounts of their lives that highlight the lords' virtues and dedication to the city. The four completed scenes in Francesco Novello's volume depict the family's commitment to Padua in action and portray the Carrara at the centre of Paduan communal history.

The Carrara portrayed in the secular scenes of the *Gesta magnifica* enact their own 'great deeds'. For instance, the first illustration (f. 1v) shows the Holy Roman Emperor, Frederick II (1194–1250), restraining the earliest recorded

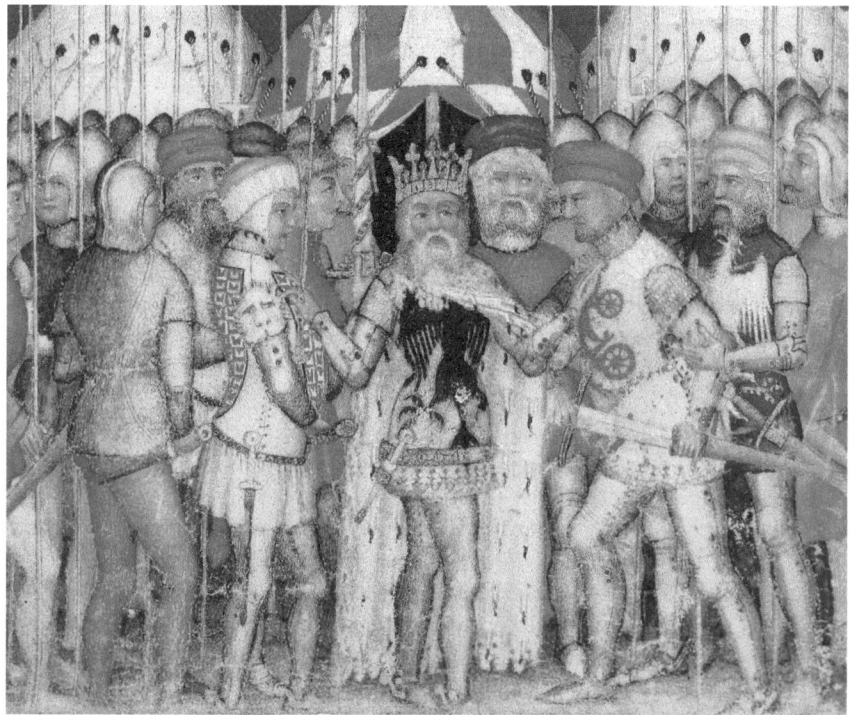

Figure 6.3 Scene of Giacomo da Carrara defying Ezzelino da Romano

Gesta magnifica domus Carrariensibus
Venice, Biblioteca Nazionale Marciana, lat. X, 381 (coll. 2802), f. 1v
Folio 58 × 43 cm, Padua, ca. 1390

Photo credit: © DeA Picture Library / Art Resource, NY

Carrara family member, Giacomo da Carrara (d. 1240), from attacking Ezzelino da Romano (1194–1259), the infamous tyrant of Padua (Figure 6.3). The following illustration on the interior column of the facing page (f. 2r) portrays Giacomo's death at Ezzelino's hands (Plate 8). In the execution scene, the artist portrayed Giacomo surrounded by Ezzelino's knights and hemmed in by their spears. Giacomo lies face down on the ground, his hands tied behind his back, and blood streaming from his wounds. The executioner stands above him, poised to strike the killing blow. A Franciscan monk kneels beside Giacomo and looks at Ezzelino as the lord lowers his sceptre, giving the order for Giacomo's death.

As art historians Giordana Mariani Canova and Luca Baggio have discussed, despite different narrative emphases, the execution scene in the *Gesta magnifica* borrowed recognisable compositional elements from Altichiero's scene of the martyrdom of Saint George in the Oratory of San Giorgio, a scene in which Altichiero also portrayed the elder Francesco as a witness.[23] The execution scenes in both fresco and codex feature a prominent clerical figure who blesses the protagonist, a ring of armed soldiers that directs our attention to the action at the centre of the scene, and an authority figure who points a sceptre to signal the execution.

The arrangement of these compositional elements varies slightly between the manuscript and the fresco: where Giacomo lies on the ground, Saint George kneels. Saint George faces the right side of the fresco, while Giacomo faces the left side of the illustration. The priest in the fresco stands and wears a white stole with yellow stripes over a long, green-blue robe, while his counterpart in the book illustration kneels and wears the brown habit of the Franciscan order. Baggio argues that Altichiero's fresco may have been a pictorial source for the *Gesta magnifica* illustration primarily because of this figure of the Franciscan: there is no mention of a monk's benediction in the textual account of Giacomo's execution, so, the illustrator turned away from the text for this detail.[24] Rather than copying the scene of Saint George's martyrdom directly, the illustrator of the *Gesta magnifica* seems to have combined elements from Altichiero's narrative scene with this episode in the family's history in order to lend a recognisable aura of martyrdom to Giacomo's execution.[25]

The subsequent scene in the *Gesta magnifica* at the base of the neighbouring exterior column shows the investiture ceremony of Giacomo 'il Grande' (r. 1318–1319), the first elected lord of Padua, who shared the name of his ancestor (allegedly) martyred for Padua's freedom (Plate 9).[26] The anonymous illustrator portrayed Giacomo il Grande elegantly dressed in a blue cloak, standing in profile at the head of a crowd of elite Paduans and the communal council of *Anziani* (elders) in the town hall. Within the *Gesta magnifica*, the images of the two Giacomos are pendants: the sacrifice of the first Giacomo at the hands of Padua's enemy evidenced the family's commitment to the commune, a commitment that later would support Giacomo il Grande's election and his family's subsequent rule of Padua.

The final illustration in the *Gesta magnifica* shows the election of Marsilio 'il Grande' in 1337.[27] The scene of Marsilio's investiture ceremony mirrors the scene of his predecessor's in form and content, but it is better preserved (Figure 6.4). In both investiture scenes, the artist showed the Carrara lord in profile receiving the banner of the commune – a white flag with a red cross – from the *podestà* (the city's chief magistrate), who stands slightly above the lord on a dais in front of an ornate throne. Trumpets hung with banners emblazoned with the *carro* stretch out above the congregation, while well-dressed onlookers clap and cheer to express their support. The portrayal of Marsilio's supporters is reminiscent of Galeazzo Gatari's description of the reception Marsilio received when he reclaimed Padua from the della Scala on 3 August 1337. According to the *Cronaca Carrarese*, the Paduan people cheered Marsilio in the streets crying: 'Viva misser Marsilio e la cha' da Charara!' ('Long live lord Marsilio and the house of Carrara!').[28] The visual continuity of the two investiture scenes suggests the political continuity of the *signoria*, despite the 18 years between the elections.

The investiture scenes in the *Gesta magnifica* show Giacomo and Marsilio actively involved in historic moments significant to the Carrara seigniory. Their portraits within these scenes, however, share the same elegant clothing and dignified poses as those contained in another of Francesco Novello's illustrated

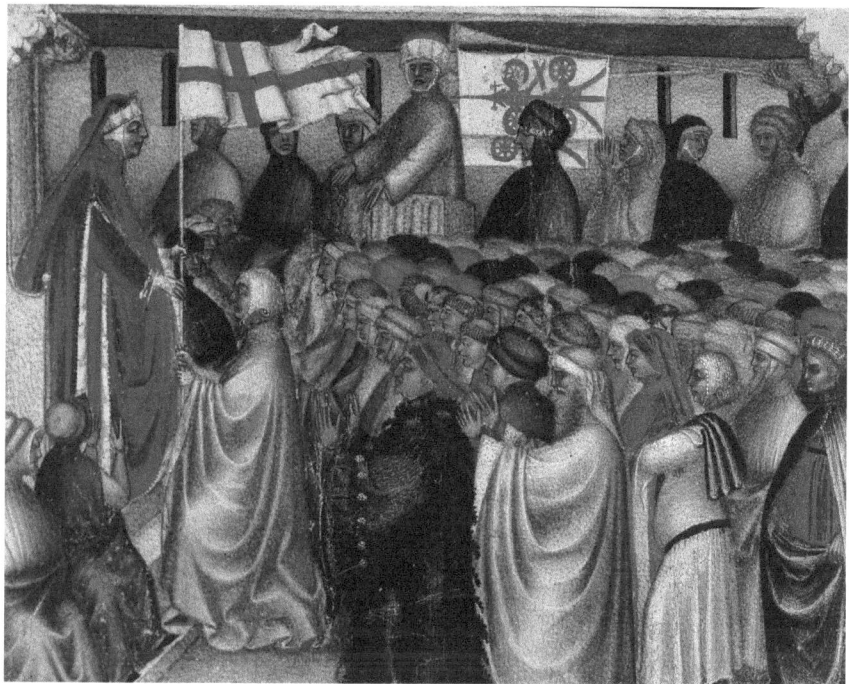

Figure 6.4 Scene of the election of Marsilio 'il Grande' da Carrara in 1337

Gesta magnifica domus Carrariensibus
Venice, Biblioteca Nazionale Marciana, lat. X, 381 (coll. 2802), f. 6r
Folio 58 × 43 cm, Padua, ca. 1390

Photo credit: Gianni Dagli Orti / The Art Archive at Art Resource, NY

books – the *Liber de principibus Carrariensibus et gestis eorum* (*The Book of the Carrara Princes and Their Deeds*) by Pier Paolo Vergerio.[29] The *Liber de principibus* is likely the book recorded on Zago's inventory as the *Libro de li nomi de li magnifici segnore da Carrara* (*Book of the Names of the Magnificent Lords of Carrara*).[30] Like the *Gesta magnifica*, this codex is large (34.2 × 24.8 cm), with 45 parchment folios. Completed around 1400, the manuscript contains full-length, *grisaille* (greyscale) profile portraits of the Carrara lords holding the flag of the commune and standing beneath representations of their shields of arms (*cimieri*). These non-narrative portraits, each isolated on its own page, introduce the celebratory biographies of the six Carrara lords that preceded Francesco il Vecchio (plus the biography of the elder Francesco's exiled grandfather, Niccolò [d. 1344]).[31]

Despite their differences in colouration and setting, the formal similarities between the portraits of the lords in these two manuscripts suggest a common model.[32] They likely imitate or directly copy the portraits of the lords found in a non-narrative fresco cycle commissioned by Francesco il Vecchio. Executed by

Altichiero in the *pozuolo*, or loggia, outside of the *Sala virorum illustrium*, the cycle portrayed the Carrara lords in the tradition of exemplary men.[33] Although the fresco cycle is now lost, Venetian nobleman Marcantonio Michiel (1484–1552), known as the 'Anonimo', described the portraits' location as well as their large size and colouration in his *Notizia d'opere del disegno* (*Notices on Works of Art [from Northern Italian Collections]*) (ca. 1530). Michiel wrote: 'The balcony at the back [of the *Sala virorum illustrium*] . . . [is] where the *Signori* of Padua are portrayed life-size in *verde* [*grisaille*]'.[34]

From the *Pozuolo* to Francesco's books

As life-sized figures 'standing' outside of the *Sala virorum illustrium*, the portraits of the *signori* guarded the entrance to Francesco il Vecchio's hall of state. They provided a contemporary lens through which the fourteenth-century viewer could interpret the fresco cycle inside. With the Carrara lords' portraits fresh in their minds, viewers mentally juxtaposed the iconography of the *viri illustres* on the interior with the bodies of the Carrara lords on the exterior. Thus, the heroes of the past were compared with the rulers (read: heroes) of the present.

The *Sala virorum illustrium*, as we have seen, contained two different types of representation of Petrarch's illustrious men.[35] The upper register showed the heroes in colourful, larger than life-sized portraits, which served as metaphorical portraits (or imagined likenesses) for Francesco il Vecchio's personal character. The *dado*, the lower register of the fresco cycle executed in *grisaille*, contained scenes of the heroes in action – that is, it showed the great deeds of the men identified in the full-length portraits above. This juxtaposition provides a template for reading not only the relationship between the ancient heroes in the *Sala virorum illustrium* and the Carrara lords portrayed in the *pozuolo* but also the narrative scenes and non-narrative portraits in the *Gesta magnifica* and the *Liber de principibus*.

The use of *grisaille* in the *dado* of the fresco cycle in the *Sala virorum illustrium* provided visual continuity that connected the interior fresco cycle to the corresponding exterior cycle. In addition, it tied the interpretation of the *grisaille* portraits of the Carrara lords to representations of exemplary deeds of illustrious men inside. As a visual prelude to the *Sala virorum illustrium*, the *grisaille* portraits in the *pozuolo* demonstrate the relationship between modern rulers and ancient heroes that Petrarch set out to cultivate in the readers of *De viris illustribus* (*On Famous Men*). The palace itself was the visible, architectural body associated with the Carrara dynasty and their rule. The exterior depicted the face of the dynasty in portrait images of Francesco il Vecchio's ancestors, while the interior portrayed the heroes whose inner qualities Petrarch longed to see epitomised in contemporary rulers.

Together, the fresco cycles formed a visible *Speculum principis*, a mirror of princes, activated by the viewer. Seen one after the other, the two cycles visually recreated the exemplary relationship between history's great men and the Carrara princes that Petrarch encouraged in his letter to Francesco il Vecchio[36] and in the prefaces to *De viris illustribus*.[37] In the heart of the city, the palace's fresco cycles related the internal, invisible qualities of the ancient heroes to the external, tangible bodies of the Carrara. Viewers orchestrated the connection between the illustrious men of the ancient world and those of Trecento Padua as they walked from the exterior to the interior of the palace.[38]

With their celebratory biographies, the portraits of the Carrara family members in both the *Gesta magnifica* and the *Liber de principibus* render the *Sala virorum illustrium*'s exemplary heroes into the context of the family's history in Padua. In both examples, the portraits in Francesco's books appropriate different elements of Petrarch's teachings as visualised in the *Sala virorum illustrium*, which focused on the emulation of characters from an imagined past and redirected them to the Paduan present and to the (imagined) role of the Carrara *signore* and his family in recent Paduan history.

The translation of the lords' portraits from fresco to book illustration in the *Gesta magnifica* points to a new negotiation of local narrative and non-narrative portrait traditions. Rather than connecting the *signori* to portraits of ancient heroes and scenes of their great deeds or to accounts of saints' lives, the appearance of their portraits in the *Gesta magnifica* activates the lord's 'hero' portraits with their own 'great deeds' recorded in Francesco Novello's book. By bringing together the non-narrative profile portraits of the lords from the loggia with visual and textual narratives that recount the lords' historic actions, the *Gesta magnifica* conflated a specifically Petrarchan ideal of exemplarity, focussed on the distant past, with a new ideal focussed on the recent history of the Carrara.

Likewise, the translation of the loggia portraits into Francesco Novello's copy of Vergerio's *Liber de principibus* demonstrates the association between 'heroic bodies' and 'great deeds' that the viewer was meant to infer from Francesco il Vecchio's juxtaposition of the *viri illustres* and the Carrara at the Reggia (Plate 10 and Figure 6.5). Vergerio wrote the *Liber de principibus* in the tradition of Petrarch's *De viris illustribus*, and, like Petrarch, he believed that history could teach the principles of moral philosophy. For his biography of the Carrara lords, however, Vergerio emphasised general moral principles from particular chapters in the family's history in order to promote good leadership and to shape the civic values of his ideal reader – the next generation of Carrara princes.[39] The *Liber de principibus* was a new type of *Speculum principis*, invoking its Petrarchan predecessor in form but using the historic 'heroic deeds' of the Carrara to ennoble the family and to guide its future leaders.

'Living statues'

In addition to their engagement with the Petrarchan rhetoric of exemplarity, the portraits of the Carrara in the *pozuolo* and in the *Liber de principibus* allude to the commemorative portrait tradition seen in tomb statuary and relief sculpture in Padua. Represented in *grisaille*, the lords appear as illusionary 'statues', and as such they commemorate the Carrara family and their rule in a manner similar to their sculptural effigies (see Figures 5.2 and 5.3).[40] However, unlike the memorialising function of portraiture in the tomb sculptures (portrait traditions that lauded *past* achievements), these portraits borrowed the association between body, heraldry and character to reveal a new ideal of living, present-day exemplars. In the

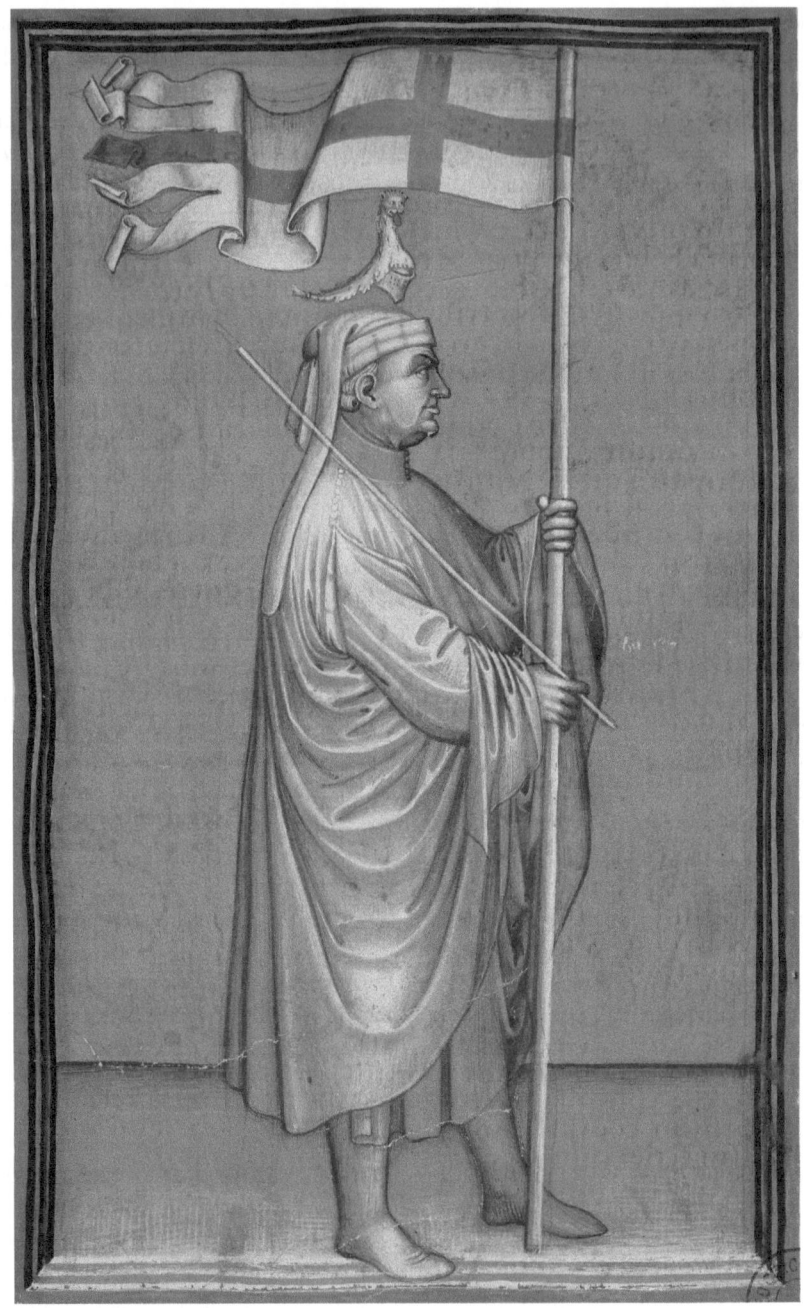

Figure 6.5 After Altichiero (?), portrait of Marsilio 'il Grande' da Carrara

Liber de principibus Carrariensibus
Padua, Biblioteca Civica, B.P. 158, f. 16v
Folio 34.2 × 24.8 cm, Padua, ca. 1402

Su gentile concessione del Comune di Padova – Assessorato Cultura e Turismo

Liber de principibus, both Vergerio and the anonymous artist portrayed the Carrara lords – in text and in image – as *living* members of a heroic community rather than as noble ancestors commemorated in death. Although rendered in *grisaille*, and thus suggestive of commemorative statuary, the portraits of the Carrara show the lords as *living* statues beneath the more colourful representations of their personal heraldic devices. The lords' eyes are open, brightly accented with white paint, and their upright stances suggest living strength rather than death's repose (see Plate 10 and Figure 6.5). One of the results of this combination of visual cues was that the lords' bodies assumed the connotations of family history and commemoration while they simultaneously provided living role models for their viewers – the current Carrara lord and his court. Vergerio wrote his biographies to effect a similar perception. They provide animated details of the lords' lives, persons and characters while also serving to memorialise them.

Vergerio's treatise on education, *De ingenuis moribus et liberalibus adulescentiae studiis* (*On the Character and Studies Befitting a Free-Born Youth*),[41] addressed to Francesco Novello's youngest son, Ubertino 'Fiorentino' da Carrara (1390–1407), provides a potential context within which to view the seemingly incongruent relationship between 'living' statues and the exemplary (historic) Carrara body. Written around 1402, *De ingenuis moribus* demonstrates how the moral advice of the *Speculum principis* tradition, as understood by Francesco il Vecchio, was brought together with the practice of physiognomy in medicine and the visual arts in Padua under Francesco Novello. The educational treatise, much like Vergerio's *Liber de principibus* and his orations,[42] combined historic Carrara patronage interests and channelled them into Francesco Novello's preferences. This treatise complements the didactic use of biography in the *Liber de principibus* and illuminates the compositional choice to imitate the *grisaille* fresco portraits of the lords in its illustration.

Like Petrarch and other humanists, Vergerio believed that education spurred virtue and was central to successful participation in the life of the city, a view of education seemingly upheld by the Carrara lords in their support of the university and the *studia humanitatis*.[43] However, Vergerio added a contemporary twist to Petrarch's view of ancient history as *magistra vitae* (as a guide to living life), one that revealed the younger humanist's educational theory as particularly Paduan. Alongside the honing of the mind through the study of history and rhetoric, moral and natural philosophy (and even medicine), and the honing of the body through the discipline of arms, Vergerio advocated that princes observe and emulate living role models. He wrote,[44]

> Socrates used to give good advice, that young men should often look at their own image in a mirror. His reasoning evidently was that those who had a fine appearance would not dishonour it with vices, while those whose appearance was more irregular would take care to make themselves attractive through their virtues.
>
> But perhaps they will have better success if they will contemplate, not [just] their own image, but the behaviour of someone else of high character, a *living mirror*. For if Publius Scipio and Quintus Fabius used to say that they were deeply inspired by gazing upon the images of famous men – an

experience common to nearly all noble minds – if Julius Caesar was spurred on to supreme power after seeing the image of Alexander the Great, what, in all reason, is bound to occur when someone can gaze on *a living effigy* and an example [of virtue] that is still breathing?

Vergerio's use of mirror imagery immediately locates this passage within the *Speculum principis* tradition and recalls Vergerio's debt to Petrarch in particular. Less obviously, however, this passage also recalls Vergerio's use of sculpture and architecture as metaphors for the development of a boy into a prince, metaphors he used frequently in his educational treatise. Vergerio claimed that humanists were 'educational artists', to borrow John McManamon's term, and that the study of the liberal arts would polish students' minds and bodies.[45] For Vergerio, the education of a prince was the conclusion of a process in which the promising 'raw material' of youth was roughly cut into a basic shape (by grammarians) and then refined and polished to brilliance (by humanists), making the man a great work of art.[46]

For Vergerio, reference to the importance of sculpture as a metaphor for learning and character development and as a visual cue to history's role as *magistra vitae* first appeared in a letter he wrote in response to the destruction of a statue of Virgil in the nearby town of Mantua. The letter was a declaration – a veritable 'manifesto'[47] – of Vergerio's beliefs about portraiture and education later recorded in his educational treatise and in his biographies of the Carrara lords. On 28 August 1397, the *signore* of Rimini, Carlos Malatesta (1368–1429), reclaimed Mantua from Giangaleazzo Visconti (1350–1402) for the anti-Visconti league, of which Francesco Novello was a member. This was a great victory for the league; however, it was marred by Malatesta's destruction of the statue of Mantua's most famous son, the poet Virgil.

On 18 September 1397, Vergerio wrote a letter to Ludovico degli Alidosi (d. 1430), papal vicar of Imola (a city in the Romagna), which conveyed his reproach for the Malatesta *signore* and defended the importance of poetry and oratory.[48] Paralleling his belief in the rhetorical power of vision, Vergerio's critique of Malatesta emphasised the importance of Virgil's statue as a visible memory.[49] Vergerio connected the representation of Virgil's body to the city of Mantua and added that the monument was appropriate for the city since it reminded the citizens of their ancestors' past greatness and so prompted them to strive for greatness in their present lives. In his letter, then, Vergerio connected commemorative, figural statuary with exemplarity, ancestry and inspiration to civic virtue. The *grisaille* portraits of the Carrara lords – in the palace loggia and in Vergerio's *Liber de principibus* – and their funerary *arche* address these same themes; however, the *grisaille* portraits, unlike the *arche*, emphasise the aliveness – the continued living presence – of the Carrara lords.

Returning to Francesco Novello's books, the portraits in Vergerio's *Liber de principibus* complemented the humanist's lessons in his education manual, *De ingenuis moribus*, while tapping into the Paduan use of physiognomy in medical, humanistic and artistic contexts. In its illustration and in its content, the *Liber de principibus* provided an avenue of expression for Vergerio's ideas about exemplarity and imitation, ideas closely related to his theory of vision's (and art's) role in education and to the practice of physiognomy and its attendant metaphors. Vergerio advocated that one should imitate both living and historic exemplars, and in the case of Ubertino, the principal reader of the *Liber de principibus*, the immediate living exemplar was his father, Francesco Novello. By upholding Francesco as a living exemplar, Vergerio's work furthered the lord's self-image as a new *vir illustris* in the tradition of his ancestors. Yet, for Vergerio, the portraits of Francesco's ancestors would also have served as 'living' statuary, not only recommending them to the reader as exemplars of past generations but connecting them to the current moral 'health' of the city as well. The *grisaille* portraits of the Carrara princes (much like the statue of Virgil) served as living memorials of Padua's illustrious past and as testaments to its present greatness that would spur the city's citizens on to future great deeds.

Physiognomy, portraiture and the *Carrara Herbal*

The connection between the Carrara lords' physical bodies, heraldry and personal characters visualised in the *Liber de principibus* and in Francesco Novello's other illustrated chronicles and biographies offers insight into the prince's collection of medical texts, in general, and into the *Carrara Herbal*, in particular. Together with Serapion's text, the plant imagery in the *Herbal* functions emblematically as a type of 'portrait', providing information about the plants' medical functions and their historical modes of representation. Like the relationship between lords' figural portraits and their heraldry described in Francesco's other books, the plant images are associated not just with the medicinal qualities of the plants represented but also with the physical body that they are capable of healing. Unlike the figural portraits and heraldry, however, the plants are not signs for the body or for personal characteristics; rather, their representations remind the viewer of the healthy body that their use – in the hands of a capable physician – can accomplish, uses Serapion's text amply explicates.

As principal reader of the *Herbal*, Francesco Novello became the possessor of this knowledge. In an environment in which the visible body was a sign of invisible character, and the healthy body of the lord a sign for a healthy body of state, Francesco's possession of knowledge associated with the advancement of physical health assumes a heightened significance. The knowledge contained in the *Carrara Herbal* taught Francesco how to heal the body; that is, the *Herbal* literalised a necessary (though insufficient) component of the metaphorical physiognomy visualised in the portraits and heraldry and discussed in chronicles and humanistic treatises. Moreover, owning the *Herbal* gave Francesco agency in establishing the metaphorical system. In many ways, the medical knowledge at Francesco's fingertips was the fulcrum on which the associations between the physical body, moral character and the healthy body of state rested: it facilitated the bodily health that underpinned the central metaphors in the Petrarchan rhetoric of exemplarity. The *Carrara Herbal* both alluded to the humanistic ideals in the patronage of Francesco Novello's ancestors and superseded them, relocating – quite literally – a key to their notions of exemplarity into Francesco Novello's hands. Francesco further stressed this connection through his collection of other medical texts, his support for the University of Padua and his patronage of physicians.

In Francesco's library, then, the *Carrara Herbal* consolidated the themes of exemplarity and commemoration addressed in the chronicles and biographies and in the family's fresco cycles and tomb sculptures with the themes of health and healing addressed in his medical texts. Commissioning an illustrated version of Serapion's pharmacopeia, Francesco Novello signalled his ability, as Padua's prince, to heal the physical bodies of his citizens. Because of his ancestors' application in their own patronage of humanistic metaphors premised on the idea of the healthy body, an application acknowledged in part by the presence of their heraldry on the frontispiece of the *Carrara Herbal*, the *Herbal* also signalled Francesco's ability to perceive the moral characteristics associated with the physical body. By presenting Francesco as both a physician with the ability to understand and heal the physical body and as a prince versed in the important metaphorical association between bodily health and morality and between a lord's healthy body and a healthy body of state, the *Carrara Herbal* marked Francesco as a defining member of the new *viri illustri* in Padua. Owning it emphasised Francesco's status not only as a positive exemplar for his people to follow but also as a new Carrara saviour and 'healer' of the body of state so recently infected by the bad government of Giangaleazzo Visconti.

In its form and content, the *Carrara Herbal* materialised Francesco's identity as the new 'health-giving' prince of Padua, the incarnation of the past, present and future of salvific Carrara leaders. While the illustrated chronicles locate Francesco as the product of the family's past triumphs, and his current book collection and patronage of the university show him as the present embodiment of the family's innovative and good leadership, the combination of these views in the *Carrara Herbal* reveal Francesco as the hope for the city's healthy future. The book actualised Francesco's ideal self. Like the prince, the medical uses of the plants illustrated and discussed in the *Herbal* result from past traditions, and, reenacted in innovative ways in a new context (orchestrated by Francesco himself), they secure the future health of Padua and its citizens.

Notes

1 On Zago's inventory (Venice, Biblioteca Nazionale Marciana, lat. XIV, 93 [coll. 4530], f. 147r), see Introduction, p. 13n3. Scholars have identified 24 illustrated or otherwise ornamented (with rubrication, gold-accented borders and decorative initials) manuscripts believed to have been produced during Francesco Novello's seigniory, including the six from Zago's list. See Mariani Canova et al. (1999: 149–206).
2 This manuscript is now Padua, Biblioteca Civica, B.P. 408/I. See Lazzarini (1901–1902: 30), and Calligari and Dal Santo (1999).
3 This manuscript is now Padua, Accademia Galileiana di Scienze, Lettere ed Arti, Archivio Papafava, Cod. 38. See Granata (1999). On Gatari and his sons, see Introduction, p. 19n45 and Chapter 3, p. 108n34.
4 On the fresco cycles, see Chapter 4.
5 This manuscript has been identified as the book bearing the same title now Padua, Biblioteca Civica, B.P. 124, XXII.
6 Cozzi (1999). On the decoration of these rooms, see Chapter 4, pp. 120–21.
7 See Chapter 5, pp. 157–8.
8 On relationship of the verses in the *Liber cimeriorum* to the *Cronaca Carrarese*, see Cozzi (1999).

9 'Ternus Vbertinus patanorum carriger heroc [herorum] / Cornigerum gessit maurum trudendo seueros. / Hic tenuit gestus aule tenuit quo[que] mores. / Carrigere simul auxit honores. / Hostibus infidias animo vigilante parauit. / Quos uidetesse truculente ubiq[ue] necauit' (*Liber cimeriorum*, Padua, Biblioteca Civica, B.P. 124, XXII, f. 16r; unpublished tr. Margaret Musgrove, personal correspondence).

10 This manuscript is now Paris, Bibliothèque nationale de France, lat. 6468. The treatise was among the manuscripts taken from Padua by Giangaleazzo Visconti in 1388 and is listed in the Visconti-Sforza library inventories of 1459, 1488 and 1490 (Gousset 1999: 136).

11 Richards (2007: 71–3) considers the diagram of the *carro* as a '*riposte* to the wheel of fortune', and, following Gousset (1999: 136), locates the diagram's iconography within the illustrative traditions of the *Psychomachia* (*Battle of the Spirits*), the Latin allegory of the epic battle between virtues and vices for the human soul, by Prudentius (ca. 348–405).

12 This manuscript is now Venice, Biblioteca Nazionale Marciana, lat. X, 381 (coll. 2802).

13 The *Gesta magnifica* is bound together with an unillustrated, vernacular account of the border war with Venice, *Storia della guerra dei confine*, written by the chancellor of the Paduan court, Nicholetto d'Alessio (ca. 1320–1393), and an unillustrated anonymous biography of Francesco Novello, the *Ystoria de mesier Francesco Zovene*, also written in the vernacular. For a complete codicological description of the codex, see Baggio (1999).

14 Mariani Canova (1994: 29–30); Baggio (1999: 192); and Richards (2007: 70).

15 For a summary of the debate on the portraits' identification, see Schmitt (1974). For individual positions, see Medin (1908); Rizzoli (1932); Gorini (1974); and Mardersteig (1974).

16 On the identifications of these portraits, see Plant (1981: 414). Francesco il Vecchio is portrayed similarly on commemorative medals, lending validity to this identification.

17 For an introduction to the artistic programme of the Lupi chapel in 'Il Santo', see Plant (1981); Richards (2000: 135–76); and Kohl (2002).

18 On the political allegory, see Plant (1981), and Norman (1995d). On the details of the Carrara alliance with Louis of Hungary, see Kohl (1998: 103–31).

19 On the iconography of this chapel and its particular significance to the Lupi family, see Plant (1981).

20 Plant (1981: 414n38). Francesco il Vecchio may appear in the *Adoration of the Magi* scene in San Giorgio, as well. On this identification, see Bobisut and Salomoni (2002: 67).

21 On Giusto de' Menabuoi's iconographical programme for the Baptistery, see, most recently, Derbes (2013).

22 Norman (1995b: 1.169); Warr (1996); and Kohl (2001). In addition, and with less certainty, scholars have identified portraits by Jacopo da Verona (1355–ca. 1443) of Francesco Novello, Francesco il Vecchio and six previous Carrara *signori*, as well as portraits of Petrarch and members of the Bovi family, in the family chapel of Pietro Bovi (fl. late fourteenth century) at the Church of San Michele (ca. 1397). The *signori*, poet, and Bovi family members witness scenes of the Magi adoring the Christ-child and the funeral of the Virgin. The Bovi were staunch Carrara supporters and worked at the mint under both the elder and younger Francesco, creating the currency that bore the visual signs (arms and devices) of the Carrara and the medals that bore their portraits. On the Bovi chapel and identification of portraits, see the classic study by Medin (1908: 100–4), and, much more recently, Saccocci (2014: 195–7). Saccocci identifies the Carrara lords by comparing their portraits in the San Michele frescoes with those in the *Liber de principibus Carrariensibus* (Padua, Biblioteca Civica, B.P. 158). For the identification of Francesco il Vecchio, in particular, Saccocci (2014: 197) analyses the representations of the lord's heraldic devices, which in the fresco adorn his vestments (and which were used by his son as well, prompting confusion in earlier identifications of the figure), and the devices represented on the medals and coins the elder Francesco

commissioned during his rule. Saccocci argues that the portrait of a 'young' Francesco il Vecchio, who holds the hand of one of the Magi and precedes the group of six Carrara lords in the scene of the Magi adoring the Christ-child, is a portrait of the lord's soul, which departed his body only four years before the fresco cycle's creation in 1397. On Jacopo da Verona, a student of Altichiero, see Pallucchini (1964: 150–2). On the production of the Carrara mint and the cast medals and currency, see Cessi (1974); Gorini (1974 and 2005); and Saccocci (2005).

23 Mariani Canova (1994: 29–30), and Baggio (1999: 191–2).

24 Baggio (1999: 191).

25 Mariani Canova (1994: 29–30), and Baggio (1999: 191).

26 For a brief discussion of Giacomo's rule of Padua and his abdication 18 months after his investiture, see Chapter 4, p. 118.

27 For a summary of the events in the intervening years between the elections, see Chapter 4, pp. 118–9. For a more detailed account of the transition of power to Marsilio, see Kohl (1998: 68–71).

28 Gatari, *Cronaca*, 2–3 agosto 1337 (eds Medin and Tolomei 1931: 22–3); my translation.

29 Baggio (1999: 191), and Richards (2000: 214–15).

30 This manuscript is now Padua, Biblioteca Civica, B.P. 158. See Lazzarini (1901–1902: 31).

31 The original late-Trecento portraits in the manuscript follow the chronology of the family and include Giacomo il Grande (r. 1318–1320), Marsilio il Grande (r. 1328–1338), Ubertino (r. 1338–1345), Niccolò, and Giacomo II (r. 1345–1350). Although he was not *signore* of Padua, the work includes the biography and portrait of Niccolò da Carrara, father of Giacomo II and Giacomino (d. 1373). Ubertino and Marsilio il Grande exiled Niccolò from Padua when he betrayed the family and joined forces with the della Scala in 1327 (see Chapter 4, p. 138n36). In the *Liber de principibus*, Niccolò is not represented as the lord of Padua but rather is shown with his hands bound, perhaps to suggest that he was prevented from taking his rightful place as *signore*. While he does not hold the banner of the commune, the white flag with a red cross, Niccolò carries the sceptre or rod, a marker of power carried by all the other lords, which further suggests the legitimacy of the leadership he was denied. Notably, the other portraits in the *Liber de principibus* – of Marsiglietto Papafava (r. 1345), Giacomino (Giacomo II's brother and co-ruler of Padua with Francesco il Vecchio from 1350–1355), and the elder and younger Francesco (without accompanying biographies) – are Quattrocento additions. Francesco il Vecchio and Francesco Novello are shown carrying flags that bear their personal mottos, rather than the banner of the commune.

32 Baggio (1999: 191).

33 Richards (2000: 214–15) attributes the original cycle to Altichiero on account of the techniques seen in the portrait copies found in Vergerio's *Liber de principibus*. Richards compares the portraits of Giacomo il Grande and Marsilio il Grande in the *Liber de principibus* with those in Altichiero's depiction of the funeral of Saint Lucy in the Oratory of San Giorgio. He argues that whether or not earlier scholars' attributions of the book's miniatures to Jacopo da Verona, Altichiero's pupil, are accepted, viewers can still understand the book's portraits as copies of another lost fresco cycle by Altichiero (Richards 2000: 215).

34 'Il pozuolo da driedo, ove sono li Signori de Padoa ritratti al naturale de verde' (Michiel, *Notizia*, I.20, 'Nel palazzo del capitanio' [ed. Frizzoni 1884: 79; tr. Mussi 1903: 38]). For further discussion of this passage, see Gasparotto (1966–1967: 107 and 107n124); Norman (1995b: 1.164n28); Baggio (1999: 191); and Richards (2007: 63). To my knowledge, all published editions and translations of Michiel's work derive from the autograph manuscript now Venice, Biblioteca Nazionale Marciana, ital. XI, 67 (coll. 7351), which dates from 1521 to 1543.

35 See Chapter 4, pp. 127–9.

36 *Rerum Senilium* XIV.1 (eds Nota and Dotti 2002–2013: 4.228–313; tr. Bernardo et al. 1992: 2.521–52). See Chapter 4, pp. 132–3 and 147n118.

37 Ed. Martellotti (1955: 218–27) ('long' preface, 1351–1353), and ed. Martellotti (1964: 3–5) ('short' preface, 1371–1374); tr. Kohl (1974: 138–42 and 142–4), respectively. See Chapter 4, p. 132.

38 My interpretation of viewer perception and the development of meaning through bodily experience is indebted to Johnson (1995), and Shusterman (1999 and 2008). More recently, Terry-Fritsch (2012), a historian of Renaissance art exploring Shusterman's theory of somaesthetics, charted what she calls an 'embodied activation' of architecture (270) in relation to secular spectators' experiences of the frescoes at the convent of San Marcos, Florence, created by Fra Angelico (1395–1455) between 1439 and 1444. Currently, she is completing a book project on the somaesthetic experience in Renaissance Florence.

39 McManamon (1996: 110–11).

40 On the tomb sculptures, see Chapter 5, pp. 158–61.

41 Ed. and tr. Kallendorf (2002: 2–91).

42 On Vergerio's orations and their synthesis of the patronage interests of the elder and younger Francescos, see Chapter 3, p. 103.

43 For example, early in his treatise, Vergerio wrote: 'For parents can provide their children with no more dependable protection in life than instruction in honorable arts and liberal disciplines. With such an endowment, children can usually overcome and bring distinction to [even] obscure family origins and humble homelands' ('Neque enim opes ullas firmiores aut certiora praesidia vitae parare filiis genitores possunt quam si eos exhibeant honestis artibus et liberalibus disciplinis instructos, quibus rebus praediti et obscura suae gentis nomina et humiles patrias attollere atque illustrare consueverunt') (Vergerio, *De ingenuis moribus*, 'Praefatio', §2 [ed. and tr. Kallendorf 2002: 4–5]).

44 'Hinc bene praecipiebatur a Socrate, ut adulescentes in speculo suam imaginem crebro contemplarentur, ea scilicet ratione, ut hi quibus inesset speciei dignitas, vitiis illam non dehonestarent; qui vero deformiori specie viderentur, formosos se ex virtutibus reddere curarent. [10] Magis autem id ipsum consequi fortasse poterunt, si non tam suam speciem quam alienos probati hominis mores et *vivum speculum* intuebuntur. Nam si P. Scipio et Q. Fabius (quod omnibus fere generosis mentibus usu evenit) illustrium virorum contemplandis imaginibus excitari se magnopere dicebant – quae res Iulium quoque Caesarem visa magni Alexandri imagine ad summam rerum accendit – quid consentaneum est evenire, cum ipsam *vivam effigiem* et adhuc spirans exemplum intueri licet?' (Vergerio, *De ingenuis moribus*, 'Signa liberalis ingenii', §9–10 [ed. and tr. Kallendorf 2002: 12–13; my emphasis]).

45 McManamon (1996: 101).

46 McManamon (1996: 101). Vergerio suggested this ideal in many areas of his treatise. For instance, he wrote, 'In youth, therefore, the *foundations* for living well are to be laid, and the mind must be trained to virtue while it is young and *impressionable*, for the mind will preserve throughout life the impressions it takes on now' ('Iacienda sunt igitur in hac aetate *fundamenta* bene vivendi et conformandus ad virtutem animus, dum tener est et facilis quamlibet *impressionem* admittere: quae ut nunc erit, ita et in reliqua vita servabitur') (Vergerio, *De ingenuis moribus*, 'Praefatio', §2 [ed. and tr. Kallendorf 2002: 4–5; my emphasis]).

47 McManamon (1996: 73).

48 Vergerio, *Epistolario* 81 (ed. Smith 1934: 189–202). For further analysis of Vergerio's response to the destruction of the Virgil statue, and the responses of other contemporary humanists, see McManamon (1996: 72–80).

49 Vergerio, *Epistolario* 81 (ed. Smith 1934: 195–6). McManamon (1996: 75) examines the significance of what he terms the 'visible memorial' to Vergerio's conception of humanism and the role of humanists. For a detailed study of vision's centrality to Vergerio's theory of education and rhetorical practice, see McManamon (1996: especially Chapters 3, 5 and 6).

Conclusion

> The world that revealed itself in the book and the book itself were never, at any price, to be divided. So with each book its content, too, its world, was palpably there, at hand. But equally, this content and the world transfigured every part of the book. They burned within it, blazed from it.[1]
>
> ~ Walter Benjamin, 'A Berlin Chronicle'

Let us return briefly to Pier Paolo Vergerio, Francesco Novello's court humanist and teacher of his children, who described the important role of books in a way that illuminates Francesco's commission of the *Carrara Herbal*. In *De ingenuis moribus et liberalibus adulescentiae studiis* (*On the Character and Studies Befitting a Free-Born Youth*, ca. 1402),[2] written for Francesco's youngest son, Vergerio called books an ideal 'second memory' ('secundae memoriae').[3] This description is a fitting one for Francesco's illustrated chronicles and biographies, which, in both their textual and visual contents, combined and refined ancestral memories and histories. But it is also a fitting description for the *Carrara Herbal*, which, in its textual and visual contents, re-enacted medical traditions and transformed humanistic ones in a contemporary Paduan context. In *De ingenuis moribus*, Vergerio writes:[4]

> Cicero says, What a happy family books make! Absolutely honest and well-behaved! A family that does not fuss or shout, that is neither rapacious, voracious or contumacious, that speaks or remains silent as it is bidden, that always stands ready to execute your every command, and that you never hear saying anything you don't want to hear, and that only says as much as you want to hear. So, since our memory cannot hold everything and indeed retains very little, scarcely enough for particular purposes, books, in my view, should be acquired and preserved as a kind of second memory.

Of course, Vergerio's comment speaks as much to the selective reading practiced by readers and the selective writing practiced by writers as to books' roles as repositories for knowledge. To be an ideal 'happy family' (perhaps especially for princes), books tell readers what they want to hear: they 'execute your every command'. A book helps its readers to remember or forget as they shape an understanding of the knowledge conveyed by the book and map it onto their wider perception of the world. This kind of persuasive power is part of what made books so alluring to the *signori* of Padua.

Despite any potential criticism of books' powers of persuasion and readers' sometimes wilful lack of objectivity, Vergerio pointed to the physical and mental engagement with books in the building of knowledge and, more importantly, in the distillation of meaning from that knowledge. It is this idea of books' agency that most resonates with Francesco Novello's book-collecting practices. Like other illustrated books, the *Carrara Herbal* is a repository of visual and textual information. It keeps this information at hand and serves as a potential site for structuring knowledge and consolidating memory. Yet the book's content, the way its content is presented and the book object itself also have histories and participate in other histories – histories of translation and transmission and of ownership and collection, for instance – which inform their meaning.

Commissioning and owning the *Carrara Herbal* was part of Francesco Novello's history, part of his chronicle as prince of Padua. Certainly, as one his books, the *Herbal* served as an attribute for the prince. Its presence in Francesco's library recorded for posterity an idealised aspect of his knowledge, taste and sense of familial identity. In this way, the *Carrara Herbal* was a 'second memory' not just for Francesco Novello: it was a link for future generations to the family's past as well. Through its complementarity with family patronage interests, the *Herbal* pointed to the cultivated identities of Francesco's father and his father's father. It entered Francesco's patronage into conversation with a history of collecting illustrated books, with Carrara support of the University of Padua, and with a vision of self and family inaugurated by his ancestors. The *Herbal* provided a point of continuity within the family's history – through these connections to traditional patterns of patronage – and a point of discontinuity or rupture that stressed Francesco's individual identity as *signore*. The point of discontinuity – chiefly, the differences in subject matter and format between the *Herbal* and the books traditionally collected by earlier Carrara lords – demonstrated Francesco Novello's awareness of the changes to the studies and practices of medicine and humanism in Padua and his ability to structure his self-representation in response both to those changes and to his family's history.

This mutability, what art historians Alexander Nagel and Christopher Wood might call the book's 'temporal flexibility',[5] is evident not just in the *Herbal*'s role in Francesco's library or its place in the family's history of patronage. It is wrought into the fabric of the book itself, in both its text and imagery. When Jacobus Philippus translated Serapion's treatise from Latin into Paduan dialect, he added to the history of Serapion's work and activated it in an entirely new time and context, just as Simon of Genoa had done when he translated the treatise from Arabic into Latin in the late thirteenth century. Both translators enabled Serapion's work to grow in influence, to become a site of knowledge and history accessed by a wider readership, which, in turn, opened new avenues for future interpretations. Likewise, for the anonymous artist. In his plant imagery, he reflected on past models and innovated new ones, and doing so, he nested another site for the construction of knowledge, memory and history within the book object. By crafting the past, the artist imagined – opened up – a future for his illustrations.[6]

For the *Carrara Herbal*, its connection to past authorities (textual, visual and familial) legitimised the book's presence in Francesco's library. Its newness, however, made it novel and distinctive and so imagined its place in the future of illustrated books of *materia medica* and in princes' – or others' – book collections (a future quickly realised by the translation, virtually wholesale, of the artist's illustrations into the so-called *Roccabonella Herbal* in the middle of the fifteenth century).[7] Considered in this way, the *Carrara Herbal* becomes not simply a site of medical and botanical knowledge or of aesthetic pleasure, not simply part of a genealogy of illustrated books of *materia medica* or of a prince's library. Rather, as this study has sought to show, the *Herbal* becomes a site where identities and knowledge are negotiated, consolidated and exchanged – the identities of plants and knowledge of their medicinal values, certainly, but also those of the prince, his family and of an ideal future reader. By looking to the *Carrara Herbal*'s engagement with medicine and humanism, I have sought to track the *Herbal*'s ability to enable such exchange. Through its very nature as an illustrated book about medicine central to bodily health and its place as a book in the prince's library, the *Herbal* engaged commonplaces about health and reading in circulation at court and at the University of Padua. These commonplaces – such as the advice to seek out useful and pleasant knowledge to cultivate health or to look to the physical body for clues to a person's character – are points of continuity between the discourses of medicine and humanism and their more popular understanding at the close of the fourteenth century.

The *Herbal* evidences this continuity through its dual nature. It contains prescriptions for healing vetted by ancient medical authorities and their more recent Arabic counterparts, prescriptions that associate the book with curricula at the medical schools of Padua. Yet the *Herbal* presents this information in a way that simultaneously connects it to traditions of active reading associated with preserving the health of the body and soul (of elite readers), traditions vetted by humanist authorities, like Petrarch, with ties to the history of Padua and the Carrara dynasty. Thus, through its subject matter and its very identity as an illustrated book, the *Herbal* responds both to the popularity of Arabic medicine at the university and to humanists' metaphorical use of medicine in their glosses of civil history and in their 'prescriptions' for meditative reading and the care of the soul (*anima cura*). This particular affinity to humanistic discourses on health and education aligned the *Herbal* with the celebration of Petrarch and the use of the poet's rhetoric of exemplarity in the patterns of self-making practiced by Francesco Novello's ancestors and assumed into Francesco's other illustrated books.

Humanists provided the metaphorical medicine to ensure the healthy moral body (the soul), while physicians provided the literal medicine to ensure the healthy physical one, the necessary seat of its moral counterpart. Artists and humanists in Padua visualised and described the healthy moral body by analogy to an idealised healthy, physical body. Portraits of the Carrara lords commissioned for the family palace and translated into Francesco Novello's illustrated chronicles and biographies (in text and image) reflect this understanding of the body. Considered in light of the complementary (and interdisciplinary) relationship between literal and metaphorical health, the tools contained in the *Carrara Herbal* for ensuring the physical health of the body take on a heightened significance.

The medical knowledge in the *Carrara Herbal* facilitates an alternative perception of the 'healthy' bodies presented in the lords' portraits. The medicines and their judicious application, as described in the *Herbal*, have the power to nurture a literal healthy body, without which the humanists' metaphorical healthy body would have no place to manifest. In other words, the health-giving and health-promoting knowledge in the *Herbal* made its reader – Francesco Novello – the architect of the literal foundation upon which humanists and artists built their use of a healthy body as a metaphor for a healthy moral character and – in a ruler – for a healthy state.

Within this system, the relationship between the identities of the plants in the *Herbal* and the accompanying information about their medicinal values parallels that between the portraits of the Carrara lords and the accounts of their histories preserved in Francesco Novello's other illustrated books. Like the Carrara portraits that accompany and embody accounts of the lords' 'great deeds', the plants' 'portraits' in the *Herbal* accompany and embody Serapion's account of their 'great deeds' – their ability to heal and to cure the physical body of disease. Through his book collection, Francesco Novello came to possess both the medical knowledge to heal the physical body and the humanistic knowledge to cultivate the healthy moral body. As the reader and owner of these books and the knowledge therein, Francesco united past traditions and present innovations in medicine and humanism under the aegis of his own ideal leadership. He became the 'healthy' head of Padua's civic body and the 'prince physician' of the *res publica*.

Accordingly, the power of the *Carrara Herbal* – what Vergerio would call its role as a 'second memory' – speaks in relative terms to what Nagel and Wood recognise as the power of a historical object, especially an art object, to 'fold time'.[8] As they describe it, the historical object exists in its moment of creation and in a flexible sense of past and future. As a creation, the object necessarily responds to what came before it – it did not appear *ex nihilo*. By alluding to past influences or by eschewing them, the object charges the viewers' present experience, directing their attention both backward in time (to an older model or artefact as site of imitation or rupture) and forward to new beholders who, as Nagel and Wood argue, 'will activate and reactivate' its meaning in other historical moments.[9] Considered in this way, the *Carrara Herbal* is at once old and new. By pointing its viewers and readers simultaneously backward and forward in time, the *Herbal* facilitated distinct impressions both of its form and content and of its owner. It honoured past knowledge traditions, artistic practices and princely identities while generating innovative new ones that complemented Francesco Novello's vision of self as the harbinger of 'health' to Padua and its citizens – present and future.

Notes

1   Benjamin, 'A Berlin Chronicle' (tr. Jephcott and Shorter 1979: 341).
2   Ed. and tr. Kallendorf (2002: 2–91).

3 Vergerio, *De ingenuis moribus*, 'Excellens studium tractat, armorum scilicet et litterarum', §38 (ed. and tr. Kallendorf 2002: 44, 46–7).
4 'O iucundam familiam [librorum]! ut recte Cicero appellat, utique et frugi et bene morigeram! Non enim obstrepit, non inclamat; non est rapax, non vorax, non contumax; iussi loquuntur et item iussi tacent; semperque ad omne imperium praesto sunt; a quibus nihil umquam, nisi quod velis et quantum velis, audias. [38] Eos igitur (quoniam nostra memoria non est omnium capax ac paucorum quidem tenax et vix ad singula sufficit) secundae memoriae loco habendos asservandosque censeo' (Vergerio, *De ingenuis moribus*, 'Excellens studium tractat, armorum scilicet et litterarum', §37–8 [ed. and tr. Kallendorf 2002: 44–7]).
5 Nagel and Wood (2010: 9).
6 On the relationship between artistic novelty and authority as ties to past and future, see Nagel and Wood (2010: 11–12).
7 This manuscript is now Venice, Biblioteca Nazionale Marciana, lat. VI, 59 (coll. 2548). On the *Roccabonella Herbal* and the artist's, Andrea Amadio, copying of the *Carrara Herbal*'s imagery, see Baumann (1974: 126–8); Mariani Canova (1988: 25–6); Paganelli and Cappelletti (1996: 111–16); Collins (2000: 281), and their relevant bibliographies.
8 Nagel and Wood (2010: 13).
9 Nagel and Wood (2010: 9–11).

Appendix

List of the 61 manuscripts from Francesco Zago's inventory, 1404 (Venice, Biblioteca Nazionale Marciana, lat. XIV, 93 [coll. 4530], fol. 147r).[1]

List of 57 manuscripts given to Francesco Zago, the gastaldo camerlengo, *on 9 May 1404*

1. Primus liber Rasis (Rhazes, ca. 854–925 or 935), de capite
2. Secundus liber Rasis, de occulis
3. Tertuys liber Rasis
4. Quartus liber Rasis
5. Quintus liber Rasis, de stomacho
6. Sextus liber Rasis, de euacuationibus
7. Septimus liber Rasis
8. Octauus liber Rasis
9. Nonus liber Rasis
10. Decimus liber Rasis
11. Undecimus liber Rasis
12. Duodecimus liber Rasis, de podagra (gout)
13. Teritus decimus liber Rasis
14. Quartus decimus liber Rasis
15. Decimus sextus liber Rasis
16. Decimus septimus liber Rasis
17. Decimus octauus liber Rasis
18. Decimus nonus liber Rasis
19. Vigessimus liber Rasis
20. Vigessimus liber primus Rasis
21. Vigessimus secundus liber Rasis
22. Vigessimus tertius liber Rasis
23. Vigessimus quartus liber Rasis
24. Vigessimus quintus liber Rasis
25. Tertia pars Auicene (Avicenna, 980–1037)
26. Prima pars Nicolai
27. Secunda pars Nicolai[2]

28 Liber de remedijs utriusque fortune[3]
29 Libro de multi remedij per le gotte, cum .ij. croxe negre su[4]
30 Libro de le passione de zonture, cum una stella rossa[5]
31 Cronica del Mussato per letra[6]
32 Primus liber Auicene, copertus curamine albo
33 Libro del chataro[7]
34 Libro del le consolatione de le medixine, in carta de banbaxina[8]
35 Libro de diuersi vini medicinale
36 Libro del coneyo de maist. Marsilio de Sancta Sofia[9]
37 Libro de Constantino[10]
38 Libro de li dicti de maist. Piero da Pernumia[11]
39 Libro de menerijs
40 Libro grande de le ribaldarie
41 Libro pecenin de le ribaldarie
42 Methaura de Aristotile[12]
43 Libro de la raxon de la luna[13]
44 Libro de li nomi de li Magni. Segnore da Carrara[14]
45 Liber Jntroitus Magni. Dominj[15]
46 Liber Cimeriorum dominorum de Carraria[16]
47 Libro de Mauricio in franzoxe[17]
48 Serapiom in volgare[18]
49 El segondo de Auicena in volgare
50 Libro grande da la croxe[19]
51 Libro da li inçegni
52 Libro di morti
53 Tesaurus pauperum in volgare[20]
54 Extrato de Auicena, pecenin, couerto de rosso
55 Libro de la generale cura del stomago, couerto de carta de caureo
56 Cura cólere frigide, copertus de carta capreti
57 Quaderno uno de cançon destexe, couerto de carta de caureo

Books added to inventory by the priests Cristoforo and Brussano

58 Quinterni .vj. de Auicena nuouo
59 Libro quinto de Auicena nuouo – R[ecepi] die xij Jullij
60 Libro che se chiama psalmista – R. die xvj augusti
61 a Bresano R. Quinterni .v. del libro de infantia Saluatoris – R. die ultimo augusti

Notes

1 Pélissier (1899: 6.177–80) published a transcription of the *consegna*, the list of consignment, which includes the inventory of Francesco Novello's library. Lazzarini (1901)
   published the inventory separately, identified several of the works, their authors and/or
   potential subject matter, and connected six of Zago's entries to actual manuscripts from
   the Carrara library. See Introduction, p. 13n3. My identifications of the manuscripts
   follow Lazzarini's.

2 Both works by Nicolai likely derive from the *Antidotarium Nicolai* (*Nicholas's Anti-dotes*), by Nicholas of Salerno (fl. ca. 1150). This compilation became compulsory reading at the University of Paris during the thirteenth century.

3 This manuscript, *De remediis utriusque fortunae* (*On the Remedies for Different For-tunes*), is the sole Petrarchan work inventoried by Zago.

4 An insignia of a black cross adorns this manuscript, which contains a treatise on rem-edies for gout.

5 An insignia of a red star adorns this manuscript, which contains a treatise on arthritis (*dolore di zonture*; for identification of the condition, see Roscoe 1799: 2.168, note 'b').

6 This manuscript is likely the account of communal Padua and its citizens, *De traditione Padue ad Canem Grandem anno 1328 mense septembri et causis precedentibus* (*On Paduan Tradition until Cangrande [della Scala's Usurpation] in September 1328 and its Preceding Causes*), by Albertino Mussato (1261–1329). It is now Padua, Biblioteca Civica, B.P. 408/I.

7 This manuscript is likely the chronicle of seigniorial Padua by Galeazzo Gatari (1344–1405) and his sons Andrea (ca. 1370–d. after 1454) and Bartolomeo (1380–1439). It is now Padua, Accademia Galileiana di Scienze, Lettere ed Arti, Archivio Papafava, Cod. 38.

8 This manuscript may be the treatise by Mesue (ca. 777–857), *De consolatione medici-narum simplicium.*

9 Marsilio da Santa Sofia (d. 1405) was a local Paduan physician.

10 This manuscript likely contains a work by the influential Salernitan doctor and transla-tor, Constantine 'the African' (d. ca. 1078).

11 Piero da Pernumia (d. after 1393) was Francesco il Vecchio's personal physician.

12 *Methaura* is a fourteenth-century vernacular redaction of parts of Aristotle's *Meteo-rologica* (*Meteorology*). Its contents mostly derive from commentaries on the original Aristotelian text by Thomas Aquinas (ca. 1225–1274) and Albertus Magnus (ca. 1200–1280).

13 This manuscript may be an alchemical treatise.

14 This manuscript is the *Liber de principibus Carrariensibus et gestis eorum* (*The Book of the Carrara Princes and Their Deeds*), an illustrated book of the Carrara genealogy by Pier Paolo Vergerio (ca. 1369–1444). It is now Padua, Biblioteca Civica, B.P. 158.

15 This manuscript is the anonymous *Gesta magnifica domus Carrariensis* (*The Magnifi-cent Deeds of the Carrara House*), now Venice, Biblioteca Nazionale Marciana, lat. X, 381 (coll. 2802).

16 *Liber cimeriorum dominorum de Carraria* (*The Book of the Carrara Lords' Cimieri*) is the work of Lazzaro de' Malrotondi (fl. 1376–1405). It is now Padua, Biblioteca Civica, B.P. 124, XXII.

17 This manuscript contains the sole French treatise in the collection.

18 This manuscript is the translation into Paduan dialect of Serapion the Younger's (fl. mid-thirteenth century) *Liber Serapionis aggregatus in medicinis simplicibus* (*Serapion's Book of Aggregated Simple Medicines*), the *Libro agregà de Serapiom*, now the *Carrara Herbal*, London, British Library, Egerton 2020.

19 This manuscript may contain a devotional text or meditation on the cross.

20 This manuscript is likely a translation into Paduan dialect of the *Thesaurus pauperum*, by Peter of Spain (fl. thirteenth century).

Bibliography

Illustrative sources

Codex Vindobonensis (also known as *Vienna Dioscorides*): Vienna, Österreichische Nationalbibliothek, *medicus graecus* 1.

Gesta magnifica domus Carrariensis: Venice, Biblioteca Nazionale Marciana, lat. X, 381 (coll. 2803).

Herbarium Apuleii Platonici:
- Florence, Biblioteca Medicea Laurenziana, plut. 73.16.
- Vienna, Österreichische Nationalbibliothek, lat. 93.

Liber cimeriorum dominorum de Carraria: Padua, Biblioteca Civica, B.P. 124, XXII.

Tacuinum Sanitatis:
- Rome, Biblioteca Casanatense, 459 (also known as *Historia Plantarum*).
- Vienna, Österreichische Nationalbibliothek, series nova 2644.

Tractatus de herbis:
- London, British Library, Egerton 747.
- London, British Library, Sloane 4016.
- Paris, Bibliothèque de l'Ecole des Beaux-Arts, Masson 116.

Tractatus liber de herbis et plantis (also known as *Herbal of Manfred de Monte Imperiale*): Paris, Bibliothèque nationale de France, lat. 6823.

Caronelli, Francesco. *De Currus Carrariensis moraliter descriptus*: Paris, Bibliothèque nationale de France, lat. 6468.

de' Grassi, Giovannino. *Taccuino di disegni*: Bergamo, Biblioteca Civica, 'A. Mai', Cassaforte 1.21 (facsimile edition: *Giovannino de' Grassi, Taccuino di disegni: Codice della Biblioteca Civica di Bergamo* [Monumenta Bergomensia 5]. Bergamo: Edizioni Monumenta Bergomensia, 1961).

Roccabonella, Niccolò. *Liber de simplicibus* (also known as *Roccabonella Herbal*): Venice, Biblioteca Nazionale Marciana, lat. VI, 59 (coll. 2548).

Serapion. *Libro agregà de Serapiom* (also known as *Carrara Herbal*): London, British Library, Egerton 2020.

Vergerio, Pier Paolo. *De principibus Carrariensibus et gestis eorum*: Padua, Biblioteca Civica, B.P. 158.

Archival sources

Atti notarili, Codice 35: Padua, Accademia Patavina, Archivio Papafava dei Carraresi.

Manuscript sources

da Nono, Giovanni. *De generatione aliquorum civium urbis Padue*: Padua, Biblioteca del Seminario vescovile, 11.

Primary sources

1. Anonymous works

Gesta magnifica. R. Cessi (ed.), *Gesta magnifica domus Carrariensis*, in *Rerum Italicarum Scriptores*, new ed., vol. 17, pt. 1, tome 2. Bologna: Zanichelli, 1942–1948.
La guerra da Trivixo. R. Cessi (ed.), *La guerra da Trivixo (1383)*, in *Rerum Italicarum Scriptores*, new ed., vol. 17, pt. 1, tome 3. Bologna: Zanichelli, 1964, pp. 227–66.
Thebaid. M. West (ed. and tr.), *Thebaid*, in *The Greek Epic Fragments from the Seventh to the Fifth Centuries BC* (Loeb Classical Library 497). Cambridge, MA, and London: Harvard University Press, 2003, pp. 42–57.
Ystoria de mesier Francesco Zovene. R. Cessi (ed.), *Ystoria de mesier Francesco Zovene*, in *Rerum Italicarum Scriptores*, new ed., vol. 17, pt. 1, tome 3. Bologna: Zanichelli, 1964, pp. 173–226.

2. Authored works

Aeschylus, *Seven Against Thebes*. A.H. Sommerstein (ed. and tr.), *Aeschylus*, 'Seven Against Thebes', in A.H. Sommerstein (ed. and tr.), *Aeschylus, Persians. Seven Against Thebes. Suppliants. Prometheus Bound* (Loeb Classical Library 145). Cambridge, MA, and London: Harvard University Press, 2009, pp. 152–275.
Alberti, *Della pittura*. J. Spencer (ed. and tr.), *Leon Battista Alberti, On Painting*. New Haven and London: Yale University Press, 1956.
Albertus Magnus, *De animalibus libri XXVI*. H. Stadler (ed.), *Albertus Magnus, De animalibus libri XXVI. Nach der Cölner Urschrift*, 2 vols (Beiträge zur Geschichte der Philosophie des Mittelalters 15–16). Münster: Aschendorffsche, 1916–1920.
Alderotti, *Consilia*. P.P. Giorgi and G.F. Pasini (eds), *Consilia di Taddeo Alderotti*. Bologna: Istituto per la storia dell'Università di Bologna, 1997.
Al-Ḥarīrī, *Maqamat*. O. Grabar (ed. and tr.), *Maqamat Al-Hariri*, 2 vols. London: Touch@ rt, 2003.
Anselm of Laon, *I Thessalonians 5.19–21*. J.P. Migne and A.G. Hamman (eds), *Anselm of Laon* (attrib.), 'I Thessalonians 5: 19–21', in *Biblia Latina cum glossa ordinaria* (Patrologiae cursus completus, Series Latina 114). Paris: Migne, 1852, col. 620.
Aquinas, *Ethicorum Aristotelis ad Nichomachum expositio*. R.M. Spiazzi (ed.), *S. Thomae Aquinatis in Decem Libros Ethicorum Aristotelis ad Nichomachum expositio*. Turin: Marietti, 1949 (English translation: C.I. Litzinger, *Commentary on the Nicomachean Ethics*, 2 vols. Chicago: Henry Regnery, 1964).
Aristotle, *Analytica priora*. H. Tredennick (ed. and tr.), *Aristotle*, 'Prior Analytics', in H.P. Cooke and H. Tredennick (eds and tr.), *Aristotle, The Categories. On Interpretation. Prior Analytics* (Loeb Classical Library 325). Cambridge, MA: Harvard University Press, and London: W. Heinemann, 1938, pp. 198–532.
Aristotle, *Ethica ad Nicomachum*. J. Henderson (ed.) and H. Rackham (tr.), *Aristotle, Nicomachean Ethics* (Loeb Classical Library 73). Cambridge, MA: Harvard University Press, and London: W. Heinemann, 1926.

Aristotle, ***Physiognomica***. T.E. Page, E. Capps, W.H.D. Rouse, L.A. Post and E.H. Warmington (eds) and W.S. Hett (tr.), *Aristotle*, 'Physiognomics', in T.E. Page, E. Capps, W.H.D. Rouse, L.A. Post and E.H. Warmington (eds) and W.S. Hett (tr.), *Aristotle, Minor Works* (Loeb Classical Library 307). Cambridge, MA: Harvard University Press, and London: W. Heinemann, 1936, pp. 84–140.

Aristotle, ***Problemata***. J. Henderson (ed.) and W.S. Hett (tr.), *Aristotle*, 'Problems: Books 32–38', in J. Henderson (ed.), W.S. Hett (tr.) and H. Rackham (tr.), *Aristotle, Problems: Books 32–38. Rhetorica ad Alexandrum* (Loeb Classical Library 317). Cambridge, MA: Harvard University Press, and London: W. Heinemann, 1937, pp. 2–255.

Augustine, ***Confessiones***. J.J. O'Donnell (ed. and tr.), *Augustine, Confessions*, 3 vols. Oxford: Oxford University Press, 1992.

Avicenna, ***Liber canonis. De medicinis cordialibus. Cantica***. A. Alpago, N. Massa and B. Rinio (eds), and G. Cremonensis, A. Villanovanus and A. Blasius (tr.), *Auicennae medicorum Arabum principis, Liber Canonis, De medicinis cordialibus, et Cantica*. Basileae: Per Joannes Hervagios, 1556.

Avicenna, ***Liber canonis. De medicinis cordialibus. Cantica***. A. Alpago, N. Massa and B. Rinio (eds), and G. Cremonensis, A. Villanovanus and A. Blasius (tr.), *Avicennae Liber canonis. De medicinis cordialibus. Cantica. De removendis nocumentis in regimine sanitatis. De syrupo acetoso*. Venetiis: apud Iuntas, 1582.

Avicenna, ***Liber canonis***. G. Cremonensis (tr.), *Avicennae Liber canonis*. Venetiis: per Paganinum de Paganinis, 1507 (facsimile edition Hildesheim: G. Olms, 1964; partial English translation [book 1 only]: O.C. Gruner, *A Treatise on the Canon of Medicine of Avicenna, Incorporating a Translation of the First Book*. London: Luzac, 1930; M. Abu-Asab, H. Amri and M.S. Micozzi, *Avicenna's Medicine: A New Translation of the 11th-Century Canon with Practical Applications for Integrative Health Care*. Rochester, VT: Healing Arts Press, 2013).

Bacon, ***Secretum secretorum***. R. Steele (ed.), *Secretum secretorum cum glossis et notulis tractatus brevis et utilis ad declarandum quedam obscure dicta Fratris Rogeri* (Opera hactenus inedita Rogeri Baconi 5). Oxford: Oxford University Press, 1920.

Barberino, ***I Documenti d'Amore***. F. Egidi (ed.), *I Documenti d'Amore di Francesco da Barberino*, 4 vols in 3. Rome: la Società Filologica Romana, 1905–1927.

Bartholomaeus Mini (attrib.), ***Tractatus de herbis***. I. Ventura (ed.), *Bartholomaeus Mini de Sensis, Tractatus de herbis: MS London, British Library, Egerton 747* (Edizione nazionale: La Scuola Medica Salernitana 5). Florence: SISMEL Edizioni del Galluzzo, 2009.

Blasius, ***Cantica Avicennae***. H. Jahier and A. Noureddine (eds and tr. French), *Poème de la médecine. Urğūza fī 't-tibb. Cantica Avicennae. Texte arabe, traduction francaise, traduction latine du XIIIe siècle avec introductions, notes et index*. Paris: Belles Lettres, 1956.

Bruni, ***De studiis et litteris liber***. C. Kallendorf (ed. and tr.), 'Leonardo Bruni, *De studiis et litteris liber (The Study of Literature)*', in C. Kallendorf (ed.), *Humanist Educational Treatises* (The I Tatti Renaissance Library 5). Cambridge, MA, and London: Harvard University Press, 2002, pp. 92–125.

Cennini, ***Il libro dell'arte***. D. Thompson (tr.), *Cennino Cennini, The Craftsman's Handbook 'Il Libro dell'Arte'*. New Haven: Yale University Press, 1969.

Cicero, ***De officiis***. W. Miller (ed. and tr.), *Cicero, De officiis (On Duties)* (Loeb Classical Library 30). Cambridge, MA: Harvard University Press, and London: W. Heinemann, 1913.

Cicero, *De oratore*. E. Sutton and H. Rackham (eds and tr.), *Cicero, De oratore (On the Orator)*, 2 vols (Loeb Classical Library 348 and 349). Cambridge, MA: Harvard University Press, and London: W. Heinemann, 1942.

Conversini, *De dilectione regnantium*. B. Kohl and J. Day (eds and tr.), 'Giovanni Conversini da Ravenna, *De dilectione regnantium (On the Proper Love Due Princes)*', in B. Kohl and J. Day (eds), *Two Court Treatises*. Munich: Wilhelm Fink, 1987, pp. 93–249.

Conversini, *De primo eius introitu ad aulam*. B. Kohl and J. Day (eds and tr.), 'Giovanni Conversini da Ravenna, *De primo eius introitu ad aulam, 13 September 1385 (Of His Earliest Introduction to Court)*', in B. Kohl and J. Day (eds), *Two Court Treatises*. Munich: Wilhelm Fink, 1987, pp. 21–83.

Cortusi, *Chronica*. B. Pagnin (ed.), *Guglielmo Cortusi, Chronica de novitatibus Padue et Lombardie*, in *Rerum Italicarum Scriptores*, new ed., vol. 12, pt. 5. Bologna: Zanichelli, 1941.

da Nono, *Visio Egidii Regis Patavie*. G. Fabris (ed.), *Giovanni da Nono, Visio Egidii Regis Patavie*, in *Bolletino del Museo Civico di Padova* 10–11 (1934–1939), pp. 1–20 (repr. in Fabris [ed.] 1977, *Cronache e cronisti padovani*, Padua: Rebellato, pp. 139–58).

de Premierfait, *Prologue*. G. di Stefano (ed.), *Laurent de Premierfait*, 'Prologue du translateur du *Livre des Cent Nouvelles* de Jehan Bocace de Certald', in G. di Stefano (ed.) and L. de Premierfait (tr.), *Giovanni Boccaccio, Decameron* (Bibliothèque du moyen français 3). Montréal: CERES, 1998, pp. 1–6.

de' Crescenzi, *Ruralium commodorum*. W. Richter and R. Richter-Bergmeier (eds), *Pietro de' Crescenzi, Ruralia commoda: das Wissen des vollkommenen Landwirts um 1300*, 4 vols (Editiones Heidelbergenses 26). Heidelberg: C. Winter, 1995–1998.

Dioscorides, *De materia medica*. M. Wellmann (ed.), *Pedanii Dioscuridis Anazarbei de materia medica libri quinque*, 3 vols. Berlin: Weidmann, 1906–1914 (English translation: L.Y. Beck, *Dioscorides. De Materia Medica* [Altertumswissenschaftliche Texte und Studien 38]. Hildesheim: Olms, 2005; English translation of the preface: J. Scarborough and V. Nutton, 'Dioscorides, *On Materia Medica. Preface*', in J. Scarborough and V. Nutton (eds), 'The Preface to Dioscorides' *Materia Medica*: Introduction, Translation, and Commentary', *Transactions and Studies of the College of Physicians of Philadelphia*, ser. 5, 4 [1982], pp. 195–7).

Galen, *Ars medica*. C.G. Kühn (ed. and Latin tr.), 'Galeni, *Ars medica*', in C.G. Kühn (ed.), *Claudii Galeni Opera Omnia* (Medicorum Graecorum Opera quae exstant 1–20), 22 vols. Lipsiae: C. Cnobloch, 1821–1833, 1:305–412 (English translation: P.N. Singer, 'The art of medicine', in P.N. Singer [ed.], *Galen. Selected Works*. Oxford and New York: Oxford University Press, 1997, pp. 345–96).

Galen, *De complexionibus*. R.J. Durling (ed.), *Burgundio of Pisa's Translation of Galen's Peri kraseōn "De complexionibus"* (Galenus Latinus I). Berlin: De Gruyter, 1976.

Gatari, *Cronaca*. A. Medin and G. Tolomei (eds), *Galeazzo, Bartolomeo* and *Andrea Gatari, Cronaca Carrarese*, in *Rerum Italicarum Scriptores*, new ed., vol. 17, pt. 1. Bologna: Zanichelli, 1931 (Partial English translation: D. Symes, *The Fortunes of Francesco Novello da Carrara Lord of Padua, an Historical Tale of the Fourteenth Century, from The Chronicles of Gataro, with Notes*. Edinburgh: Constable, 1830).

Guarino, *De ordine docendi ac studendi*. C. Kallendorf (ed. and tr.), 'Battista Guarino, *De ordine docendi ac studendi (A Program of Teaching and Learning)*', in C. Kallendorf (ed.), *Humanist Educational Treatises* (The I Tatti Renaissance Library 5). Cambridge, MA, and London: Harvard University Press, 2002, pp. 260–310.

Livy, *Ab urbe condita*. B. Foster (ed. and tr. vols. I–V); F.G. Moore (ed. and tr. vols. VI–VIII); E.T. Sage (ed. and tr. vols. IX–XI); E.T. Sage and A.C. Schlesinger (eds and tr.

vols. XII); A.C. Schlesinger (ed. and tr. vol. XIII); A.C. Schlesinger and J. Obsequens (ed. and tr. vol. XIV), *Livy, Ab urbe condita (History of Rome)*, 14 vols (Loeb Classical Library 114, 133, 172, 191, 233, 295, 301, 313, 332, 355, 367, 396, 404). Cambridge, MA: Harvard University Press, and London: W. Heinemann, 1919–1959.

Michiel, *Notizia*. G. Frizzoni (ed.), *Marcantonio Michiel, Notizia d'Opere di Disegno, pubblicata e illustrata da D. Jacopo Morelli*, 2nd edn. Bologna: Zanichelli, 1884 (English translation: P. Mussi and G.C. Williamson, *The Anonimo: Notes on Pictures and Works of Art in Italy Made By an Anonymous Writer in the Sixteenth Century*. London: G. Bell and Sons, 1903).

Mussato, *De traditione Patavii*. L.A. Muratori (ed.), *Albertino Mussato, De traditione Patavii ad Canem Grandem anno 1328 mense septembris et causis precedentibus*, in *Rerum Italicarum Scriptores*, vol. 10. Milan: Typographia Societatis palatinae, 1727, cols 715–68.

Mussato, *Opera*. L. Pignoria (ed.), *Albertino Mussato, Historia augusta Henrici VII caesaris et alia quae extant opera*. Venetiis: Ex Typographia Ducali Pinelliana, 1636.

Mussato, *Sette libri inediti del De gestis Italicorum*. L. Padrin (ed.), *Albertino Mussato, Sette libri inediti del De gestis italicorum post Henricum VII* (Monumenti storici, ser. 3. Cronache e diarii). Venice: A spese della Società, 1903.

Petrarch, *De remediis utriusque fortunae*. E. Fenzi (ed.), G. Fortunato and L. Alfinito (tr.), *Francesco Petrarca, De remediis utriusque fortunae (Rimedi all'una e all'altra fortuna)* (Umanesimo e Rinascimento 1). Naples: La scuola di Pitagora Editrice, 2009 (English translation: C.H. Rawski, *Remedies for Fortune Fair and Foul: A Modern English Translation of* De Remediis Utriusque Fortune, *with a Commentary*, 5 vols. Bloomington: Indiana University Press, 1991).

Petrarch, *De sui ipsius et multorum ignorantia*. L.M. Capelli (ed.), *Francesco Petrarca, De sui ipsius et multorum ignorantia*. Paris: Champion, 1906 (English translation: D. Marsh, 'On His Own Ignorance and that of Many Others', in D. Marsh [ed.], *Invectives* [The I Tatti Renaissance Library 11]. Cambridge, MA, and London: Harvard University Press, 2008, pp. 113–83).

Petrarch, *De viris illustribus*. G. Martellotti (ed.), *Francesco Petrarca, De viris illustribus* (Edizione nationale delle opere di Francesco Petrarca 2). Florence: Sansoni, 1964 (with Italian translation: L. Razzolini [ed.] and D. Albanzani [tr.], *Le vite degli uomini illustri di Francesco Petrarca. Volgarizzate da Donato degli Albanzani da Pratovecchio. Ora per la prima volta messe in luce secondo un codice Laurenziano citato dagli Accademici della Crusca*, 2 vols in 3 [Collezione di opere inedite o rare dei primi tre secoli della lingua 34–36]. Bologna: Presso Gaetano Romagnoli, 1874; and S. Ferrone, C. Malta and P. de Capua [eds and tr.], *De viris illustribus*, 4 vols [Edizione nazionale delle opere di Francesco Petrarca 3, Opere storiche]. Florence: Le Lettere, 2006–2012; partial English translation [of prefaces only]: B. Kohl, 'Petrarch's Prefaces to *De viris illustribus*', *History and Theory* 13 [1974], pp. 138–44 [repr. in B. Kohl (ed.), *Culture and Politics in Renaissance Padua*, section I, Aldershot: Ashgate Variorum, 2001]).

Petrarch, *Invective contra medicum*. D. Marsh (ed. and tr.), *Francesco Petrarca, Invective contra medicum (Invectives against a Physician)*, in D. Marsh (ed.), *Invectives* (The I Tatti Renaissance Library 11). Cambridge, MA, and London: Harvard University Press, 2003, pp. 2–179.

Petrarch, *Prose*. G. Martellotti (ed.), *Francesco Petrarca, Prose* (La Letteratura Italiana: storia e testi 7). Milan: Ricciardi, 1955.

Petrarch, *Rerum familiarium.* V. Rossi (ed. vols. 1–3) and U. Bosco (ed. vol. 4), *Francesco Petrarca, Le Familiari* (*Rerum familiarium*), 4 vols (Edizione nazionale delle opere di Francesco Petrarca 10–13). Florence: Sansoni, 1933–1942, repr. Florence: Le Lettere, 1997 (English translation: A.S. Bernardo, *Letters on Familiar Matters: Rerum Familiarium Libri I–XXIV*, 3 vols. Baltimore: Johns Hopkins University Press, 1975–1985; repr. New York: Italica, 2005).

Petrarch, *Rerum senilium.* E. Nota and U. Dotti (eds), and F. Castelli, P. Laurens, J.-Y. Boriaud, C. Laurens, F. Fabre, F. La Brasca, A. de Rosny and L. Schebat (tr.), *Francesco Petrarca, Lettres de la vieillesse (Rerum Senilium)*, 5 vols (Les Classiques de l'Humanisme 14, 16, 21, 26 and 42). Paris: Belles Lettres, 2002–2013 (English translation: A.S. Bernardo, R.A. Bernardo and S. Levin, *Letters of Old Age: Rerum Senilium Libri I–XVIII*, 2 vols. Baltimore: Johns Hopkins University Press, 1992; repr. New York: Italica, 2005).

Petrarch, *Testamentum.* T.E. Mommsen (ed. and tr.), 'Francesco Petrarca, *Testamentum*', in T.E. Mommsen, *Petrarch's Testament*. Ithaca, NY: Cornell University Press, 1957, pp. 68–93.

Pietro d'Abano, *Conciliator.* Petrus Abanensis, *Conciliator controversiarum, quae inter philosophos et medicos versantur.* Venetiis: Apud Iuntas, 1565 (facsimile edition with commentary: E. Riondato and L. Oliveri [eds.], *Pietro d'Abano, Conciliator. Ristampa fotomeccanica dell'edizione Venetiis apud Iuntas 1565* [I Filosofi Veneti, Sezione II: Ristampe 1]. Padua: Antenore, 1985).

Pietro d'Abano, *Expositio problematum Aristotelis.* Petrus Abanensis, *Expositio problematum Aristotelis cum textu.* Mantua: Paulus de Butzbach, 1475 (Partial English translation with commentary: J. Thomann, 'Pietro d'Abano, *Expositio in Problematibus Aristotelis*, xxxvi, 1', in J. Thomann, 'Pietro d'Abano on Giotto', *Journal of the Warburg and Courtauld Institutes* 54 [1991], pp. 242–3).

Pietro d'Abano, *Liber compilationis phisonomie.* Petrus Abanensis, *Liber compilationis phisonomie.* Padua: Maufer, 1474.

Platearius, *Circa Instans.* G. Malandin (ed. and tr.), F. Avril and P. Lietaghi (commentary), *Matthaeus Platéarius, Le livre des simples médecines, d'après le manuscrit Français 12322 de la Bibliothèque nationale de Paris.* Paris: Ozalid, 1986.

Pliny (the Elder), *Naturalis historia.* L. von Jan and K.F.T. Mayhoff (eds), *C. Plinii Secundi, Naturalis Historia, Libri XXXVII*, 6 vols. Lipsiae: Teubner, 1892–1898 (English translations: J. Bostock and H.T. Riley, *The Natural History of Pliny*, 6 vols. London: Bohn, 1855–1857; and H. Rackham [vols. 1–5 and 9], W.H.S. Jones [vols. 6, 7 (with A.C. Andrews), 8] and D.E. Eichholz [vol. 10], *Natural History*, 10 vols [Loeb Classical Library 330, 352–3, 370–71, 392–4, 418–19]. Cambridge, MA: Harvard University Press, and London: W. Heinemann, 1938–1963).

Pliny (the Younger), *Epistulae.* W. Melmoth (ed. and tr.) and W.M.L. Hutchinson (rev. edn.), *Pliny the Younger, Letters (Epistulae)*, 2 vols (Loeb Classical Library 55 and 59). New York: Macmillan, and London: W. Heinemann, 1915 (Alternative English translation: P.G. Walsh, *Complete Letters*. Oxford: Oxford University Press, 2006).

Poliziano, *Opera.* S. Gryphius (ed.), *Angeli Politiani opera: quorum primus hic tomus complectitur Epistolarum libros XII*, 3 vols in 2. Lyon: Gryphium, 1533.

Portenari, *Della felicità di Padova.* Angelo Portenari, *Della felicità di Padova.* Padua: P.P. Tozzi, 1623.

Reguardati, *Pulcherrimum & utilissimum opus ad sanitatis conseruationem.* Benedetto Reguardati, *Pulcherrimum & utilissimu[m] opus ad sanitatis co[n]seruationem æditu[m] ab eximio artium & medicine professore magistro Benedicto de Nursia.* Bologna: De Lapis, 1477.

Saladino da Ascoli, *Compendium aromatariorum.* Bologna: Benedictus Hectoris, 1488 (German translation: L. Zimmermann, *Saladini de Asculo, Serenitatis principis Tarēti physici principalis, Compendium aromatariorum. Zum ersten Male ins Deutsche übertragen, eingeleitet, erklärt und mit dem lateinischen.* Lipsiae: J.A. Barth, 1919).

Savonarola, *Del felice progresso di Borso d'Este.* M.A. Mastronardi (ed.), *Michele Savonarola, Del felice progresso di Borso d'Este.* Bari: Palomar, 1996.

Savonarola, *Libellus de magnificis ornamentis regie civitatis Padue.* A. Segarizzi (ed.), *Michele Savonarola, Libellus de magnificis ornamentis regie civitatis Padue,* in *Rerum Italicarum Scriptores,* new ed., vol. 24, pt. 15. Città di Castello: S. Lapi, 1902.

Savonarola, *Libreto de tutte le cose.* J. Nystedt (ed.), *Michele Savonarola, Libreto de tutte le cose che se magnano: un'opera di dietetica del sec. XV.* Stockholm: Almqvist & Wiksell International, 1988.

Seneca, *De clementia.* K. Hosius (ed.), *L. Annaei Senecae, De beneficiis libri VII, De clementia libri II,* Lipsiae: Teubner, 1914 (English translation: J.W. Basore, 'On Mercy [*De clementia*]', in J.W. Basore [ed.], *Moral Essays,* 3 vols [Loeb Classical Library 214, 254 and 310]. Cambridge, MA: Harvard University Press, and London: W. Heinemann, 1928–1935, vol. 1, pp. 357–447).

Serapion, *Liber aggregatus in medicinis simplicibus.* G. Ineichen (ed.), *Serapion, El libro agregà de Serapiom, volgarizzamento di frater Jacobus Philippus de Padua,* 2 vols. Venice and Rome: Istituto per la collaborazione culturale, 1962–1966.

Statius, *Thebaid.* D.R. Shackleton Bailey (ed. and tr.), *Statius, Thebaid,* 2 vols (Loeb Classical Library 207 [vol. 1, Books 1–7] and 498 [vol. 2, Books 8–12]). Cambridge, MA, and London: Harvard University Press, 2003.

Theophanes, *Chronographia.* C. de Boor (ed.), *Theophanis Chronographia,* 2 vols. Lipsiae: B.G. Teubnneri, 1883–1885.

Theophrastus, *Historia plantarum.* Sir A. Hort (ed. and tr.), *Theophrastus, Enquiry into Plants,* 2 vols (Loeb Classical Library 70 and 79). Cambridge, MA: Harvard University Press, and London: W. Heinemann, 1916–1926.

Vergerio, *Ad Franciscum Juniorem de Carraria.* L.A. Muratori (ed.), *Pier Paolo Vergerio, Ad Franciscum Juniorem de Carraria,* in *Rerum Italicarum Scriptores,* vol. 16. Milan: Ex Typographia societatis Palatinae in Regia Curia, 1730, cols 204A–215C.

Vergerio, *De dignissimo funebri apparatu.* L.A. Muratori (ed.), *Pier Paolo Vergerio, De dignissimo funebri apparatu in exequiis clarissimi omnium principis Francisci Senioris de Carraria,* in *Rerum Italicarum Scriptores,* vol. 16. Milan: Ex Typographia societatis Palatinae in Regia Curia, 1730, cols 189A–194A.

Vergerio, *De ingenuis moribus.* C. Kallendorf (ed. and tr.), 'Pier Paolo Vergerio, De ingenuis moribus et liberalibus adulescentiae studiis (*The Character and Studies Befitting a Free-Born Youth*)', in C. Kallendorf (ed.), *Humanist Educational Treatises* (The I Tatti Renaissance Library 5). Cambridge, MA, and London: Harvard University Press, 2002, pp. 2–91.

Vergerio, *De principibus.* A. Gnesotto (ed.), '*Pier Paolo Vergerio, De principibus Carrariensibus et gestis eorum*', *Atti e memorie dell'Accademia Patavina di scienze, lettere ed arti* 41 (1924), pp. 327–475.

Vergerio, *Epistolario.* L. Smith (ed. and tr.), *Pier Paolo Vergerio, Epistolario (148 Letters)* (Fonti per la Storia d'Italia 74). Rome: Tipografia del Senato, 1934.

Vergerio, *Oratorio in funere Francisci Senioris de Carraria.* L.A. Muratori (ed.), *Pier Paolo Vergerio, Oratorio in funere Francisci Senioris de Carraria, Patavii Principis,* in *Rerum Italicarum Scriptores,* vol. 16. Milan: Ex Typographia societatis Palatinae in Regia Curia, 1730, cols 194B–198C.

Secondary literature

Agrimi and Crisciani 1994. J. Agrimi and C. Crisciani, *Les Consilia médicaux* (Typologie des sources du Moyen Âge Occidental 69). Turnhout: Brepols.

Alessio 1976. F. Alesso, 'Filosofia e Scienza: Pietro d'Abano', in G. Folena (ed.), *Storia della cultura Veneta*, vol. 2: *Il Trecento*. Vicenza: Neri Pozza, pp. 171–206.

Alexander 1992. J.J.G. Alexander, *Medieval Illuminators and their Methods of Work*. New Haven: Yale University Press.

Alexander 1994. J.J.G. Alexander, 'Patrons, Libraries and Illuminators in the Italian Renaissance', in J.J.G. Alexander (ed.), *The Painted Page: Italian Renaissance Illumination, 1450–1550*. New York: Prestel, pp. 11–20.

Alexander 2002. J.J.G. Alexander, *Studies in Italian Manuscript Illumination*. London: Pindar Press.

Ambrosoli 1992. M. Ambrosoli, *Scienziati, contadini e proprietari: botanica e agricoltura nell' Europa occidentale 1350–1850*. Turin: Giulio Einaudi (English translation cited here: M. McCann Salvatorelli, *The Wild and the Sown: Botany and Agriculture in Western Europe, 1350–1850*. Cambridge: Cambridge University Press, 1997).

Aminrazavi 1997. M. Aminrazavi, 'Ibn Sīnā (Avicenna)', in H. Selin (ed.), *Encyclopedia of the History of Science, Technology, and Medicine in Non-Western Cultures*. London, Boston, Dordrecht: Kluwer Academic Publishers, pp. 434–6.

Arnaldez 1978. R. Arnaldez, 'Isṭifan b. Basīl', in P.J. Bearman, Th. Bianquis, C.E. Bosworth, E. van Donzel and W.P. Heinrichs (eds), *The Encyclopaedia of Islam*, 2nd ed. Leiden: Brill, vol. 4, pp. 254–5.

Arnaldez 1997. R. Arnaldez, 'Ibn Buṭlān', in H. Selin (ed.), *Encyclopedia of the History of Science, Technology, and Medicine in Non-Western Cultures*. London, Boston, Dordrecht: Kluwer Academic Publishers, pp. 417–18.

Anderson 1977. F. Anderson, *An Illustrated History of the Herbals*. New York: Columbia University Press.

Arber 1912. A. Arber, *Herbals: Their Origin and Evolution: A Chapter in the History of Botany, 1470–1670*. Cambridge: Cambridge University Press.

Armstrong 1983. L. Armstrong, 'The Illustrations of Pliny's *Historia naturalis*: Manuscripts before 1430', *Journal of the Warburg and Courtauld Institutes* 46, pp. 19–39.

Armstrong 1999. L. Armstrong, 'Copie di miniature del *Libro degli Uomini Famosi*, Poiano 1476, di Francesco Petrarca, e il ciclo perduto di affreschi nella Reggia Carrarese di Padova', in G. Mariani Canova, G. Baldissin Molli and F. Toniolo (eds), *Parole Dipinte. La Miniatura a Padova dal Medioevo al Settecento*. Modena: Franco Cosimo Panini, pp. 513–23 (English translation: 'Miniatures in Copies of Francesco Petrarca, *Libro degli Uomini Famosi*, Poiano, 1476 and the Lost Fresco Cycles in the Reggia Carrarese of Padua', in L. Armstrong, *Studies of Renaissance Miniaturists in Venice*, 2 vols. London: Pindar Press, 2003, vol. 1, pp. 175–212).

Arslan 1963. E. Arslan, 'Riflessioni sulla pittura gotica "Internazionale" in Lombardia nel tardo Trecento', *Arte Lombarda* 8, pp. 25–66.

Avril 1984. F. Avril, *Dix siècles d'enluminure Italienne: VIe–XVIe siècles*. Paris: Bibliothèque nationale de France.

Avril 1986. F. Avril, 'Etude codicologique et artistique', in G. Malandin (ed. and tr.), F. Avril and P. Lietaghi (commentary), *Platéarius, Le livre des simples médecines: d'après le manuscrit français 12322 de la Bibliothèque nationale de Paris*. Paris: Ozalid, pp. 268–83.

Baggio 1999. L. Baggio, '*Chronica de Carrariensibus* (*Gesta magnifica domus Carrariensis*; Nicoletto d'Alessio, *Storia della confine*), No. 69', in G. Mariani Canova,

G. Baldissin Molli and F. Toniolo (eds), *Parole Dipinte. La Miniatura a Padova dal Medioevo al Settecento*. Modena: Panini, pp. 190–2.

Balty-Guesdon 1996. M.-G. Balty-Guesdon, 'Le livre médical et son illustration', in É. Delpont (ed.), *La médecine au temps des califes. À l'ombre d'Avicenne: exposition présentée du 18 novembre 1996 au 2 mars 1997 (Paris, l'Institut du monde arabe)*. Gand: Snoeck-Ducaju & Zoon, and Paris: Institut du monde arabe, pp. 230–7.

Barbour 2004. J.D. Barbour, *The Value of Solitude: The Ethics and Spirituality of Aloneness in Autobiography*. Charlottesville, VA, and London: University of Virginia Press.

Barton 1994. T.S. Barton, *Power and Knowledge: Astrology, Medicine and Physiognomics Under the Roman Empire*. Ann Arbor: University of Michigan Press.

Barzon 1924. A. Barzon, *I cieli e la loro influenza negli affreschi del salone in Padova*. Padua: Seminario.

Bauman 2002. J. Bauman, 'Tradition and Transformation: The Pleasure Garden in Piero de' Crescenzi's *Liber Ruralium Commodorum*', *Studies in the History of Gardens and Designed Landscapes* 22, pp. 99–141.

Baumann 1974. F.A, Baumann, *Das Erbario Carrarese und die Bildtradition des Tractatus de Herbis. Ein Beitrag zur Geschichte der Pflanzendarstellung im Übergang von Spätmittelalter zur Frührenaissance*. Bern: Benteli.

Beagon 1992. M. Beagon, *Roman Nature: The Thought of Pliny the Elder*. Oxford and New York: Oxford University Press.

Belloni et al. 1958. G. Belloni, R. Cipriani, and M.L. Ferrari, *Arte Lombarda dai Visconti agli Sforza, Palazzo reale, Milano, aprile-giugno 1958*. Milano: Silvana.

Benjamin 1970. W. Benjamin and G. Scholem (ed.), *Berliner Chronik* (Bibliothek Suhrkamp 251). Frankfurt-am-Main: Suhrkamp (English translation cited here: E. Jephcott and K. Shorter, 'A Berlin Chronicle', in W. Benjamin, E. Jephcott (tr.) and K. Shorter (tr.), *One Way Street and Other Writings*. London: Verso, 1979, pp. 293–346).

Bertiz 2003. A.A. Bertiz, *Picturing Health: The Garden and Courtiers at Play in the Late Fourteenth-Century Illuminated* Tacuinum Sanitatis. Los Angeles: University of Southern California. Unpublished PhD thesis.

Bettini 1974. S. Bettini, 'Le miniature del "*Libro agregà de Serapion*" nella cultura artistica del tardo Trecento', in L. Grossato (ed.), *Da Giotto al Mantegna*. Milano: Electa, pp. 55–60.

Billanovich 1951. G. Billanovich, 'Petrarch and the Textual Tradition of Livy', *Journal of the Warburg and Courtauld Institutes* 14, pp. 137–208.

Blair-Dixon 2004. C. Blair-Dixon, *Schism and the Politics of Memory: Constructing Authority from Hippolytus through the Laurentian Schism*. Manchester: University of Manchester. Unpublished PhD thesis.

Blanchard 2001. S. Blanchard, 'Petrarch and the Genealogy of Asceticism', *Journal of the History of Ideas* 62, pp. 401–23.

Blunt and Raphael 1979. W. Blunt and S. Raphael, *The Illustrated Herbal*. New York: Thames and Hudson.

Bobisut and Salomoni 2002. D. Bobisut and L.G. Salomoni, *Altichiero da Zevio: The Chapel of St. James and the Oratory of St. George*. Padua: Messaggero Padova.

Bodin and Hedlund 2013. H. Bodin and R. Hedlund (eds), *Byzantine Gardens and Beyond* (Acta Universitatis Upsaliensis. Studia Byzantina Upsaliensia 13). Uppsala: Uppsala Universitet.

Bodon 2009. G. Bodon, *Heroum imagines: la Sala dei Giganti a Padova. Un monumento della tradizione classica e della cultura antiquaria (Studi di arte veneta 16)*. Venice: Istituto Veneto di scienze, lettere ed arti.

Bolland 1996. A. Bolland, 'Art and Humanism in Early Renaissance Padua: Cennini, Vergerio and Petrarch on Imitation', *Renaissance Quarterly* 49, pp. 469–87.

Booton 1994. D. Booton, *Pictorial Seasons: A Cultural Study of the Cycle of Calendar Paintings in the Torre dell'Aquila*. New York: New York University. Unpublished PhD thesis.

Boulton 1990. D'A.J.D. Boulton, 'Insignia of Power: The Use of Heraldic and Paraheraldic Devices by Italian Princes, c. 1350–1500', in C. Rosenberg (ed.), *Art and Politics in Late Medieval and Early Renaissance Italy: 1250–1500*. London and Notre Dame: Notre Dame University Press, pp. 103–27.

Briggs 1999. C. Briggs, *Giles of Rome's* De Regimine Principum*: Reading and Writing Politics at Court and University, ca. 1275–ca. 1525*. Cambridge: Cambridge University Press.

Britton 2002. P.D.G. Britton, 'The Signs of Faces: Leonardo on Physiognomic Science and the "Four Universal States of Man"', *Renaissance Studies* 16, pp. 143–62.

Brockelmann 1927. C. Brockelmann, 'Kalila Wa Dimna', in M.Th. Houtsma (ed.), *The Encyclopaedia of Islam*, 1st ed. Leiden: Brill, vol. 4, pp. 694–98.

Brooks 2008. G. Brooks. *People of the Book: A Novel*. New York and London: Penguin.

Brubaker 1997. L. Brubaker, 'Memories of Helena: Patterns in Imperial Female Matron-age in the Fourth and Fifth Centuries', in E. James (ed.), *Women, Men, Eunuchs. Gender in Byzantium*. London: Routledge, pp. 52–75.

Brubaker 2002. L. Brubaker, 'The *Vienna Dioscorides* and Anicia Juliana', in A. Little-wood, H. Maguire, and J. Wolschke-Bulmahn (eds), *Byzantine Garden Culture*. Washington, DC: Dumbarton Oaks, pp. 189–214.

Buberl 1937. P. Buberl, *Die byzantinischen Handschriften: 1. Der Wiener Dioskurides und die Wiener Genesis*. Leipzig: Hiersemann.

Buettner 1992. B. Buettner, 'Profane Illuminations, Secular Illusions: Manuscripts in Late Medieval Courtly Society', *Art Bulletin* 74, pp. 75–90.

Buettner 2001. B. Buettner, 'Past Presents: New Year's Gifts at the Valois Courts, ca. 1400', *Art Bulletin* 83, pp. 598–625.

Burckhardt 2005. J. Burckhardt, *Italian Renaissance Paintings According to Genres (Die Malerei nach Inhalt und Aufgaben)*, tr. D. Britt and C. Beamish (Texts and Documents). Los Angeles, CA: Getty Publications.

Burnett 1995. C. Burnett, '"Magister Iohannes Hispalensis et Limiensis' and Qusta ibn Luqa's *De differentia spiritus et animae*: A Portuguese Contribution to the Arts Curriculum?', *Mediaevalia. Textos e estudos* 7–8, pp. 221–67.

Burnett 2005. C. Burnett, 'Gerard of Cremona', in T. Glick, F. Wallis and S.J. Livesey (eds), *Medieval Science, Technology and Medicine: An Encyclopedia*. New York: Rout-ledge, pp. 191–2.

Bushnell 1996. R.W. Bushnell, *A Culture of Teaching: Early Modern Humanism in Theory and Practice*. Ithaca, NY: Cornell University Press.

Calcaterra 1939–1940. C. Calcaterra, 'La concezione storica del Petrarca', *Annali della Cattedra Petrarchesca* 9, pp. 3–25.

Calkins 1986. R. Calkins, 'Piero de' Crescenzi and the Medieval Garden', in E. MacDou-gall (ed.), *Medieval Gardens* (Dumbarton Oaks Colloquium on the History of Landscape Architecture IX). Washington, DC: Dumbarton Oaks, pp. 155–75.

Calligari and Dal Santo 1999. M. Calligari and V. Dal Santo, 'Alberino Mussato, *De tra-ditione Padue ad Canem Grandem anno 1328 mense septembri et causis precedentibus*, No. 55', in G. Mariani Canova, G. Baldissin Molli and F. Toniolo (eds), *Parole Dipinte. La Miniatura a Padova dal Medioevo al Settecento*. Modena: Panini, p. 158.

Campbell 2008. C.J. Campbell, *The Commonwealth of Nature: Art and Poetic Community in the Age of Dante*. University Park: Pennsylvania State University Press.

Campbell 2004. S.J. Campbell, *The Cabinet of Eros: Renaissance Mythological Painting and the Studiolo of Isabella d'Este*. New Haven: Yale University Press.

Capo 1976. L. Capo, 'I cronisti dei Carraresi', in G. Folena and G. Arnaldi (eds), *Storia della cultura Veneta*, 5 vols. Vicenza: Neri Pozza, vol. 2 (*Il Trecento*), pp. 311–37.

Castellini 1993. P. Castellini, 'Architettura e decorazione nel Palazzo della Ragione di Padova', *Scienza e Storia* 9, pp. 89–97.

Cessi 1974. F. Cessi, 'Monetazione e medaglistica dei Carraresi', in L. Grossato (ed.), *Da Giotto al Mantegna*. Milan: Electa, pp. 86–90.

Cessi 1985. R. Cessi, *Padova Medioevale: studi e documenti*, 2 vols. D. Gallo and P. Sambin (eds). Padua: Erredici.

Cittadella 1842. G. Cittadella, *Storia della dominazione Carrarese in Padova*, 2 vols. Padua: Seminario.

Cogliati Arano 1976. L. Cogliati Arano, *The Medieval Health Handbook Tacuinum Sanitatis (Ibn Botlân)*. New York: G. Braziller.

Cogliati Arano 1988. L. Cogliati Arano, 'Tacuinum Sanitatis', in R. Bussi (ed.), *Di sana pianta: erbari e taccuini di sanità. Le radici storiche della nuova farmacologia*. Modena: Panini, pp. 13–20.

Colle 1824–1825. F.M. Colle, *Storia Scientifico-Letteraria dello Studio di Padova*, 4 vols. Padua: Minerva.

Collins 2000. M. Collins, *Medieval Herbals: The Illustrative Traditions*. Toronto: University of Toronto Press.

Collins 2010. M. Collins, 'Miscellaneous Medical and Pharmacological Texts', in G. d'Andiran (ed.), *Early Medicine: From the Body to the Stars*. Basel: Schwabe, p. 169.

Collins and Raphael 2003. M. Collins and S. Raphael, *A Medieval Herbal: A Facsimile of British Library Egerton MS 747*. London: British Library.

Conner 1999. C.L. Conner, 'The Epigram in the Church of Hagios Polyeuktos in Constantinople and its Byzantine Response', *Byzantion* 69, pp. 479–527.

Cozzi 1999. E. Cozzi, '*Liber cimeriorum dominorum de Carraria*, No. 52', in G. Mariani Canova, G. Baldissin Molli and F. Toniolo (eds), *Parole Dipinte. La Miniatura a Padova dal Medioevo al Settecento*. Modena: Panini, p. 151.

Crisciani 1990. C. Crisciani, 'History, Novelty, and Progress in Scholastic Medicine', *Osiris*, 2nd Series 6 (M.R. McVaugh and N.G. Siraisi [eds], *Renaissance Medical Learning: Evolution of a Tradition*). Philadelphia: History of Science Society, pp. 118–39.

Crisciani 2003. C. Crisciani, 'Michele Savonarola, Medico: tra università e corte, tra Latino e volgare', in N. Bray and L. Sturlese (eds), *Filosofia in volgare nel Medioevo*. Louvain-la-Neuve: FIDEM, pp. 433–49.

Crisciani 2005. C. Crisciani, 'Histories, Stories, Exempla, and Anecdotes: Michele Savonarola from Latin to Vernacular', in G. Pomata and N. Siraisi (eds), *Historia: Empiricism and Erudition in Early Modern Europe*. Cambridge, MA, and London: MIT Press, pp. 297–324.

Crisciani and Zuccolin 2011. C. Crisciani and G. Zuccolin (eds), *Michele Savonarola: medicina e cultura di corte* (Micrologus' Library 37). Florence: SISMEL Edizioni del Galluzzo.

d'Adda 1875–1879. G. d'Adda, *Indagini storiche, artistiche e bibliografiche sulla libreria visconteo-sforzesca del Castello di Pavia*. Milan: G. Brigola.

d'Alverny 1952. M.-T. d'Alverny, 'Notes sur les traductions médiévales des oeuvres philosophiques d'Avicenne', *Archives d'histoire doctrinale et littéraire du Moyen Âge* 19, pp. 337–58.

d'Andiran 2010. G. d'Andiran (ed.), *Early Medicine: From the Body to the Stars*. Basel: Schwabe.

Daston and Park 2001. L. Daston and K. Park, *Wonders and the Order of Nature, 1150–1750*. New York: Zone.

Degenhart and Schmitt 1968–1980. B. Degenhart and A. Schmitt (eds), *Corpus der Italienischen Zeichnungen 1300–1450*, 2 vols. Berlin: Gebr. Mann.

Delisle 1868–1881. L. Delisle, *Le cabinet des manuscrits de la Bibliothèque impériale-nationale*, 3 vols. Paris: Imprimerie impériale.

Delisle 1884. L. Delisle, 'Notice sur deux livres ayant appartenu au roi Charles V', *Notices et Extraits des Manuscrits de la Bibliothèque nationale* 31, pp. 1–31.

Delisle 1896. L. Delisle, 'Notice sur un livre annoté par Pétrarque (ms. latin 2201 de la Bibliothèque nationale)', *Notices et Extraits des Manuscrits de la Bibliothèque nationale* 35, pp. 393–408.

Denieul-Cormier 1956. A. Denieul-Cormier, 'La très ancienne physiognomonie et Michel Savonarole', *La Biologie Médicale* 45, pp. 1–107.

Derbes 2013. A. Derbes, 'Patronage, Gender & Generation in Late Medieval Italy: Fina Buzzacarini and the Baptistery of Padua', in C. Hourihane (ed.), *Patronage: Power and Agency in Medieval Art* (Index of Christian Art 15). University Park: University of Pennsylvania Press, pp. 119–50.

Derbes and Sandona 2008. A. Derbes and M. Sandona, *The Usurer's Heart: Giotto, Enrico Scrovegni, and the Arena Chapel in Padua*. University Park: Pennsylvania State University Press.

Dilg 1999. P. Dilg, 'The *Liber aggregatus in medicinis simplicibus* of Pseudo-Serapion: An Influential Work of Medical Arabism', in C. Burnett and A. Contadini (eds), *Islam and the Italian Renaissance*. London: Warburg Institute (London University Press), pp. 221–31.

Dixon 1990. A. Dixon, 'The Morgan Model Drawings and the Genesis of the *Tacuinum Sanitatis* Illustrations', *Arte Lombarda* 92–3, pp. 9–20.

Dunlop 2009. A. Dunlop, *Painted Palaces: The Rise of Secular Art in Early Renaissance Italy*. New Haven: Yale University Press.

Eamon 1994. W. Eamon, *Science and the Secrets of Nature: Books of Secrets in Medieval and Early Modern Culture*. Princeton: Princeton University Press.

El-Bizri 2006. N. El-Bizri, 'Ibn Sina, or Avicenna', in J. Meri (ed.), *Medieval Islamic Civilization: An Encyclopedia*, 2 vols. New York: Routledge, vol. 1, pp. 369–70.

Elkhadem 1990. H. Elkhadem, 'Le Taqwīm al-Ṣiḥḥa (Tacuini Sanitatis) d'Ibn Buṭlān: Histoire du texte', *Acta Belgica Historiae Medicinae* 3, pp. 139–46.

Ettinghausen 1962. R. Ettinghausen, *Arab Painting*. Geneva: Skira.

Evans 1945. E.C. Evans, 'Galen the Physician as Physiognomist', *Transactions and Proceedings of the American Philological Association* 76, pp. 287–98.

Fabris 1932–1933. G. Fabris, 'La cronaca di Giovanni da Nono', *Bolletino del Museo Civico di Padova* 8, pp. 1–33, and 9, pp. 167–200.

Fabris 1977. G. Fabris, *Cronache e cronisti Padovani*. Cittadella: Rebellato.

Findlen 1994. P. Findlen, *Possessing Nature: Museums, Collecting, and Scientific Culture in Early Modern Italy*. Berkeley: University of California Press.

Foligno 1910. C. Foligno, *The Story of Padua*. London: J.M. Dent & Sons, Ltd.

Forster 2006. R. Forster, *Das Geheimnis der Geheimnisse: die arabischen und deutschen Fassungen des pseudo-aristotelischen 'Sirr al-asrār, Secretum secretorum'* (Wissensliteratur im Mittelalter 43). Wiesbaden: Reichert.

Forster 2010. R. Forster, 'Transmission of Knowledge through Literature: The Literary Frames of the Pseudo-Aristotelian *Sirr al-Asrār* and *Kitāb al-Tuffāḥa*', *Eos* 97, pp. 101–17.

Fortenbaugh 1992–1993. W.W. Fortenbaugh, *Theophrastus of Eresus: Sources for his Life, Writings, Thought, and Influence*, 2 vols (Philosophia Antiqua 54). Leiden: Brill.

French 2001. R.K. French, *Canonical Medicine: Gentile da Foligno and Scholasticism*. Leiden: Brill.

Frojmovič 1996. E. Frojmovič, 'Giotto's Allegories of Justice and the Commune in the Palazzo della Ragione in Padua: A Reconstruction', *Journal of the Warburg and Courtauld Institutes* 59, pp. 24–47.

Frojmovič 2007. E. Frojmovič, 'Giotto's Circumspection', *The Art Bulletin* 89, pp. 195–210.

Gamillscheg 2007. E. Gamillscheg, 'Das Geschenk für Juliana Anicia: Überlegungen zu Struktur und Entstehung des *Wiener Dioskurides*', in K. Belke and E. Kislinger (eds), *Byzantina Mediterranea: Festschrift für Johannes Koder zum 65. Geburtstag*. Vienna: Bohlau, pp. 187–95.

Ganguzza Billanovich 1977a. M.C. Ganguzza Billanovich, 'Carrara, Francesco da, il Novello', *Dizionario Biografico degli Italiani*, vol. 20, pp. 656–62.

Ganguzza Billanovich 1977b. M.C. Ganguzza Billanovich, 'Carrara, Giacomo da [d. ca. 1240]', *Dizionario Biografico degli Italiani*, vol. 20, pp. 671–3.

Ganguzza Billanovich 1977c. M.C. Ganguzza Billanovich, 'Carrara, Giacomo da [d. 1324]', *Dizionario Biografico degli Italiani*, vol. 20, pp. 673–5.

Ganguzza Billanovich 1977d. M.C. Ganguzza Billanovich, 'Carrara, Giacomo da [d. 1350]', *Dizionario Biografico degli Italiani*, vol. 20, pp. 675–6.

Ganguzza Billanovich 1977e. M.C. Ganguzza Billanovich, 'Carrara, Marsilietto Papafava da', *Dizionario Biografico degli Italiani*, vol. 20, pp. 688–91.

Ganguzza Billanovich 1977f. M.C. Ganguzza Billanovich, 'Carrara, Marsilio da [d. ca. 1292]', *Dizionario Biografico degli Italiani*, vol. 20, pp. 691–3.

Ganguzza Billanovich 1977g. M.C. Ganguzza Billanovich, 'Carrara, Marsilio da [d. 1338]', *Dizionario Biografico degli Italiani*, vol. 20, pp. 693–5.

Ganguzza Billanovich 1977h. M.C. Ganguzza Billanovich, 'Carrara, Nicolò da', *Dizionario Biografico degli Italiani*, vol. 20, pp. 696–8.

Ganguzza Billanovich 1977i. M.C. Ganguzza Billanovich, 'Carrara, Ubertino da', *Dizionario Biografico degli Italiani*, vol. 20, pp. 700–2.

Garin 1947. E. Garin (ed.), *La disputa delle arti nel Quattrocento* (Edizione nazionale dei classici del pensiero Italiano 9). Florence: Vallecchi.

Garin 1961. E. Garin, 'Gli umanisti e la scienza', *Rivista di filosofia* 52, pp. 259–78.

Garin 1965. E. Garin, *Scienza e vita civile nel Rinascimento italiano*. Bari: Laterza (English translation cited here: P. Munz, *Science and Civic Life in the Italian Renaissance*. Garden City, NY: Anchor, 1969).

Gardner 2011. J. Gardner, *Giotto and His Publics: Three Paradigms of Patronage*. Cambridge, MA: Harvard University Press.

Gasparotto 1966–1967. C. Gasparotto, 'La reggia dei da Carrara, il Palazzo di Ubertino e le nuove stanze dell'Accademia Patavina', *Atti e memorie dell'Accademia Patavina di scienze, lettere ed arti* 79, pp. 71–116.

Gasparotto 1968–1969. C. Gasparotto, 'Gli ultimi affreschi venuti in luce nella reggia dei da Carrara e una documentazione inedita sulla camera di Camillo', *Atti e memorie dell'Accademia Patavina di scienze, lettere ed arti* 81, pp. 243–61.

Gerstinger 1970. H. Gerstinger, *Dioscurides. Codex Vindobonensis med. gr. 1 der Österreichischen Nationalbibliothek*, 2 vols (Codices selecti phototypice impressi 12). Graz: Akademische Druck- und Verlagsanstalt.

Gibson and Morello 2011. R.K. Gibson and R. Morello (eds), *Pliny the Elder: Themes and Contexts*. Leiden: Brill.

Gibson and Morello 2012. R.K. Gibson and R. Morello, *Reading the Letters of Pliny the Younger: An Introduction*. Cambridge: Cambridge University Press.

Gilbert 1928. A.H. Gilbert, 'Notes on the Influence of the *Secretum Secretorum*', *Speculum* 3, pp. 84–98.

Givens 2005. J. Givens, *Observation and Image-Making in Gothic Art*. Cambridge: Cambridge University Press.

Givens 2006. J. Givens, 'Reading and Writing the Illustrated *Tractatus de herbis*, 1280–1526', in J. Givens, K. Reeds and A. Touwaide (eds), *Visualizing Medieval Medicine and Natural History, 1200–1550* (AVISTA Studies in the History of Medieval Technology, Science and Art 5). Aldershot: Ashgate, pp. 115–46.

Givens et al. 2006. J. Givens, K. Reeds and A. Touwaide (eds), *Visualizing Medieval Medicine and Natural History, 1200–1550* (AVISTA Studies in the History of Medieval Technology, Science and Art 5). Aldershot: Ashgate.

Gloria 1878. A. Gloria (ed.), *Documenti inediti intorno al Petrarca con alcuni cenni della casa di lui in Arquà e della Reggia dei da Carrara in Padova (discorso tenuto per l'inaugurazione del Museo Petrarchesco di Arquà)*. Padua: Museo Civico.

Gloria 1884. A. Gloria (ed.), *Monumenti della Università di Padova (1222–1318)*, 2 vols. Venice: Segreteria del R. Istituto (repr. Bologna: Forni, 1972).

Gloria 1888. A. Gloria (ed.), *Monumenti della Università di Padova (1318–1405)*, 2 vols. Padua: Seminario (repr. Bologna: Forni, 1972).

Godman 1998. P. Godman, *From Poliziano to Machiavelli: Florentine Humanism in the High Renaissance*. Princeton: Princeton University Press.

Goichon 1999. A.-M. Goichon, 'Ibn Sīnā', in P.J. Bearman, Th. Bianquis, C.E. Bosworth, E. van Donzel and W.P. Heinrichs (eds), *The Encyclopaedia of Islam*, 2nd ed. Leiden: Brill, vol. 3, pp. 941–7.

Gorini 1974. G. Gorini, 'Iconografia monetale e cultura figurativa a Padova nei secoli XIV e XV', in L. Grossato (ed.), *Da Giotto al Mantegna*. Milan: Electa, pp. 81–5.

Gorini 2005. G. Gorini, 'Le medaglie carraresi: genesi e fortuna', in O. Longo (ed.), *Padova Carrarese*. Padua: Il Poligrafo, pp. 259–67.

Gousset 1999. M.-T. Gousset, 'Franciscus de Caronellis, *De Curru Carrariensis*, No. 45', in G. Mariani Canova, G. Baldissin Molli and F. Toniolo (eds), *Parole Dipinte. La Miniatura a Padova dal Medioevo al Settecento*. Modena: Panini, p. 136.

Grabar 2006. O. Grabar, 'Pictures or Commentaries: The Illustrations of the *Maqamat* of Al-Hariri', in *Islamic Visual Culture, 1100–1800* (Constructing the Study of Islamic Art 2). Aldershot: Ashgate, pp. 187–206.

Grafton and Jardine 1986. A. Grafton and L. Jardine. *From Humanism to the Humanities: Education and the Liberal Arts in Fifteenth and Sixteenth-Century Europe*. London: Duckworth.

Grafton and Siraisi 1999. A. Grafton and N.G. Siraisi (eds), *Natural Particulars: Nature and the Disciplines in Renaissance Europe*. Cambridge, MA: MIT Press.

Granata 1999. L. Granata, '*Cronaca Carrarese*, No. 56', in G. Mariani Canova, G. Baldissin Molli and F. Toniolo (eds), *Parole Dipinte. La Miniatura a Padova dal Medioevo al Settecento*. Modena: Panini, p. 159.

Green 2005. M.H. Green, 'Constantine the African', in T. Glick, F. Wallis and S.J. Livesey (eds), *Medieval Science, Technology and Medicine: An Encyclopedia*. New York: Routledge, pp. 145–7.

Greene 1982. T. Greene, *The Light in Troy: Imitation and Discovery in Renaissance Poetry*. New Haven: Yale University Press.

Greene 1989. T. Greene, 'Petrarch and the Humanist Hermeneutic', in H. Bloom (ed.), *Petrarch* (Modern Critical Views). New York: Chelsea House, pp. 103–24.

Grendler 2002. P.F. Grendler, *The Universities of the Italian Renaissance*. Baltimore: Johns Hopkins University Press.

Grossato 1964. L. Grossato, 'La decorazione pittorica del salone', in C.G. Mor (ed.), *Il Palazzo della Ragione di Padova*. Venice: Neri Pozza, pp. 47–67.

Grossato 1974. L. Grossato (ed.), *Da Giotto al Mantegna*. Milan: Electa.

Gunzburg 2013. D. Gunzburg, 'Giotto's Sky: The fresco paintings of the first floor Salone of the Palazzo della Ragione, Padua, Italy', *Journal for the Study of Religion, Nature and Culture* 7, pp. 407–33.

Hampton 1990. T. Hampton, *Writing from History: The Rhetoric of Exemplarity in Renaissance Literature*. Ithaca: Cornell University Press.

Harvey 2008. E.R. Harvey, 'Ibn Sarābī', in H. Selin (ed.), *Encyclopedia of the History of Science, Technology, and Medicine in Non-Western Cultures*, 2nd ed., 2 vols. New York: Springer, vol. 1, pp. 1118–19.

Hoeniger 2006. C. Hoeniger, 'The Illuminated *Tacuinum Sanitatis* Manuscripts from Northern Italy ca. 1380–1400: Sources, Patrons, and the Creation of a New Pictorial Genre', in J. Givens, K. Reeds and A. Touwaide (eds), *Visualizing Medieval Medicine and Natural History, 1200–1550* (AVISTA Studies in the History of Medieval Technology, Science and Art 5). Aldershot: Ashgate, pp. 51–82.

Hopkins 1971. J.F.P Hopkins, 'Ibn Wāfid', in P.J. Bearman, Th. Bianquis, C.E. Bosworth, E. van Donzel and W.P. Heinrichs (eds), *The Encyclopaedia of Islam*, 2nd ed. Leiden: Brill, vol. 3, p. 987.

Huguet-Termes 2008. T. Huguet-Termes, 'Islamic Pharmacology and Pharmacy in the Latin West: An Approach to Early Pharmacopoeias', *European Review* 16, pp. 229–39.

Hyde 1966a. J.K. Hyde, 'Medieval Descriptions of Cities', *Bulletin of the John Rylands Library* 48, pp. 308–40.

Hyde 1966b. J.K. Hyde, *Padua in the Age of Dante*. Manchester: University of Manchester Press.

Hyde 1993. J.K. Hyde, *Literacy and Its Uses: Studies on Late Medieval Italy*. D. Waley (ed.). New York: St. Martin's Press.

Ineichen 1962–1966. G. Ineichen (ed.), *El Libro agregà de Serapiom, volgarizzamento di Frater Jacobus Philippus de Padua*, 2 vols. Venice and Rome: Istituto per la collaborazione culturale.

Iskandar 1997. A. Iskandar, 'Ḥunayn ibn Isḥāq', in H. Selin (ed.), *Encyclopedia of the History of Science, Technology, and Medicine in Non-Western Cultures*. London, Boston, Dordrecht: Kluwer Academic Publishers, pp. 399–400.

Ivanoff 1964. N. Ivanoff, 'Il problema iconologico degli affreschi', in C.G. Mor (ed.), *Il Palazzo della Ragione di Padova*. Venice: Neri Pozza, pp. 71–84.

Jacobus 1999. L. Jacobus, 'Giotto's Annunciation in the Arena Chapel, Padua', *The Art Bulletin* 81, pp. 93–107.

Jacquart 1990. D. Jacquart, 'Theory, Everyday Practice, and Three Fifteenth-Century Physicians', *Osiris*, 2nd Series 6 (M.R. McVaugh and N.G. Siraisi [eds], *Renaissance Medical Learning: Evolution of a Tradition*), pp. 140–60.

Jacquart 1996. D. Jacquart, 'The Influence of Arabic Medicine in the Medieval West', in R. Rashed (ed.), *Encyclopedia of the History of Arabic Science*, 3 vols. London and New York: Routledge, vol. 3, pp. 963–84.

Jacquart 2010. D. Jacquart, 'Between East and West: The Medieval Foundations of European Medicine', in G. d'Andiran (ed.), *Early Medicine: From the Body to the Stars*. Basel: Schwabe, pp. 75–8.

Jacquart and Paravicini Bagliani 2007. D. Jacquart and A. Paravicini Bagliani (eds), *La scuola medica salernitana: gli autori e testi* (Edizione nazionale: La Scuola Medica Salernitana 1). Florence: SISMEL Edizioni del Galluzzo.

Johnson 1995. G.A. Johnson, 'Activating the Effigy: Donatello's Pecci Tomb in Siena Cathedral', *Art Bulletin* 77, pp. 445–59.

Johnson 2010. W.A. Johnson, *Readers and Reading Culture in the High Roman Empire: A Study of Elite Communities*. Oxford and New York: Oxford University Press.

Kádár 1978. Z. Kádár, *Survivals of Greek Zoological Illuminations in Byzantine Manuscripts*. Budapest: Akadémiai Kiadó.

Kahn 1989. V. Kahn, 'The Figure of the Reader in Petrarch's *Secretum*', in H. Bloom (ed.), *Petrarch* (Modern Critical Views). New York: Chelsea House, pp. 139–58.

Kallendorf 1999. C. Kallendorf, *Virgil and the Myth of Venice: Books and Readers in the Italian Renaissance*. Oxford and New York: Oxford University Press.

Kallendorf 2002. C. Kallendorf (ed.), *Humanist Educational Treatises*. Cambridge, MA, and London: Harvard University Press.

Keith-Falconer 1885. I. Keith-Falconer, 'Introduction', in I. Keith-Falconer (ed. and tr.), *Kalīlah and Dimnah or the Fables of Bidpai*. London: Cambridge University Press, pp. xxxiii–lxxxv.

Kerner 2004. J. Kerner, 'Art in the Name of Science: Illustrated Manuscripts of the Kita Al-Diyaq'. New York: New York University. Unpublished PhD thesis.

Kibre 1962. P. Kibre, *Scholarly Privileges in the Middle Ages; the Rights, Privileges, and Immunities of Scholars and Universities at Bologna, Padua, Paris, and Oxford*. Cambridge, MA: Mediaeval Academy of America.

Kibre 1984. P. Kibre, 'Arts and Medicine in the Universities in the Later Middle Ages', in P. Kibre, *Studies in Medieval Science: Alchemy, Astrology, Mathematics and Medicine*. London: Hambledon Press, pp. 213–27.

Kiilerich 2001. B. Kiilerich, 'The Image of Anicia Juliana in the *Vienna Dioscorides*: Flattery or Appropriation of Imperial Imagery?', *Symbolae Osloenses* 76, pp. 169–90.

Kirkham 2009a. V. Kirkham, 'Chronology of Petrarch's Life and Works', in V. Kirkham and A. Maggi (eds), *Petrarch: A Critical Guide to the Complete Works*. Chicago: Chicago University Press, pp. xv–xxii.

Kirkham 2009b. V. Kirkham, 'Petrarch the Courtier: Five Public Speeches (*Arenga fact Venecijs, Arringa facta Mediolani, Arenga facta in civitate Novarie, Collatio brevis coram Iohanne Francorum rege, Orazione per la seconda ambasceria veneziana*)', in V. Kirkham and A. Maggi (eds), *Petrarch: A Critical Guide to the Complete Works*. Chicago: Chicago University Press, pp. 141–50.

Klemm and De Leemens 2005. M. Klemm and P. De Leemens, 'Pietro d'Abano', in T. Glick, F. Wallis and S.J. Livesey (eds), *Medieval Science, Technology and Medicine: An Encyclopedia*. New York: Routledge, pp. 404–5.

Knuuttila 2004. S. Knuuttila, *Emotions in Ancient and Medieval Philosophy*. Oxford: Oxford University Press.

Kohl 1968. B.G. Kohl, 'The Signoria of Francesco Il Vecchio da Carrara in Padua, 1350–1388'. Baltimore: Johns Hopkins University. Unpublished PhD thesis.

Kohl 1974. B.G. Kohl, 'Petrarch's Prefaces to *De viris illustribus*', *History and Theory* 13, pp. 132–44.

Kohl 1977. B.G. Kohl, 'Carrara, Francesco da, Il Vecchio', *Dizionario Biografico degli Italiani*, vol. 20, pp. 649–56.

Kohl 1983. B.G. Kohl, 'Conversini, Giovanni', *Dizionario Biografico degli Italiani*, vol. 28, pp. 574–8.

Kohl 1989. B.G. Kohl, 'Giusto de' Menabuoi e il mecentismo artistico', in A.M. Spiazzi (ed.), *Giusto de' Menabuoi nel Battistero di Padova*. Trieste: Lint, pp. 24–6.

Kohl 1998. B.G. Kohl, *Padua under the Carrara, 1318–1405*. Baltimore: Johns Hopkins University Press.

Kohl 2001. B.G. Kohl, 'Fina da Carrara, née Buzzacarini: Consort, Mother, and Patron of Art in Trecento Padua', in S. Reiss and D. Wilkins (eds), *Beyond Isabella: Secular Women Patrons of Art in Renaissance Italy* (Sixteenth-Century Essays and Studies 54). Kirksville, MO: Truman State University Press, pp. 19–37.

Kohl 2002. B.G. Kohl, 'La Corte Carrarese, i Lupi di Soragna e la committenza artistica al Santo', *Il Santo* 42, pp. 317–27.

Kohl 2007. B.G. Kohl, 'Chronicles into Legends and Lives: Two Humanist Accounts of the Carrara Dynasty in Padua', in S. Dale, A. Williams Lewin and D.J. Osheim (eds), *Chronicling History: Chroniclers and Historians in Medieval and Renaissance Italy*. University Park: Pennsylvania State University Press, pp. 223–48.

Kraye 2005. J. Kraye, 'Pseudo-Aristotle', in T. Glick, F. Wallis and S.J. Livesey (eds), *Medieval Science, Technology and Medicine: An Encyclopedia*. New York: Routledge, pp. 423–5.

Kristeller 1978. P.O. Kristeller, 'Philosophy and Medicine in Medieval and Renaissance Italy', in S.F. Spicker (ed.), *Organism, Medicine, and Metaphysics: Essays in Honor of Hans Jonas on His 75th Birthday, May 10, 1978* (Philosophy and Medicine 7). Dordrecht: Springer Netherlands, pp. 29–40.

Kristeller 1979. P.O. Kristeller, *Renaissance Thought and Its Sources*. New York: Columbia University Press.

Kristeller 1988. P.O. Kristeller, 'Humanism', in C.B. Schmitt, Q. Skinner and E. Kessler (eds), *The Cambridge History of Renaissance Philosophy*. Cambridge: Cambridge University Press, pp. 113–37.

Kyle 2010. S.R. Kyle, 'The *Carrara Herbal* in Context: Imitation, Exemplarity, and Invention in Late Fourteenth-Century Padua'. Atlanta: Emory University. Unpublished PhD thesis.

Kyle 2014. S.R. Kyle, 'A New Heraldry: Vision and Rhetoric in the *Carrara Herbal*', in W.S. Melion, M. Weeman and B. Rothstein (eds), *The Anthropomorphic Lens: Anthropomorphism, Microcosmism and Analogy in Early Modern Thought and Visual Arts* (Intersections 34). Leiden: Brill, pp. 231–50.

Kyle 2015. S.R. Kyle, 'Ancestral Memory and Petrarch's *De Remediis utriusque fortunae* in Carrara Padua', *Mediaevalia* 35, pp. 177–92.

Lazzarini 1901–1902. V. Lazzarini, 'Libri di Francesco Novello da Carrara', *Atti e memorie dell'Accademia Patavina di scienze, lettere ed arti* 18, pp. 25–36.

Lazzarini 1934. V. Lazzarini, 'Statuto che conferisce la Signoria a Francesco I da Carrara', *Archivio Veneto*, ser. 5, 16, pp. 284–90.

Littlewood et al. 2002. A. Littlewood, H. Maguire and J. Wolschke-Bulmahn (eds), *Byzantine Garden Culture*. Washington, DC: Dumbarton Oaks.

Lockwood 1951. D.P. Lockwood, *Ugo Benzi, Medieval Philosopher and Physician, 1376–1439*. Chicago: University of Chicago Press.

Lorenzoni 1977. G. Lorenzoni, 'L'intervenuto dei Carraresi, la Reggia e il Castello', in L. Puppi and F. Zuliani (eds), *Padova: case e palazzi*. Vicenza: Neri Pozza, pp. 29–45.

MacLaren 2010. S. MacLaren, 'Giotto's Envy and Francesco da Barberino's Renown: Naturalism, Personification, and Artistic Innovation', paper presented at the annual meeting for the College Art Association. Chicago, Illinois, February 10–13.

Maggiulli and Buffa Giolito 1996. G. Maggiulli and M.F. Buffa Giolito, *L'altro Apuleio: problemi aperti per una nuova edizione dell'Herbarius*. Naples: Loffredo.

Malagola 1888. C. Malagola (ed.), *Statuti delle Università e dei collegi dello studio bolognese*. Bologna: Zanichelli.

Manca 2001. J. Manca, 'Moral Stance in Italian Renaissance Art: Images, Text, and Meaning', *Artibus et Historiae* 22, pp. 51–76.

Mango and Ševčenko 1961. C. Mango and I. Ševčenko, 'Remains of the Church of St. Polyeuktos at Constantinople', *Dumbarton Oaks Papers* 15, pp. 243–7.

Manzalaoui 1961. M.A. Manzalaoui, 'The *Secreta secretorum*. The Medieval European Version of *Kitāb Sirr ul-Asrār*', *Bulletin of the Faculty of Arts* (Alexandria) 15, pp. 83–107.

Manzalaoui 1974. M.A. Manzalaoui, 'The Pseudo-Aristotelian *Kitab Sirr Al-Asrar*: Facts and Problems', *Oriens* 23–24, pp. 147–257.

Manzalaoui 1977. M.A. Manzalaoui (ed.), *Secretum Secretorum: Nine English Versions*. Oxford: Oxford University Press.

Mardersteig 1974. G. Mardersteig, 'I ritratti del Petrarca e dei suoi amici di Padova', *Italia medioevale e umanistica* 17, pp. 251–80.

Mariani Canova 1988. G. Mariani Canova, 'La traduzione europea degli erbari miniati e la scuolo veneta', in R. Bussi (ed.), *Di sana pianta: erbari e taccuini di sanità. Le radici storiche della nuova farmacologia*. Modena: Panini, pp. 21–8.

Mariani Canova 1994. G. Mariani Canova, 'La miniatura Padovano nel periodo Carrarese', in A.M. Spiazzi (ed.), *Attorno a Giusto de' Menabuoi: Aggiornamenti e studi sulla pittura a Padova nel Trecento: atti della giornata di studio 18 dicembre 1990*. Treviso: Zoppelli, pp. 19–40.

Mariani Canova 1999. G. Mariani Canova, 'Serapion il Giovane, *Liber Agregà*', in G. Mariani Canova, G. Baldissin Molli and F. Toniolo (eds), *Parole Dipinte. La Miniatura a Padova dal Medioevo al Settecento*. Modena: Panini, pp. 154–7.

Mariani Canova et al. 1999. G. Mariani Canova, G. Baldissin Molli and F. Toniolo (eds), *Parole Dipinte. La miniatura a Padova dal Medioevo al Settecento*. Modena: Panini.

Martellotti 1949. G. Martellotti, 'Linee di sviluppo dell'umanesimo petrarchesco', *Studi Petrarcheschi* 2, pp. 51–80.

Marti 1960. M. Marti, 'Aldobrandino da Siena', *Dizionario Biografico degli Italiani*, vol. 2, p. 115.

Marvin 1880. W.T.R. Marvin, *The Carrara Medals with Notices of the Dukes of Padua Whose Effigies They Bear*. With some additions and changes from the original printing in the *American Journal of Numismatics*, January 1880 ed. Boston: The Author.

Mazal 1981. O. Mazal, *Pflanzen, Wurzeln, Säfte, Samen: antike Heilkunst in Miniaturen des Wiener Dioskurides*. Graz: Akademische Druck- und Verlagsanstalt.

Mazal 1998. O Mazal (ed.), *Der Wiener Dioskurides. Codex medicus Graecus 1 der Österreichen Nationalbibliothek*, 2 vols (Glanzlichter der Buchkunst 8). Graz: Akademische Druck- und Verlagsanstalt.

Mazzatini 1886a. G, Mazzatini, 'Alcuni codici latini Visconteo-Sforzeschi della Biblioteca Nazionale di Parigi', *Archivio storico Lombardo* 13, pp. 17–58.

Mazzatini 1886b. G, Mazzatini, *Inventario dei manoscritti italiani dei biblioteche di Francia*, vol. 1, *Manoscritti italiani della Biblioteca Nazionale di Parigi*. Rome: Presso i principali Librai.

Matter 1997. E.A. Matter, 'The Church Fathers and the *Glossa Ordinaria*', in I. Backus (ed.), *The Reception of the Church Fathers in the West: From the Carolingians to the Maurists*. Leiden: Brill, pp. 83–112.

McManamon 1996. J.M. McManamon, *Pierpaolo Vergerio the Elder: The Humanist as Orator* (Medieval and Renaissance Texts & Studies 163). Binghamton, NY: MRTS.

McVaugh 1971. M. McVaugh, 'Constantine the African', in C.C. Gillespie (ed.), *Dictionary of Scientific Biography*, vol. 3, pp. 393–5.

Medin 1908. A. Medin, 'I ritratti autentici di Francesco il Vecchio e di Francesco Novello da Carrara', *Bolletino del Museo civico di Padova* 11, pp. 100–4.

Mellini 1965. G.L. Mellini, *Altichiero e Jacopo Avanzi*. Milan: Edizioni di Comunità.

Meri 2006. J. Meri (ed.), *Medieval Islamic Civilization: An Encyclopedia*, 2 vols. New York: Routledge.

Minio-Paluello 1949. L. Minio-Paluello, 'Il "Fedone" Latino con note autografe del Petrarca', *Accademia Nazionale dei Lincei: Rendiconti della Classe di Scienze Morali* 8, pp. 107–13.

Moly Mariotti 1993. F. Moly Mariotti, 'Contribution à la connaissance des *Tacuina Sanitatis* Lombards', *Arte Lombarda* n.s. 104, pp. 32–9.

Mommsen 1952. T.E. Mommsen, 'Petrarch and the Decoration of the Sala Virorum Illustrium in Padua', *Art Bulletin* 34, pp. 95–116.

Mommsen 1957. T.E. Mommsen, *Petrarch's Testament*. Ithaca, NY: Cornell University Press.

Mor 1964a. C.G. Mor (ed.), *Il Palazzo della Ragione di Padova*. Venice: Neri Pozza.

Mor 1964b. C.G. Mor, 'Il Palazzo della Ragione nella vita di Padova', in C.G. Mor (ed.), *Il Palazzo della Ragione di Padova*. Venice: Neri Pozza, pp. 1–20.

Müller 2012. A.E. Müller, 'Ein vermeintlich fester Anker. Das Jahr 512 als zeitlicher Ansatz des "Wiener Dioskurides"', *Jahrbuch der Österreichischen Byzantinistik* 62, pp. 103–9.

Murray 1953. P. Murray, 'Notes on Some Early Giotto Sources', *Journal of the Warburg and Courtauld Institutes* 16, pp. 58–80.

Nagel and Wood 2010. A. Nagel and C.S. Wood, *Anachronic Renaissance*. New York: Zone Books.

Nathan 2010. G. Nathan, 'The *Vienna Dioscorides*' Dedicatio to Anicia Juliana: A Usurpation of Imperial Patronage?', *Byzantina Australiensa* 17 (G. Nathan [ed.], *Basileia. Imperium and Culture in Byzantium. Papers in Honour of Elizabeth and Michael Jeffreys*), pp. 95–102.

Nolhac 1891. P. de Nolhac, 'Le *De Viris Illustribus* de Pétrarque: notice sur les manuscrits originaux, suivie de fragments inédits', *Notices et extraits des manuscrits de la Bibliothèque nationale et autres bibliothèques, publiés par l'institut national de France* 34, pp. 61–148.

Nolhac 1907. P. de Nolhac, *Pétrarque et l'humanisme*, 2 vols. Paris: Honoré Champion (Abridged English translation: *Petrarch and the Ancient World*. Boston: D.B. Updike, 1907).

Norman 1995a. D. Norman, 'Astrology, Antiquity and Empiricism: Art and Learning', in D. Norman (ed.), *Siena, Florence and Padua: Art, Society and Religion 1280–1400*, 2 vols. New Haven: Yale University Press, vol. 1 (Interpretative Essays), pp. 197–216.

Norman 1995b. D. Norman, '"Splendid Models and Examples from the Past": Carrara Patronage of Art', in D. Norman (ed.), *Siena, Florence and Padua: Art, Society and Religion 1280–1400*, 2 vols. New Haven: Yale University Press, vol. 1 (Interpretative Essays), pp. 155–76.

Norman 1995c. D. Norman, '"The Glorious Deeds of the Commune": Civic Patronage of Art', in D. Norman (ed.), *Siena, Florence and Padua: Art, Society and Religion 1280–1400*, 2 vols. New Haven: Yale University Press, vol. 1 (Interpretative Essays), pp. 134–53.

Norman 1995d. D. Norman, 'Those Who Pay, Those Who Pray and Those Who Paint: Two Funerary Chapels', in D. Norman (ed.), *Siena, Florence and Padua: Art, Society and Religion 1280–1400*, 2 vols. New Haven: Yale University Press, vol. 2 (Case Studies), pp. 169–94.

Nutton 1985a. V. Nutton, 'Humanistic Surgery', in A. Wear, R.K. French and I.M. Lonie (eds), *The Medical Renaissance of the Sixteenth Century*. Cambridge: Cambridge University Press, pp. 75–99.

Nutton 1985b. V. Nutton, 'John Caius and the Eton Galen: Medical Philology in the Renaissance', *Medizenhistorisches Journal* 20, pp. 227–52.

Nutton 1988. V. Nutton, 'Prisci Dissectionum Professores: Greek Texts and Renaissance Anatomists', in A.C. Dionisotti, A. Grafton and J. Kraye (eds), *The Uses of Greek and Latin: Historical Essays*. London: Warburg Institute, pp. 111–26.

Nutton 1995a. V. Nutton, 'Medicine in the Medieval West', in L.I. Conrad, M. Neve, R. Porter and A. Wear (eds), *The Western Medical Tradition: 800 BC to AD 1800*, 1st ed. Cambridge: Cambridge University Press, pp. 139–205.

Nutton 1995b. V. Nutton, 'The Changing Language of Medicine, 1450–1550', in O. Weijers (ed.), *Vocabulary of Teaching and Research between Middle Ages and Renaissance: Proceedings of the Colloquium, London, Warburg Institute, 11–12 March 1994* (Études sur le vocabulaire intellectuel du Moyen Âge 8). Turnhout: Brepols, pp. 184–98.

Nutton 1997. V. Nutton, 'The Rise of Medical Humanism: Ferrara, 1464–1555', *Renaissance Studies* 11, pp. 2–19.

Nutton 2004. V. Nutton, 'Galen of Pergamum', in H. Cancik, H. Schneider and C.F. Salazar (eds), *Brill's New Pauly: Encyclopaedia of the Ancient World*. Leiden: Brill, vol. 5, cols 654–61.

Nutton 2008. V Nutton, 'Focus: Islamic Medicine and Pharmacy: Ancient Mediterranean Pharmacology and Cultural Transfer', *European Review* 16, pp. 211–17.

Nutton 2013. V. Nutton, *Ancient Medicine*, 2nd ed. New York: Routledge.

O'Kane 2003. B. O'Kane, *Early Persian Painting: Kalila and Dimna Manuscripts of the Late Fourteenth Century*. New York: I.B. Tauris.

Ogilvie 2005. B.W. Ogilvie, 'Natural History, Ethics, and Physio-Theology', in G. Pomata and N.G. Siraisi (eds), *Historia: Empiricism and Erudition in Early Modern Europe*. Cambridge, MA: MIT Press, pp. 75–103.

Ogilvie 2006. B.W. Ogilvie, *The Science of Describing: Natural History in Renaissance Europe*. Chicago: University of Chicago Press.

Olivi 1888. L. Olivi, 'Del matrimonio del marchese Nicolò III d'Este con Gigliola figlia di Francesco Novello da Carrara', *Atti e memorie della R. deputazione di storia patria di Modena e Parma*, ser. 3, 5, pp. 335–76.

Olson 1982. G. Olson, *Literature as Recreation in the Later Middle Ages*. Ithaca: Cornell University Press.

Ongaro 2005. G. Ongaro, 'La medicina durante la signoria dei Carraresi', in O. Longo (ed.), *Padova Carrarese*. Padua: Il Poligrafo, pp. 185–202.

Opsomer-Halleux 1978. C. Opsomer-Halleux, 'Un botaniste du XIVe siècle. Manfredus de Monte Imperiale', *XVth Congress of the History of Science, Abstracts of Scientific Section Papers* 38. Edinburgh: Edinburgh University Press, pp. 10–9.

Opsomer-Halleux 1991. C. Opsomer-Halleux, *L'art du vivre en santé: images et recettes du Moyen Âge (le Tacuinum Sanitatis [manuscript 1041] de la Bibliothèque de l'Université de Liège)*. Alleur (Belgique): Ed. du Perron.

Opsomer-Halleux 2003. C. Opsomer-Halleux, 'Le scribe, l'enlumineur et le commanditaire: à propos des *Tacuina sanitatis* illustrés', in H. Spilling (ed.), *La collaboration dans la production de l'écrit médiéval, Actes du XIIIe colloque international de paléographie Latine (Weingarten, 22–25 Septembre 2000)* (Matériaux pour l'histoire 4). Paris: Ecole nationale des Chartres, pp. 183–92.

Orofino 1990. G. Orofino, 'Gli erbari di età sveva', *Schede Medievali* 19, pp. 325–46.

Orofino 1991. G. Orofino, 'Dioskurides war gegen Pflanzenbilder', *Die Waage* 4, pp. 144–9.

Osler 2007. N. Osler, *Ad Infinitum: A Biography of Latin*. London: Harper Press.

Pächt 1950. O. Pächt, 'Early Italian Nature Studies and the Early Calendar Landscape', *Journal of the Warburg and Courtauld Institutes* 13, pp. 13–47.

Paganelli and Cappelletti 1996. F. Paganelli and E.M. Cappelletti, 'Il codice erbario *Roccabonella* (sec. XV) e suo contributo alla storia della farmacia', *Atti e memorie dell'Accademia Patavina di scienze, lettere ed arti* 13, pp. 111–6.

Pallucchini 1964. R. Pallucchini, *La pittura Veneziana del Trecento*. Venice: Istituto per la collaborazione culturale.

Paravicini Bagliani 1991. A. Paravicini Bagliani, *Medicina e scienze della natura alla corte dei papi nel duecento* (Società Internazionale per lo Studio del Medioevo Latino, Biblioteca di Medioevo Latino 4). Spoleto: Centro Italiano di Studi sull' Alto Medioevo.

Pardo 1997. M. Pardo, 'Giotto and the "Things Not Seen, Hidden in the Shadow of Natural Ones"', *Artibus et Historiae* 18, pp. 41–53.

Pavord 2005. A. Pavord, *The Naming of Names: The Search for Order in the World of Plants*. New York: Bloomsbury.

Pélissier 1899. L.G. Pélissier, 'La bibliothèque du seigneur de Padoue en 1404', in F. Bournon and F. Mazerolle (eds), *La Correspondance Historique et Archéologique. Organe d'informations mutuelles entre historiens et Archéologues*. Paris: Fontemoing 6, pp. 177–80.

Pellegrin 1951. E. Pellegrin, 'Nouveaux manuscrits annoté par Pétrarque à la Bibliothèque nationale de Paris', *Scriptorium* 5, pp. 265–78.

Pellegrin 1955. E. Pellegrin, *La Bibliothèque des Viscontis et des Sforza, ducs de Milan, au XVe siècle*. Paris: C.N.R.S.

Pellegrin 1969. E. Pellegrin, *La Bibliothèque des Viscontis et des Sforza, ducs de Milan, au XVe siècle. Supplement*. Paris: C.N.R.S.

Pender and Struever 2012. S. Pender and N.S. Struever (eds), *Rhetoric and Medicine in Early Modern Europe*. Burlington, VT: Ashgate.

Pesenti Marangon 1976. T. Pesenti Marangon, 'Michele Savonarola a Padova: l'ambiente, le opere, la cultura', *Quaderni per la storia dell'Università di Padova* 9–10, pp. 45–102.

Pesenti Marangon 1999. T. Pesenti Marangon, '*Studio dei farmaci e produzione di commenti nell' Università di arti e medicina di Padova nel primo ventennio del Trecento*', *Annali di storia delle università italiane*, 3, pp. 61–78.

Peterson 1993. K.E. Peterson, 'Translatio libri Avicennae *De Viribus Cordis* et *Medicinis Cordialibus* de Arnaldi de Villanova'. Cambridge, MA: Harvard University. Unpublished PhD thesis.

Petrucci 1995. A. Petrucci, *Writers and Readers in Medieval Italy: Studies in the History of Written Culture*. New Haven: Yale University Press.

Plant 1981. M. Plant, 'Portraits and Politics in Late Trecento Padua: Altichiero's Frescoes in the San Felice Chapel, San Antonio', *Art Bulletin* 63, pp. 406–25.

Plant 1987. M. Plant, 'Patronage in the Circle of the Carrara Family: Padua, 1337–1405', in F.W. Kent and P. Simons (eds), *Patronage, Art and Society in Renaissance Italy*. Oxford: Clarendon, pp. 177–200.

Pomata and Siraisi 2005. G. Pomata and N.G. Siraisi (eds), *Historia: Empiricism and Erudition in Early Modern Europe*. Cambridge, MA, and London: MIT Press.

Premerstein 1903. A. von Premerstein, 'Anicia Juliana im Wiener Dioskorides-Kodex', *Jahrbuch der Kunsthistorischen Sammlungen des Allerhöchsten Kaiserhauses* 24, pp. 105–24.

Premerstein et al. 1906. A. von Premerstein, C. Wessely and I. Mantuani, *De Codicis Dioscuridei Aniciae Iulianae picturis illustratus, nunc Vindobonensis. Med. Gr. 1. Historia, forma, scriptura, picturis*, 2 vols. Leiden: A.W. Sijthoff.

Premuda 1970. L. Premuda, 'Abano, Pietro d'', in C.C. Gillespie (ed.), *Dictionary of Scientific Bibliography*, vol. 1, pp. 4–5.

Pritchard 1989. T. Pritchard, 'Aristotle's Advice to Alexander: Two English Metrical Versions of an Alexandreis Passage', *Journal of the Warburg and Courtauld Institutes* 52, pp. 209–13.

Rajna 1875. P. Rajna, 'Le origini delle famiglie Padovane e gli eroi dei Romanzi cavallereschi', *Romania* 4, pp. 161–83.

Rawski 1991. C.H. Rawski (ed. and tr.), *Remedies for Fortune Fair and Foul: A Modern English Translation of* De Remediis Utriusque Fortune*, with a Commentary*. Bloomington: Indiana University Press.

Reeds 1976. K. Reeds, 'Medical Humanism and Botany', *Annals of Science* 33, pp. 519–42.

Reeds 1991. K. Reeds, *Botany in Medieval and Renaissance Universities*. New York: Garland.

Rice 1959. D.S. Rice, 'The Oldest Illustrated Arabic Manuscript', *Bulletin of the School of Oriental and African Studies* 22, pp. 207–20.

Richards 2000. J. Richards, *Altichiero: An Artist and His Patrons in the Italian Trecento*. Cambridge and New York: Cambridge University Press.

Richards 2007. J. Richards, *Petrarch's Influence on the Iconography of the Carrara Palace in Padua: The Conflict between Ancestral and Antique Themes in the Fourteenth Century*. Lewiston, NY: Edwin Mellen.

Richter-Bernburg 2006. L. Richter-Bernburg, 'Al-Razi, or Rhazes', in J. Meri (ed.), *Medieval Islamic Civilization: An Encyclopedia*, 2 vols. New York: Routledge, vol. 2, pp. 671–3.

Riddle 1971. J.M. Riddle, 'Dioscorides', in C.C. Gillespie (ed.), *Dictionary of Scientific Biography*, vol. 4, pp. 119–23.

Riddle 1974. J.M. Riddle, 'Theory and Practice in Medieval Medicine', *Viator* 5, pp. 157–84.

Riddle 1980. J.M. Riddle, 'Dioscorides', in P.O. Kristeller and F.E. Crantz (eds), *Catalogus translationum et commentariorum: Medieval and Renaissance Latin Translations and Commentaries. Annotated Lists and Guides*. Washington, DC: Catholic University of America Press, vol. 4, pp. 1–143.

Riddle 1981. J.M. Riddle, 'Pseudo-Dioscorides' *Ex Herbis Femininis* and Early Medieval Medical Botany', *Journal of the History of Biology* 14, pp. 43–82.

Riddle 1986. J.M. Riddle, *Dioscorides on Pharmacy and Medicine*. Austin: Texas University Press.

Riva 2001. E. Riva, 'The XV Century Venetian Illuminated Herbaria', *Acta XXXIV Congressus Internationalis Historiae Pharmaciae* (Firenze 20–23 ottobre, 1999). Piacenza: Accademia Italiana di Storia della Farmacia, unpaginated.

Rizzoli 1932. L. Rizzoli, 'Ritratti di Francesco il Vecchio e di Francesco Novello da Carrara in medaglie ed affreschi Padovani nel secolo XIV', *Bolletino del Museo Civico di Padova* 25, pp. 104–14.

Robert 2011. J.-N. Robert, *L'Empire des loisirs. L'otium des Romains* (L'antiquité par ses textes 15). Paris: Belles Lettres.

Rodgers 2002. R. Rodgers, 'Garden Making and Garden Culture in the Geoponika', in A. Littlewood, H. Maguire, and J. Wolschke-Bulmahn (eds), *Byzantine Garden Culture*. Washington, DC: Dumbarton Oaks, pp. 159–75.

Roscoe 1799. W. Roscoe, *The Life of Lorenzo de' Medici, Called the Magnificent*, 4 vols. Basil: Tourneisen.

Ruggles 2000. D.F. Ruggles, *Gardens, Landscape, and Vision in the Palaces of Islamic Spain*. University Park: Pennsylvania State University Press.

Ruska and Kahl 2000. J. Ruska and O. Kahl, 'Tifashi', in P.J. Bearman, Th. Bianquis, C.E. Bosworth, E. van Donzel and W.P. Heinrichs (eds), *The Encyclopaedia of Islam*, 2nd ed. Leiden: Brill, vol. 10, p. 476.

Saalman 1987. H. Saalman, 'Carrara Burials in the Baptistery of Padua', *Art Bulletin* 69, pp. 376–94.

Saccocci 2005. A Saccocci, '"Moneta mea nova non obstante": zecca e monete in epoca carrarese', in O. Longo (ed.), *Padova Carrarese*. Padua: Il Poligrafo, pp. 83–94.

Saccocci 2014. A. Saccocci, 'L'héraldique et l'iconographie des Carrara de Padoue sur les monnaies, les sceaux, les miniatures et les fresques (1338–1405)', in Y. Loskoutoff (ed.), *Héraldique et numismatique. Moyen Âge – Temps modernes*, 2 vols. Mont-Saint-Aignan: Publications de l'Université de Rouen et du Havre, vol. 2, pp. 181–204.

Sadek 1983. M.M. Sadek, *The Arabic Materia Medica of Dioscorides*. St-Jean-Chrysostome (QC): Les Éditions du Sphinx.

Sarton and Thorndike 1928. G. Sarton and L. Thorndike, 'Tacuinum', *Isis* 10, pp. 489–93.

Scarborough 2002. J. Scarborough, 'Herbs of the Field and Herbs of the Garden in Byzantine Medicinal Pharmacy', in A. Littlewood, H. Maguire and J. Wolschke-Bulmahn (eds), *Byzantine Garden Culture*. Washington, DC: Dumbarton Oaks, pp. 176–88.

Scarborough and Nutton 1982. J. Scarborough and V. Nutton, 'The Preface to Dioscorides' *Materia medica*: introduction, translation, and commentary', *Transactions and Studies of the College of Physicians of Philadelphia*, ser. 5, 4, pp. 187–227.

Schlosser 1895. J. von Schlosser, 'Ein Veronesisches Bilderbuch und die höfische Kunst des XIV. Jahrhunderts', *Jarhbuch der Kunsthistorischen Sammlungen des Allerhöchsten Kaiserhauses* 16, pp. 183–93.

Schmitt 1974. A. Schmitt, 'Zur Wiederbelebung der Antike im Trecento. Petrarcas Rom-Idee in ihrer Wirkung und die Paduaner Malerei', *Mitteilungen des Kunsthistorischen Institutes in Florenz* 17, pp. 167–218.

Segre Rutz 2000. V. Segre Rutz, 'Il *Tacuinum Sanitatis* di Verde Visconti e la miniature Milanese di fine Trecento', *Arte Cristiana* 88, pp. 375–90.

Segre Rutz 2002. V. Segre Rutz, '*Historia Plantarum*. Erbe, oro e medicina nei codici medievali', in V. Segre Rutz, E. Lazzarini, M. di Vito and S. Panini (eds), *Historia plantarum: Ms 459 Biblioteca Casanatense, l'enciclopedia medica dell'imperatore Venceslao*, 2 vols. Modena: Franco Cosimo Panini, vol. 2, pp. 11–202.

Segre Rutz et al. 2002. V. Segre Rutz, E. Lazzarini, M. di Vito and S. Panini (eds), *Historia plantarum: Ms 459 Biblioteca Casanatense, l'enciclopedia medica dell'imperatore Venceslao*, 2 vols. Modena: Franco Cosimo Panini.

Serrano Ruano 2006. D. Serrano Ruano, 'Al-Andalus', in J. Meri (ed.), *Medieval Islamic Civilization: An Encyclopedia*, 2 vols. New York: Routledge, vol. 1, pp. 43–4.

Shah 1966. M.H. Shah, *The General Principles of Avicenna's Canon of Medicine*. Karachi: Naveed Clinic.

Sharples 1995. R.W. Sharples, *Theophrastus of Eresus. Sources for his life, writings, thought and influence*, Commentary Volume 5: Sources on Biology (Human Physiology, Living Creatures, Botany: Texts 328–435). Leiden: Brill.

Shusterman 1999. R. Shusterman, 'Somaesthetics: A Disciplinary Proposal', *The Journal of Aesthetics and Art Criticism* 57, pp. 299–313.

Shusterman 2008. R. Shusterman, *Body Consciousness: A Philosophy of Mindfulness and Somaesthetics*. Cambridge and New York: Cambridge University Press.

Sigerist and Howald 1927. H. Sigerist and E. Howald (eds), *Apuleius Barbarus, Antonii musae de herba vettonica liber; Pseudo-Apulei herbarius; anonymi de taxone liber; sexti placiti liber medicinae ex animalibus etc* (Corpus Medicorum Latinorum 4). Leipzig: Teubner.

Sigler 1992. L.A. Sigler, 'The Genre of Gender: Images of Working Women in the *Tacuinum Sanitatis*'. Los Angeles: University of California. Unpublished PhD thesis.

Singer 1927. C. Singer, 'The Herbal in Antiquity and Its Transmission to Later Ages', *Journal of Hellenic Studies* 47, pp. 1–52.

Siraisi 1970. N.G. Siraisi, 'The *Expositio Problematum Aristotelis* of Peter of Abano', *Isis* 61, pp. 321–39.

Siraisi 1973. N.G. Siraisi, *Arts and Sciences at Padua: The Studium of Padua Before 1350*. Toronto: Pontifical Institute of Mediaeval Studies.

Siraisi 1981. N.G. Siraisi, *Taddeo Alderotti and His Pupils*. Princeton: Princeton University Press.

Siraisi 1985. N.G. Siraisi, 'Pietro d'Abano and Taddeo Alderotti: Two Modes of Medical Culture', *Medioevo* 11, pp. 138–62 (repr. as 'Two Models of Medical Culture, Pietro d'Abano and Taddeo Alderotti', in N.G. Siraisi, *Medicine and the Italian Universities 1250–1600* [Education and Society in the Middle Ages and Renaissance 12]. Leiden: Brill, 2001, pp. 79–99).

Siraisi 1987a. N.G. Siraisi, *Avicenna in Renaissance Italy: The Canon and Medical Teaching in Italian Universities after 1500*. Princeton: Princeton University Press.

Siraisi 1987b. N.G. Siraisi, 'The Physician's Task: Medical Reputations in Humanist Collective Biographies', in N.G. Siraisi and A.C. Crombie (eds), *The Rational Arts of Living* (Smith College Studies in History 50). Northampton, MA: Department of History, Smith College, pp. 105–33 (repr. in N.G. Siraisi, *Medicine and the Italian Universities 1250–1600* [Education and Society in the Middle Ages and Renaissance 12]. Leiden: Brill, 2001, pp. 157–83).

Siraisi 1990. N.G. Siraisi, *Medieval and Early Renaissance Medicine*. Chicago: Chicago University Press.

Siraisi 1994. N.G. Siraisi, 'Il Canone di Avicenna e l'insegnamento della medicina pratica in Europa', in F. Vanozzi (ed.), *L'insegnamento della medicina in Europa (secoli XIV–XIX). Atti del Convegno tenutosi a Siena in occasione delle celebrazioni del 750 anni dalla fondazione dell' Università di Siena* (Monografie di Quaderni Internazionali di Storia della Medicina e della Sanità 6). Siena: Typografia Senese, pp. 9–24 (English translation cited here: 'Avicenna and the Teaching of Practical Medicine', in N.G. Siraisi, *Medicine and the Italian Universities 1250–1600* [Education and Society in the Middle Ages and Renaissance 12]. Leiden: Brill, 2001, pp. 63–78).

Siraisi 2001a. N.G. Siraisi, Introduction to *Medicine and the Italian Universities, 1250–1600* (Education and Society in the Middle Ages and Renaissance 12). Leiden: Brill, pp. 1–10.

Siraisi 2001b. N.G. Siraisi, *Medicine and the Italian Universities, 1250–1600* (Education and Society in the Middle Ages and Renaissance 12). Leiden: Brill.

Siraisi 2003. N.G. Siraisi, 'History, Antiquarianism, and Medicine: The Case of Girolamo Mercuriale', *Journal of the History of Ideas* 64, pp. 231–51.

Siraisi 2004. N.G. Siraisi, 'Oratory and Rhetoric in Renaissance Medicine', *Journal of the History of Ideas* 65, pp. 191–211.

Siraisi 2007. N.G. Siraisi, *History, Medicine, and the Traditions of Renaissance Learning*. Ann Arbor: University of Michigan Press.

Skinner 1978. Q. Skinner, *The Foundations of Modern Political Thought*, vol. 1: The Renaissance. Cambridge and New York: Cambridge University Press.

Skinner 2002. Q. Skinner, *Visions of Politics: Renaissance Virtues*, 2 vols. Cambridge and New York: Cambridge University Press.

Smalley 1941. B. Smalley, *The Study of the Bible in the Middle Ages*. Oxford: Oxford University Press.

Stacey 2007. P. Stacey, *Roman Monarchy and the Renaissance Prince*. Cambridge and New York: Cambridge University Press.

Stannard 1999. J. Stannard, *Herbs and Herbalism in the Middle Ages and Renaissance*. Aldershot and Brookfield, VT: Ashgate Variorum.

Struever 1993. N.S. Struever, 'Petrarch's *Invective Contra Medicum*: An Early Confrontation of Rhetoric and Medicine', *Modern Language Notes* 108, pp. 659–79.

Stubblebine 1969. J.H. Stubblebine, *Giotto: The Arena Chapel Frescoes*. New York: Norton.

Sutton 1991. K. Sutton, 'Milanese Luxury Books: The Patronage of Bernabò Visconti', *Apollo* 13, pp. 322–6.

Sutton 1993. K. Sutton, 'Giangaleazzo Visconti as Patron: A Prayer Book Illuminated by Pietro da Pavia', *Apollo* 137, pp. 89–96.

Terry-Fritsch 2012. A. Terry-Fritsch, 'Florentine Convent as Practiced Place: Cosimo de' Medici, Fra Angelico and the Public Library of San Marco', *Medieval Encounters* 18, pp. 230–71.

Thomann 1991. J. Thomann, 'Pietro d'Abano on Giotto', *Journal of the Warburg and Courtauld Institutes* 54, pp. 238–44.

Thomas 1911. A. Thomas, 'Les manuscrits français et provençaux des ducs de Milan au châteaux de Pavie', *Romania* 40, pp. 571–609.

Thomas 1912. A. Thomas, 'Les manuscrits français et provençaux des ducs de Milan au châteaux de Pavie', *Romania* 41, pp. 614–15.

Thorndike 1923–1958. L. Thorndike, *A History of Magic and Experimental Science*, 8 vols. New York: Columbia University Press.

Thorndike 1959. L. Thorndike, '*Consilia* and more works in manuscript by Gentile da Foligno', *Medical History* 3, pp. 8–19.

Thorndike and Kibre 1963. L. Thorndike and P. Kibre, *A Catalogue of Incipits of Mediaeval Scientific Writings in Latin*, rev. ed. Cambridge, MA: Medieval Academy of America.

Toffanin 1988. G. Toffanin, *Cento chiese Padovane scomparse*. Padua: Editoriale Programma.

Toresella 1990. S. Toresella, *L'erbario inedito di P.A. Mattioli. Sono senesi i primi erbari figurati*. Siena: Università degli studi di Siena, Facoltà di Farmacia.

Toubert 1984. P. Toubert, 'Crescenzi, Pietro de', *Dizionario Biografico degli Italiani*, vol. 15, pp. 649–57.

Touwaide 1988. A. Touwaide, 'Les manuscrits illustrés du traité de matière médicale de Dioscoride', in *Proceedings – Congrès International d'Histoire de la Médecine, Düsseldorf, 1986*. Leverkussen: International Society for the History of Medicine, pp. 1148–51.

Touwaide 1992–1993. A. Touwaide, *Farmacopea arabe medieval: Codice Ayasofia 3703*, 4 vols. Milan: Antea.

Touwaide 1994. A. Touwaide, 'Le traité de matière médicale de Dioscorides en Italie depuis la fin de l'Empire Romain jusqu'aux débuts de l'école de Salerne: Essai de Synthèse', *PACT (Journal of the European Study Group on Physical, Chemical, Biological and Mathematical Techniques Applied to Archeology)* 34, pp. 275–305.

Touwaide 1995. A. Touwaide, 'Tradition and Innovation in Mediaeval Arabic Medicine: The Translations and the Heuristic Role of the Word', *Forum: Trends in Experimental and Clinical Medicine* 15, pp. 203–13.

Touwaide 1997. A. Touwaide, 'La thérapeutique médicamenteuse de Dioscoride à Galein: Du pharmaco-centrisme au médico-centrisme', in A. Debru (ed.), *Galen on Pharmacology: Philosophy, History, and Medicine* (Studies in Ancient Medicine 16). Leiden: Brill, pp. 255–82.

Touwaide 2003. A. Touwaide, 'Crateuas', in H. Cancik, H. Schneider and C.F. Salazar (eds), *Brill's New Pauly: Encyclopedia of the Ancient World. Antiquity*. Leiden: Brill, vol. 3, cols 921–2.

Touwaide 2005a. A. Touwaide, 'Botany', in T. Glick, F. Wallis and S.J. Livesey (eds), *Medieval Science, Technology and Medicine: An Encyclopedia*. New York: Routledge, pp. 97–8.

Touwaide 2005b. A. Touwaide, 'Pharmaceutical Handbooks', in T. Glick, F. Wallis and S.J. Livesey (eds), *Medieval Science, Technology and Medicine: An Encyclopedia*. New York: Routledge, pp. 393–4.

Touwaide 2005c. A. Touwaide, 'Pharmacology', in T. Glick, F. Wallis and S.J. Livesey (eds), *Medieval Science, Technology and Medicine: An Encyclopedia*. New York: Routledge, pp. 394–7.

Touwaide 2005d. A. Touwaide, 'Pharmacy and Materia Medica', in T. Glick, F. Wallis and S.J. Livesey (eds), *Medieval Science, Technology and Medicine: An Encyclopedia*. New York: Routledge, pp. 397–9.

Touwaide 2006a. A. Touwaide, 'Botany', in J. Meri (ed.), *Medieval Islamic Civilization: An Encyclopedia*, 2 vols. New York: Routledge, vol. 1, pp. 117–8.

Touwaide 2006b. A. Touwaide, 'Latin Crusaders, Byzantine Herbals', in J. Givens, K. Reeds and A. Touwaide (eds), *Visualizing Medieval Medicine and Natural History, 1200–1550* (AVISTA Studies in the History of Medieval Technology, Science and Art 5). Aldershot: Ashgate, pp. 25–50.

Touwaide 2006c. A. Touwaide, 'The Development of Paleologan Renaissance. An Analysis Based on Dioscorides' *De materia medica*', in M. Cacouros and M.-H. Congourdeau (eds), *Philosophie et sciences à Byzance de 1204 à 1453, Actes de la Table Ronde organisée au XXe Congrès International d'Études Byzantines (Paris, 2001)* (Orientalia Lovaniensia Analecta 146). Leuven: Peeters and Department Oosterse Studies Leuven, pp. 189–224.

Touwaide 2007a. A. Touwaide, 'Art and Sciences: Private Gardens and Botany in the Roman Empire', in M. Conan and W.J. Kress (eds), *Botanical Progress, Horticultural Innovation and Cultural Changes* (Dumbarton Oaks Colloquium on the History of Landscape Architecture 28). Washington, DC: Dumbarton Oaks, pp. 37–50.

Touwaide 2007b. A. Touwaide, 'Oribasius', in H. Cancik, H. Schneider and C.F. Salazar (eds), *Brill's New Pauly: Encyclopedia of the Ancient World. Antiquity*. Leiden: Brill, vol. 10, cols 203–205.

Touwaide 2007c. A. Touwaide, 'Pedanius Dioscorides', in H. Cancik, H. Schneider and C.F. Salazar (eds), *Brill's New Pauly: Encyclopedia of the Ancient World. Antiquity*. Leiden: Brill, vol. 10, cols 670–71.

Touwaide 2008a. A. Touwaide, 'Leoniceno, Nicolò', in N. Koertge (ed.), *New Dictionary of Scientific Biography*, vol. 4, pp. 264–7.

Touwaide 2008b. A. Touwaide, 'Manuscripts', in P.T. Keyser and G.L. Irby-Massie (eds), *The Encyclopedia of Ancient Natural Scientists: The Greek Tradition and Its Many Heirs*. New York: Routledge, pp. 934–6.

Touwaide 2008c. A. Touwaide, 'Pietro d'Abano sui veleni. Tradizione medievale e fonti greche', *Medicina nei Secoli* 20, pp. 591–605.

Touwaide 2009a. A. Touwaide, 'Fluid Picture-Making across Borders, Genres, Media. Botanical Illustration from Byzantium to Baghdad, Ninth to Thirteenth Centuries', in

J. Anderson (ed.), *Crossing Cultures: Conflict, Migration, and Convergence. The Proceedings of the 32nd International Congress in the History of Art (Comité International d'Histoire de l'Art, CIHA), The University of Melbourne, 13–18 January 2008*. Carlton, Australia: Miegunyah Press, pp. 159–63.

Touwaide 2009b. A. Touwaide, 'Pharmacology II: The Arabo-Islamic Cultural Sphere', in M. Landfester and F.G. Gentry (eds), *Brill's New Pauly: Encyclopedia of the Ancient World. Classical Traditions*. Leiden: Brill, vol. 4, cols 362–6.

Touwaide 2009c. A. Touwaide, 'Introduction', in A. Touwaide, E. König and C.M. García-Tejedor, *Tacuinum Sanitatis*. Barcelona: Moleiro, pp. 11–2.

Touwaide 2009d. A. Touwaide, 'A Way of Life', in A. Touwaide, E. König and C.M. García-Tejedor, *Tacuinum Sanitatis*. Barcelona: Moleiro, pp. 14–30.

Touwaide 2009e. A. Touwaide, 'A New Format', in A. Touwaide, E. König and C.M. García-Tejedor, *Tacuinum Sanitatis*. Barcelona: Moleiro, pp. 32–52.

Touwaide 2009f. A. Touwaide, 'Health, Disease and Therapeutics', in A. Touwaide, E. König and C.M. García-Tejedor, *Tacuinum Sanitatis*. Barcelona: Moleiro, pp. 54–74.

Touwaide 2011. A. Touwaide, 'Arabic into Greek: The Rise of an International Lexicon of Medicine in the Medieval Eastern Mediterranean?', in R. Wisnovsky, F. Wallis, J.C. Fumo and C. Fraenkel (eds), *Vehicles of Transmission, Translation, and Transformation in Medieval Textual Culture*. Turnhout: Brepols, pp. 195–222.

Touwaide 2013a. A. Touwaide, 'Forward: In Defense of Medical Tradition', in H. Amri and M.S. Micozzi (eds), *Avicenna's Medicine: A New Translation of the 11th-Century Canon with Practical Applications for Integrative Health Care*. Rochester: Healing Arts Press, pp. ix–xiii.

Touwaide 2013b. A. Touwaide, *Tractatus de Herbis. Sloane Ms. 4016*. Barcelona: Moliero.

Touwaide 2014. A. Touwaide, 'Al-Ghāfiqī's *Kitāb fī l-adwiya al-mufrada*, Dioscorides' *De materia medica*, and Mediterranean Herbal Traditions', in F.J. Ragep, F. Wallis, P. Miller and A. Gacek (eds), *The Herbal of Al-Ghāfiqī. A Facsimile Edition of MS 7508 in the Osler Library of the History of Medicine, McGill University, with Critical Essays*. Montreal and Kington, ON: McGill-Queen's University Press, pp. 84–120.

Trinkaus 1970. C. Trinkaus, *In Our Image and Likeness: Humanity and Divinity in Italian Humanist Thought*, 2 vols. Chicago: Chicago University Press.

Ullman 1923. B.L. Ullman, 'Petrarch's Favourite Books', *Transactions of the American Philological Association* 54, pp. 21–38.

Ullmann 1970. M. Ullmann, *Die Medizin Im Islam*. Leiden: Brill.

Unterkircher 1967. F. Unterkircher, *A Treasury of Illuminated Manuscripts: A Selection of Miniatures from Manuscripts in the Austrian National Library*. New York: Putnam.

Unterkircher 1986. F.Unterkircher (ed.), *Tacuinum Sanitatis in Medicina: Codex Vindobonensis series nova 2644 der Österreichen National Bibliothek*. Rome: Salerno.

Valentinelli 1870. J. Valentinelli, *Bibliotheca Manuscripta ad S. Marci Venetiarum. Codices MSS. Latini Tom. III*. Venice: Ex Typographia Commercii.

Ventura 2009. I. Ventura, 'Introduction', in I. Ventura (ed.), *Tractatus de herbis: MS London, British Library, Egerton 747* (Edizione nazionale: La Scuola Medica Salernitana 5). Florence: SISMEL Edizioni del Galluzzo, pp. 1–188.

Vernet 1971. J. Vernet, 'Ibn al-Bayṭār', in P.J. Bearman, Th. Bianquis, C.E. Bosworth, E. van Donzel and W.P. Heinrichs (eds), *The Encyclopaedia of Islam*, 2nd ed. Leiden: Brill, vol. 3, p. 737.

Vescovini 1986. G.F. Vescovini, 'Pietro d'Abano e gli affreschi astrologici del Palazzo della Ragione di Padova', *Labyrinthos* 9, pp. 50–75.

Vescovini 1996. G.F. Vescovini, 'L'individuale nella medicina tra medioevo e umanesimo: la physiognomica di Michele Savonarola', in R. Cardini and M. Regoliosi (eds), *Umanesimo e Medicina. Il problema dell'individuale* (Humanistica 17). Roma: Bulzoni, pp. 63–87.

Vescovini 2001. G.F. Vescovini, 'La medicina astrologica dello *Speculum phisionomie* di Michele Savonarola', *Kéiron* 8, pp. 152–61.

Voigts 1978. L.E. Voigts, 'The Significance of the Name Apuleius to the *Herbarium Apulei*', *Bulletin of the History of Medicine* 52, pp. 214–27.

Wallace 1988. W.A. Wallace, 'Traditional Natural Philosophy', in C.B. Schmitt, Q. Skinner and E. Kessler (eds), *The Cambridge History of Renaissance Philosophy*. Cambridge: Cambridge University Press, pp. 201–35.

Warr 1996. C. Warr, 'Painting in Late Fourteenth-Century Padua: The Patronage of Fina Buzzacarini', *Renaissance Studies* 10, pp. 139–55.

Weiss-Adamson 2005. M. Weiss-Adamson, 'Regimina Sanitatis', in T. Glick, S.J. Livesey and F. Wallis (eds), *Medieval Science, Technology and Medicine: An Encyclopedia*. New York: Routledge, pp. 438–9.

Weitzmann 1959. K. Weitzmann, *Ancient Book Illumination* (Martin Classical Lectures XVI). Cambridge, MA: Harvard University Press.

Wellmann 1903. M. Wellmann, 'Dioskurides aus Anazarbos in Kilikien', in *Paulys Realencyclopädie der classischen Altertumswissenschaft*. Stuttgart: Metzler Verlag, vol. 15, cols 1131–42.

Wetherbee 2012. W. Wetherbee, 'Learned Mythography: Plato and Martianus Capella', in R.J. Hexter and D. Townsend (eds), *The Oxford Handbook of Medieval Latin Literature*. Oxford: Oxford University Press, pp. 335–55.

Wilkins 1959. E.H. Wilkins, *Petrarch's Later Years*. Cambridge, MA: Mediaeval Academy of America.

Williams 2003. S.J. Williams, *The Secret of Secrets: The Scholarly Career of a Pseudo-Aristotelian Text in the Latin Middle Ages*. Ann Arbor: University of Michigan Press.

Williams 2008. S.J. Williams, 'The Pseudo-Aristotelian *Secretum Secretorum* as a Didactic Text', in J. Ruys (ed.), *What Nature Does Not Teach: Didactic Literature in the Medieval and Early Modern Periods*. Turnhout: Brepols, pp. 41–57.

Witt 2000. R.G. Witt, *In the Footsteps of the Ancients: The Origins of Humanism from Lovato to Bruni*. Leiden: Brill.

Witt 2009. R.G. Witt, 'The Rebirth of the Romans as Models of Character. *De viris illustribus*', in V. Kirkham and A. Maggi (eds), *Petrarch: A Critical Guide to the Complete Works*. Chicago: Chicago University Press, pp. 103–11.

Witthoft 1973. B. Witthoft, 'The *Tacuinum Sanitatis*: Studies in Secular Manuscript Illumination in Late Fourteenth-Century'. Cambridge, MA: Harvard University. Unpublished PhD thesis.

Witthoft 1978. B. Witthoft, 'The *Tacuinum Sanitatis*: A Lombard Panorama', *Gesta* 17, pp. 49–60.

Wolters 1976. W. Wolters, *La Scultura Veneziana Gothica (1300–1460)*, 2 vols. Venice: Alfieri.

Zak 2010. G. Zak, *Petrarch's Humanism and the Care of the Self*. Cambridge: Cambridge University Press.

Ziegler 2001. J. Ziegler, 'Text and Context on the Rise of Physiognomic Thought in the Later Middle Ages', in Y. Hen (ed.), *De Sion exibit lex et verbum domini de Hierusalem: Essays on Medieval Law, Liturgy, and Literature in Honour of Amnon Linder*. Turnhout: Brepols, pp. 159–82.

Ziegler 2005. J. Ziegler, 'Physiognomy', in T. Glick, S.J. Livesey and F. Wallis (eds), *Medieval Science, Technology and Medicine: An Encyclopedia*. New York: Routledge, pp. 399–402.

Ziegler 2007. J. Ziegler, 'Philosophers and Physicians on the Scientific Validity of Latin Physiognomy, 1200–1500', *Early Science & Medicine* 12, pp. 285–312.

Zuccolin 2007. G. Zuccolin, 'Princely Virtues in *De felici progressu* of Michele Savonarola, Court Physician of the House of Este', in I.P. Bejczy and C.J. Nederman (eds), *Princely Virtues in the Middle Ages, 1200–1500* (Disputatio 9). Turnhout: Brepols, pp. 237–58.

Zuccolin 2012. G. Zuccolin, 'The *Speculum Phisionomie* by Michele Savonarola', in A. Musco (ed.), *Universality of Reason. Plurality of Philosophies in the Middle Ages. XII Congresso internazionale di filosofia medievale, Palermo, 17–22 settembre 2007*. Palermo: Officina di Studi Medievali, pp. 873–86.

Index

Page numbers in *italics* indicate figures and illustrations.